Clinical Cardiology

Editors

COLIN C. SCHWARZWALD
KATHARYN J. MITCHELL

VETERINARY CLINICS OF NORTH AMERICA: EQUINE PRACTICE

www.vetequine.theclinics.com

Consulting Editor
THOMAS J. DIVERS

April 2019 • Volume 35 • Number 1

ELSEVIER

1600 John F. Kennedy Boulevard • Suite 1800 • Philadelphia, Pennsylvania, 19103-2899

http://www.vetequine.theclinics.com

VETERINARY CLINICS OF NORTH AMERICA: EQUINE PRACTICE Volume 35, Number 1
April 2019 ISSN 0749-0739, ISBN-13: 978-0-323-67835-3

Editor: Colleen Dietzler
Developmental Editor: Donald Mumford

Veterinary Clinics of North America: Equine Practice (ISSN 0749-0739) is published in April, August, and December by Elsevier Inc., 360 Park Avenue South, New York, NY 10010-1710. Business and Editorial Offices: 1600 John F. Kennedy Blvd., Suite 1800, Philadelphia, PA 19103-2899. Subscription prices are $287.00 per year (domestic individuals), $557.00 per year (domestic institutions), $100.00 per year (domestic students/residents), $334.00 per year (Canadian individuals), $702.00 per year (Canadian institutions), $365.00 per year (international individuals), $702.00 per year (international institutions), and $180.00 per year (international and Canadian students/residents). To receive student/resident rate, orders must be accompanied by name of affiliated institution, date of term, and the signature of program/residency coordinator on institution letterhead. Orders will be billed at individual rate until proof of status is received. Foreign air speed delivery is included in all *Clinics* subscription prices. All prices are subject to change without notice. **POSTMASTER:** Send address changes to *Veterinary Clinics of North America: Equine Practice*, 3251 Riverport Lane, Maryland Heights, MO 63043. Customer Service (orders, claims, online, change of address): Elsevier Health Sciences Division, Subscription **Customer Service, 3251 Riverport Lane, Maryland Heights, MO 63043. Tel: 1-800-654-2452 (U.S. and Canada); 314-447-8871 (outside U.S. and Canada). Fax: 314-447-8029. E-mail: journalscustomerservice-usa@elsevier.com (for print support);** E-mail: **journalsonlinesupport-usa@elsevier.com (for online support)**.

Reprints. For copies of 100 or more of articles in this publication, please contact the Commercial Reprints Department, Elsevier Inc., 360 Park Avenue South, New York, NY 10010-1710. Tel.: 212-633-3874; Fax: 212-633-3820; E-mail: reprints@elsevier.com.

Veterinary Clinics of North America: Equine Practice is covered in *MEDLINE/PubMed (Index Medicus)*, *Excerpta Medica*, *Current Contents/Agriculture, Biology and Environmental Sciences*, and *ISI*.

Contributors

CONSULTING EDITOR

THOMAS J. DIVERS, DVM
Diplomate, American College of Veterinary Internal Medicine; Diplomate, American College of Veterinary Emergency and Critical Care; Steffen Professor of Veterinary Medicine, Section of Large Animal Medicine, College of Veterinary Medicine, Cornell University, Ithaca, New York, USA

EDITORS

COLIN C. SCHWARZWALD, Prof Dr Med Vet, PhD
Diplomate, American College of Veterinary Internal Medicine (Large Animal Internal Medicine); Diplomate, European College of Equine Internal Medicine; Professor of Equine Internal Medicine; Director, Clinic for Equine Internal Medicine; Department Chair, Equine Department; Swiss Equine Cardiology Consulting, Vetsuisse Faculty, University of Zurich, Zurich, Switzerland

KATHARYN J. MITCHELL, BVSc, DVCS, DVM, PhD
Diplomate, American College of Veterinary Internal Medicine (Large Animal Internal Medicine); Senior Clinician and Researcher, Swiss Equine Cardiology Consulting, Clinic for Equine Internal Medicine, Equine Department, Vetsuisse Faculty, University of Zurich, Zurich, Switzerland

AUTHORS

JOHN D. BONAGURA, DVM, MS
Diplomate, American College of Veterinary Internal Medicine (Cardiology, Small Animal Internal Medicine); Associate Clinical Professor, Department of Clinical Sciences, College of Veterinary Medicine, North Carolina State University, Raleigh, North Carolina, USA; Professor Emeritus, Veterinary Clinical Sciences, The Ohio State University, Columbus, Ohio, USA

MARK BOWEN, BVetMed, MMedSci(MedEd), PhD, CertVA, CertEM(IntMed), PFHEA, FRCVS
Diplomate, American College of Veterinary Internal Medicine (Large Animal Internal Medicine); Diplomate, European College of Equine Internal Medicine; Professor, Veterinary Internal Medicine, Oakham Veterinary Hospital, University of Nottingham, School of Veterinary Medicine and Science, Sutton Bonington, United Kingdom

ANNELIES DECLOEDT, DVM, PhD
Assistant Professor, Department of Large Animal Internal Medicine, Faculty of Veterinary Medicine, Ghent University, Merelbeke, Belgium

MARY M. DURANDO, DVM, PhD
Diplomate, American College of Veterinary Internal Medicine (Large Animal Internal Medicine); Partner, Equine Sports Medicine Consultants, LLC, Newark, Delaware, USA

JOHN A. KEEN, BVetMed, PhD, Cert EM (Int Med), MRCVS
Diplomate, European College of Equine Internal Medicine; Senior Lecturer in Equine Medicine, Director of Equine Hospital and Practice, The Royal (Dick) School of Veterinary Studies, Roslin, Midlothian, United Kingdom

CELIA M. MARR, BVMS, MVM, PhD, FRCVS
Diplomate, European College of Equine Internal Medicine; Specialist, Internal Medicine, Rossdales Equine Hospital and Diagnostic Centre, Newmarket, Suffolk, United Kingdom

KATHARYN J. MITCHELL, BVSc, DVCS, DVM, PhD
Diplomate, American College of Veterinary Internal Medicine (Large Animal Internal Medicine); Senior Clinician and Researcher, Swiss Equine Cardiology Consulting, Clinic for Equine Internal Medicine, Equine Department, Vetsuisse Faculty, University of Zurich, Zurich, Switzerland

CRISTOBAL NAVAS DE SOLIS, LV, PhD
Diplomate, American College of Veterinary Internal Medicine (Large Animal Internal Medicine); Clinical Assistant Professor, Department of Large Animal Clinical Sciences, Texas A&M University, College Station, Texas, USA

ADAM REDPATH, BVMS(Hons), PGCert(VetMed), MRCVS
Clinical Teaching Associate, Equine Medicine, Oakham Veterinary Hospital, University of Nottingham, School of Veterinary Medicine and Science, Sutton Bonington, United Kingdom

VIRGINIA B. REEF, DVM
Diplomate, American College of Veterinary Internal Medicine (Large Animal Internal Medicine); Diplomate, American College of Veterinary Sports Medicine and Rehabilitation; Associate Member, European College of Veterinary Diagnostic Imaging; Mark Whittier and Lila Griswold Allam Professor of Medicine; Chief, Section of Imaging, Department of Clinical Studies,
New Bolton Center, University of Pennsylvania, Kennett Square, Pennsylvania, USA

BRIAN A. SCANSEN, DVM, MS
Diplomate, American College of Veterinary Internal Medicine (Cardiology); Associate Professor and Section Head of Cardiology & Cardiac Surgery, Department of Clinical Sciences, Colorado State University, Fort Collins, Colorado, USA

COLIN C. SCHWARZWALD, Prof Dr Med Vet, PhD
Diplomate, American College of Veterinary Internal Medicine (Large Animal Internal Medicine); Diplomate, European College of Equine Internal Medicine; Professor of Equine Internal Medicine; Director, Clinic for Equine Internal Medicine; Department Chair, Equine Department; Swiss Equine Cardiology Consulting, Vetsuisse Faculty, University of Zurich, Zurich, Switzerland

ANDRE C. SHIH, DVM
Diplomate, American College Veterinary Anesthesia and Analgesia; Diplomate, American College Veterinary Emergency and Critical Care; Service Chief, Capital Veterinary Specialist, Jacksonville, Florida, USA

GUNTHER VAN LOON, DVM, PhD
Diplomate, European College of Equine Internal Medicine; Associate Member, European College of Veterinary Diagnostic Imaging; Professor in Large Animal Internal Medicine, Department of Large Animal Internal Medicine, Faculty of Veterinary Medicine, Ghent University, Merelbeke, Belgium

Contents

 Video content accompanies this article at http://www.vetequine.
theclinics.com.

> Equine heart diseases can be categorized with morphologic, etiologic, and physiologic diagnoses and classified anatomically as diseases of the pericardium, myocardium, valves (endocardium), and great vessels. An appreciation of normal and pathologic physiology is a key to understanding diagnosis and therapy of heart disease. Pathophysiologic diagnoses include arrhythmias, congestive heart failure, and pulmonary hypertension. Heart rhythm disturbances can occur in isolation or with structural disease. Heart failure stems from decreased arterial filling owing to insufficient cardiac output. Pulmonary hypertension is associated with strenuous exercise, left heart failure, bronchopulmonary diseases, and pulmonary arteriopathies. The etiopathogenesis of these disorders are incompletely understood.

 Video content accompanies this article at http://www.vetequine.
theclinics.com.

> Despite advances, increased convenience, and availability of echocardiography and other diagnostic techniques in equine cardiology, a comprehensive history and clinical examination still forms the essential first step in any cardiac evaluation. This article summarizes the approach to the cardiac examination at rest, highlighting key areas for the clinician to assess, and stressing the importance of context for assessing the significance of any abnormalities detected. Ancillary techniques, such as blood pressure measurement and the laboratory assessment of cardiac disease in the horse, are also introduced.

 Video content accompanies this article at http://www.vetequine.
theclinics.com.

> This article provides an overview on the principles of transthoracic echocardiography in horses. Indications for echocardiography, equipment, and technical considerations are discussed and a systematic approach for a complete echocardiographic examination in horses is

described. Methods for assessment of chamber dimensions, allometric scaling of measurements, assessment of systolic and diastolic ventricular function, assessment of atrial function, hemodynamic assessment, and evaluation of valvular regurgitation are explained, focusing on traditional 2-dimensional (2D), motion-mode, and Doppler echocardiographic methods. Selected applications of newer echocardiographic methods, such as tissue Doppler imaging and 2D speckle tracking are also described.

Analyzing electrocardiographic (ECG) recordings, making a diagnosis and assessment of any arrhythmias present, is an important part of the workup of many equine cases. Accurate analysis requires a good-quality recording, free of as many artifacts as possible, with clear P-QRS-T complex morphology. For sustained arrhythmias, short-term recordings are sufficient to make the appropriate diagnosis before instigating treatment. Longer-term recordings are essential for arrhythmias that are paroxysmal, intermittent, or occurring infrequently, while exercising ECGs are required for arrhythmias associated with physical activity. A stepwise, logical approach to ECG analysis will help the observer to recognize and correctly diagnose any arrhythmias present.

Arrhythmias are common in horses. Sinus arrhythmia and first- and second-degree atrioventricular block are frequently found physiologic arrhythmias, but should immediately disappear after stress or exercise. Atrial premature depolarizations are usually not associated with poor performance, but are a potential trigger for atrial fibrillation. Atrial fibrillation results in an abnormal ventricular response during exercise and poses a risk for collapse in some horses. This arrhythmia can usually be treated by quinidine sulfate or transvenous electrical cardioversion. Ventricular premature depolarizations, especially when associated with structural heart disease, may be a risk factor for ventricular tachycardia or even ventricular fibrillation.

Congenital heart disease (CHD) represents a small proportion of horses undergoing clinical evaluation; however, both simple and complex defects occur during cardiac development leading to many unique malformations. This article reviews cardiac development and the fetal circulation, describes the morphologic method and the sequential segmental approach to CHD analysis, presents a summary of CHD in horses, and offers an overview of lesions that should be considered during evaluation of horses suspected to have CHD. For many forms of equine CHD, therapies are limited because cardiac interventions and cardiac surgery are not routinely pursued in this species.

Video content accompanies this article at http://www.vetequine.
theclinics.com.

Degenerative myxomatous disease is common and is associated with aging. Poor prognostic indicators for equine aortic regurgitation specifically include ventricular ectopy, increased pulse pressure, and hyperkinetic pulses. Valvular prolapse is a functional abnormality diagnosed echocardiographically, about which knowledge is limited. A better understanding of its role in valvular regurgitation is needed. Infective endocarditis presents with fever and other systemic signs accompanying valvular regurgitation. The prognosis is poor, warranting aggressive therapy. Other forms of valvular disease occur rarely, but often presenting with severe regurgitation. Management of horses with valvular disease is focused on assessment of severity and regular clinical, echocardiographic, and electrocardiographic monitoring.

 Video content accompanies this article at http://www.vetequine.
theclinics.com.

Pericardial, myocardial, and great vessel diseases are relatively rare in horses. The clinical signs are often nonspecific and vague, or related to the underlying cause. Physical examination usually reveals tachycardia, fever, venous distension or jugular pulsation, a weak or bounding arterial pulse, ventral edema, and abnormal cardiac auscultation such as arrhythmia, murmur, or muffled heart sounds. The prognosis depends on the underlying cause and the disease progression, and ranges from full recovery to poor prognosis for survival. This article focuses on the etiology, diagnosis, prognosis, and treatment of pericarditis, pericardial mass lesions, myocarditis, cardiomyopathy, and great vessel aneurysm or rupture.

The physiology of exercise and training is fascinating, and hundreds of interesting studies have given insight into its mechanisms. Exercise testing is a useful clinical tool that can help veterinarians assess poor performance, fitness, and performance potential and prevent injuries. The clinically applicable aspects of cardiovascular adaptions to training and exercise testing are highlighted in this review. Different exercise tests should be used to evaluate horses performing in different disciplines and levels. Exercise tests that simultaneously assess several body systems can be beneficial when assessing poor performance, because this is often a multifactorial problem with signs not detectable at rest.

Horses have a high prevalence of resting arrhythmias, cardiac murmurs, and valvular regurgitation, and training can increase the prevalence. This makes it challenging for equine veterinarians who are asked to evaluate horses for poor performance to determine the clinical relevance of some findings. In addition, cardiac disease has the potential to cause collapse or sudden death, putting both the horse and rider at risk. Further diagnostics, such as echocardiograms and resting and exercising ECGs can help to sort out the impact of an abnormality found on resting physical examination. However uncertainty over the importance of some findings continues to exist.

Arrhythmias detected on prepurchase examination should be confirmed with an ECG. Exercising ECG determines if the arrhythmia is overdriven during exercise or is a safety concern. An echocardiogram is needed in all horses with a grade 3/6 or louder mid to late systolic, holosystolic, or pansystolic murmur or any holodiastolic decrescendo murmur to identify the cardiac abnormality and its hemodynamic impact. Most horses with arrhythmias and murmurs have a normal performance career and life expectancy and are insurable. Risks for sudden death and congestive heart failure associated with the common murmurs and arrhythmias are identified, because these horses cannot be insured.

Monitoring variables of cardiac performance in horses is challenging owing to patient size, temperament, and anatomic peculiarities. Blood pressure is a major determinant of afterload, but it is not a reliable surrogate of cardiac performance and tissue perfusion. Cardiac output, together with arterial and venous oxygen content, provides insight as to the adequacy of delivery of blood and oxygen to the body as a whole and can be used to gauge the fluid responsiveness and cardiovascular status of the patient. Measurement of intracardiac pressures serves to assess cardiac filling pressures, myocardial performance, and vascular resistance.

Many cardiac therapeutics lack significant evidence of benefit in the horse, and in many cases their use is based on extrapolation of evidence from other species. In recent years there has been a push to develop a better understanding of both the pharmacodynamics and pharmacokinetics of these drugs. Recent data have described the use of antiarrhythmic agents including sotalol, flecainide, and amiodarone. Data about the use of ACE inhibitors in the management of congestive heart failure are encouraging and support their use in certain cases, wheras evidence for other medicines, such as pimobendan, remain speculative.

VETERINARY CLINICS OF NORTH AMERICA: EQUINE PRACTICE

RELATED SERIES

Veterinary Clinics of North America: Food Animal Practice

THE CLINICS ARE NOW AVAILABLE ONLINE!
Access your subscription at:
www.theclinics.com

Preface

Equine Cardiology in the Twenty-First Century

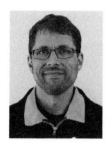
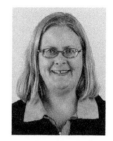

Colin C. Schwarzwald,
Prof Dr Med Vet, PhD, Dipl. ACVIM, Dipl. ECEIM

Katharyn J. Mitchell,
BVSc, DVCS, DVM, PhD, Dipl. ACVIM

Editors

In the 34 years since the first *Veterinary Clinics of North America: Equine Practice* issue focused on cardiology was published, there have been tremendous advances made in the field of equine cardiology.

At that time, in August 1985, diagnostic radiology and nuclear angiocardiography for assessment of cardiac size and function were the subjects of an entire article, while echocardiography, described in another article, had only been used in horses for less than a decade. Today, diagnostic radiology is rarely used, and nuclear imaging has completely disappeared in clinical equine cardiology. We now have fully digital echocardiography equipment that routinely performs high-quality two-dimensional (2D), M-mode, and blood-flow Doppler imaging and allows comprehensive assessment of cardiac size and function in horses of nearly all sizes and breeds. With tissue Doppler imaging, 2D speckle tracking, intracardiac imaging, and four-dimensional (ie, three-dimensional real-time) echocardiography becoming more universally available, there is an increasing focus on using these novel methods to better assess even early stages of disease or the more unusual or less commonly recognized conditions.

Another focus in recent times has been the development of improved wireless electrocardiographic (ECG) technologies, allowing continuous ECG recordings to be easily obtained at rest and during exercise and to be digitally stored and analyzed using sophisticated computer algorithms. In the upcoming years, we expect further advances in this field of research, with wearable devices and machine learning algorithms aiding in data collection and automated ECG analyses.

With the wider availability of these novel diagnostic technologies, there is increasing knowledge of the prevalence of cardiac abnormalities in the equine population and a growing awareness of the potential consequences of cardiac disease with respect to performance, collapse, and sudden death.

Vet Clin Equine 35 (2019) xi–xii
https://doi.org/10.1016/j.cveq.2019.01.002
0749-0739/19/© 2019 Published by Elsevier Inc.

vetequine.theclinics.com

This is an exciting time to be involved in equine cardiology, and several groups around the world are exploring innovative methods not only for diagnosis and monitoring but also for treatment of horses with heart disease. With one of the most exciting recent developments, transvenous electrical cardioversion, we now have access to an additional effective therapy for horses with atrial fibrillation. At the same time, our understanding and use of equine-oriented cardiovascular pharmaceuticals have also expanded. And with the most contemporary technology, even mapping of the heart's electrical activity and ablation of arrhythmogenic foci have recently become within reach. While these methods are certainly not considered routine procedures in horses and are still at their very early stages of development, in the next *Veterinary Clinics of North America: Equine Practice* issue focused on cardiology, likely a few decades from now, these might well be described as established methods for treatment of selected arrhythmias in horses.

With all these technical advances and developments, we must not forget that a thorough history-taking and physical examination, careful auscultation of heart and lungs, and conventional echocardiographic and ECG techniques are still the mainstay of any clinical examination of a horse with heart disease. Hence, they are covered in this issue in depth.

It is our great honor that two of the authors from the 1985 issue, Dr John D. Bonagura and Dr Virginia B. Reef, have also contributed articles in this most current issue. Both individuals have made a huge impact on the field of equine cardiology over the course of their illustrious careers. This lasting contribution is felt particularly through their training of newer generations of equine cardiologists, with several of the authors in this issue, including ourselves, having spent time working closely with Drs Bonagura and Reef and other authors of that first 1985 issue.

We hope that this second cardiology issue of *Veterinary Clinics of North America: Equine Practice* will be of use to many equine practitioners and provide a comprehensive update on the diagnosis and management of cardiac disease with contributions from recognized experts working in the field of equine cardiology.

Colin C. Schwarzwald, Prof Dr Med Vet, PhD, Dipl. ACVIM, Dipl. ECEIM
Swiss Equine Cardiology Consulting
Clinic for Equine Internal Medicine
Equine Department
University of Zurich
Winterthurerstrasse 260
Zurich 8057, Switzerland

Katharyn J. Mitchell, BVSc, DVCS, DVM, PhD, Dipl. ACVIM
Swiss Equine Cardiology Consulting
Clinic for Equine Internal Medicine
Equine Department
University of Zurich
Winterthurerstrasse 260
Zurich 8057, Switzerland

E-mail addresses:
cschwarzwald@vetclinics.uzh.ch (C.C. Schwarzwald)
kmitchell@vetclinics.uzh.ch (K.J. Mitchell)

Overview of Equine Cardiac Disease

John D. Bonagura, DVM, MS[a,b,*]

KEYWORDS

- Equine heart disease • Equine cardiology • Equine heart failure

KEY POINTS

- A knowledge of normal and pathologic physiology is a key to understanding equine cardiac diseases and therapy of heart failure in this species.
- Equine heart diseases can be categorized anatomically as diseases of the pericardium, myocardium, valves and endocardium, and the great vessels.
- Heart rhythm disturbances are an important functional type of heart disease and can lead to exercise intolerance or serious clinical signs, such as syncope or sudden death.
- Congestive heart failure is a pathophysiologic state resulting from insufficient arterial filling caused by underlying heart disease. It is not a specific etiologic diagnosis.
- Pulmonary hypertension is a pathophysiologic state associated with strenuous exercise, left heart failure, severe pulmonary parenchymal diseases, pulmonary arteriopathy, and functional arterial vasoconstriction.

Video content accompanies this article at http://www.vetequine.theclinics. com.

INTRODUCTION

Cardiovascular function is essential for exercise, thermoregulation, respiration, and organ function. Heart diseases are relatively common in horses, involving various congenital and acquired cardiac lesions. Fortunately, many cardiac diseases in this species are mild and well-tolerated. However, moderate to severe lesions can decrease exercise performance, reduce lifespan, or generate safely concerns for both the rider and the horse. Clinical assessment of cardiac disease is best served

Disclosure Statement: The author has no relationship with a commercial company that has a direct financial interest in this subject matter or the materials discussed in article nor with a company making a competing product.
[a] Department of Clinical Sciences, College of Veterinary Medicine, North Carolina State University, 1060 William Moore Drive, Raleigh, NC 27606, USA; [b] Veterinary Clinical Sciences, The Ohio State University, Columbus, OH, USA
* Corresponding author. Department of Clinical Sciences, College of Veterinary Medicine, North Carolina State University, 1060 William Moore Drive, Raleigh, NC 27606.
E-mail address: Bonagura.1@osu.edu

Vet Clin Equine 35 (2019) 1–22
https://doi.org/10.1016/j.cveq.2019.01.001
0749-0739/19/© 2019 Elsevier Inc. All rights reserved.

by an awareness of normal structure and function, an appreciation of pathologic physiology, and an understanding of heart diseases particularly relevant to this species. This article provides an overview of these subjects and focuses on relevant clinical pathophysiology. Often-used abbreviations for cardiac structure, disease, and dysfunction are expanded in **Box 1**.

The heart consists largely of cardiomyocytes that form the bulk of the myocardium and electrical conduction system. Passive components of the heart, including connective tissues, cardiac valves, and the pericardium, support normal cardiac function. Each of these structures represents a potential primary or secondary target of heart disease.

Normal heart function demands a recurring and coordinated sequence of electrical activity, myocyte contraction, myocardial relaxation, and movement of blood across the cardiac chambers and great vessels. Normal blood flow is guided by action of the 4 heart valves. When considering cardiac pathology and pathophysiology, potential lesions can be grouped based on anatomic structures; namely, the pericardium, myocardium, valves and endocardium, impulse-forming and conduction system, and great vessels (aorta and pulmonary trunk). Starting with this anatomic categorization, causes of cardiovascular disease can be further subdivided into morphologic, physiologic (functional), and etiologic diagnoses (**Box 2**).

Comprehensive reviews of equine cardiac anatomy, physiology, and disease have been published.[1] This review offers a high-level view of equine heart diseases, with a focus on normal structure and function, common heart pathologies,[2] and clinically relevant pathophysiology. Greater detail regarding diagnosis and management of specific disorders are provided in other articles in this issue as well as the American College of Veterinary Internal Medicine consensus report on cardiac disorders in equine athletes.[3]

ANATOMIC AND PATHOLOGIC CONSIDERATIONS

Anatomic features of the pericardial space, the myocardium and cardiac chambers, the heart valves, and the specialized impulse-forming and conduction system underpin a clinician's understanding of equine heart disease. Some of the major anatomic features of the heart, and related cardiac pathologies, are the focus of this section. Arrhythmias are discussed in Katharyn J Mitchell's article, "Equine Electrocardiography," and in Gunther van Loon's article, "Cardiac Arrhythmias in Horses," in this issue. See online Videos 1 and 2 for echocardiographic examples of some disorders.

Box 1
Abbreviations used in this article

2D, 2-dimensional	PA, pulmonary artery (arterial)
AR, aortic regurgitation	PAH, pulmonary arterial hypertension
AV, atrioventricular	PH, pulmonary hypertension
BP, blood pressure	PR, pulmonary regurgitation
CHF, congestive heart failure	RA, right atrium (atrial)
CO, cardiac output	RV, right ventricle (ventricular)
EIPH, exercised-induced pulmonary hemorrhage	SV, stroke volume
LA, left atrium (atrial)	TR, tricuspid regurgitation
LV, left ventricle (ventricular)	VHD, valvular heart disease
MR, mitral regurgitation	

Box 2
Categorization of cardiac diseases

Anatomic
  Pericardium
  Myocardium
  Valves and endocardium
  Impulse-forming and conduction system
  Great vessels

Morphologic and etiologic diagnoses
  Abnormalities of development (anomalies), genetic diseases
    Cardiac malformations
    Cell channelopathies (?)
  Myocardial diseases
    Cellular degeneration, hemorrhage, necrosis, infiltration, fibrosis, and arrhythmogenesis
    Cellular injury (eg, toxicosis, nutritional deficiencies, and ischemia)
    Metabolic diseases
    Catecholamine-induced injury
    Toxicosis
    Infiltrative diseases: neoplasia, amyloid
    Idiopathic disorders of the myocardium
  Degenerative valvular diseases
    Age-related
    Myxomatous change (idiopathic)
  Inflammatory diseases
  Infectious, immune-mediated, idiopathic
    Pericarditis
    Myocarditis
    Bacterial endocarditis
    Noninfective valvulitis (idiopathic)
    Vasculitis
  Vascular diseases affecting the heart
    Vasculitis
    Arteriosclerosis
    Hypertension
      Systemic arterial
      Pulmonary arterial
      Pulmonary venoocclusive disease
  Neoplastic diseases
    Infiltrative myocardial diseases
    Cardiac mass effect
  Traumatic injury

Physiologic diagnoses, causes of heart failure
  Ventricular dysfunction
    Systolic (contractility) dysfunction
    Diastolic (filling) dysfunction
      Pericardial diseases
    Combined systolic and diastolic ventricular dysfunction
      Cardiomyopathies (ildiopathic and secondary)
      Relentless tachyarrhythmias
  Increased cardiac workload
    Volume overload
      Shunts
      Valvular regurgitation
      High-output states (eg, anemia)
    Pressure overload
      Systemic hypertension
      Pulmonary hypertension
      Outflow tract stenosis
  Diseases of the impulse-forming and conduction system, arrhythmias
    Tachyarrhythmias
    Bradyarrhythmias

Pericardium

The pericardial space is formed by the reflection of 2 membranes, the parietal pericardium and visceral pericardium (epicardium). The epicardium is tightly adhered to the myocardium. The outer parietal pericardium includes a fibrous connective tissue layer. The pericardial space is lined by mesothelial cells that secrete a small volume of serous lubricating fluid not normally visible by echocardiography. Functionally, the pericardium influences cardiac filling and ventricular interdependence, prevents acute cardiac dilation, and creates a barrier to contiguous infection. Infective and noninfective etiologies of pericarditis (**Fig. 1**) are the most common disorders of clinical disease, with neoplasia and trauma relatively rare causes.[4] Pericardial disorders are characterized by ventricular diastolic dysfunction (see Clinical Pathophysiology). Clinical syndromes and treatment of pericardial disease are described in Annelies Decloedt's article, "Pericardial Disease, Myocardial Disease, and Great Vessel Abnormalities in Horses," in this issue.

Myocardium and Cardiac Chambers

The myocardium represents the major structural component of the atria and ventricles. The relative thicknesses of the atrial and ventricular walls reflects the pressures generated by each chamber. Specialized myocardial cells constitute the impulse-forming and conduction system of the heart. Accepting some histologic and electrophysiologic differences, nearly all cardiomyocytes demonstrate the properties of excitability, conduction of ionic currents, contraction after excitation, active relaxation, and passive elongation. Specialized myocardial cells form the sinoatrial and atrioventricular (AV) nodes, as well as the His-Purkinje system of the ventricles. These cells initiate the cardiac impulse and direct current flow across the atria and ventricles. Autonomic influences have a profound effect on myocardial cell function and the heart is richly supplied with both parasympathetic and sympathetic nerves. Intercellular junctions and connective tissues support both cellular functions and pump dynamics, influencing the electrical and mechanical properties of the heart. For example, myocardial diseases and cardiac remodeling in congestive heart failure (CHF) are not limited to cardiomyocytes, but also include intercellular junctions and cardiac connective tissues.

Normal ventricular function depends on the health of the myocardium, level of autonomic traffic, venous return and cardiac filling, the impedance to ejection of blood, and

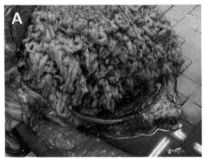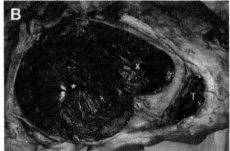

Fig. 1. Pathology of pericardial disease. Postmortem examples of pericarditis. (*A*) Proliferative reaction on the epicardium within the pericardial space. (*B*) Constrictive effusive pericardial disease. Note the thickened epicardium surrounding the compressed right (x) and left (*asterisk*) ventricles. Thrombosis (T) is evident within the residual pericardial space, which is largely obliterated by fusion of the parietal and epicardial membranes.

the frequency of cardiac activation. These physiologic variables are more commonly referred to as inotropy (contractility), preload (end-diastolic chamber volume), after-load (impedance to ejection of blood relating to wall stress), and heart rate. Regulation of the heart is well-described in standard textbooks of physiology and medicine. The modulation of myocardial function is greatly influenced by autonomic stimulation. Sympathetic nervous system input via mainly the beta-1 adrenergic receptor aug-ments heart rate (chronotropism), AV conduction (dromotropism), cellular excitability (bathmotropism), myocardial contractile state (inotropism), and myocardial relaxation (lusitropism). Vagal efferent traffic exerted through the muscarinic receptor has the opposite effects, both directly and indirectly by depressing sympathetic influence on cardiac function.

Atria

The right atrium (RA) consists of a relatively smooth cavernous chamber and a muscular, finely trabeculated appendage or auricle. This chamber receives desatu-rated systemic and coronary venous blood throughout the cardiac cycle. The RA is a complicated structure anatomically, and is best visualized through multiple imaging windows using echocardiography. Normal electrical impulses originate here from the sinoatrial node and extend into the AV node. Vagal input has a profound effect on nodal function and mechanisms for blood pressure (BP) control include vagal surges that cause sinus node depression and physiologic AV block. Right atrial pressure is a major determinant of right ventricular (RV) filling (preload) and therefore stroke volume (SV) and cardiac output (CO). The normal RV is particularly sensitive to filling, such that decreased venous return owing to dehydration, sweating, or venous pooling can significantly limit CO, BP, and exercise capacity.

The left atrium (LA) is situated to the left and caudal to the RA. The trabeculated appendage of the LA is more narrow based than for the RA, and the auricular tip is ori-ented left and cranial toward the pulmonary trunk. This chamber receives oxygenated pulmonary venous blood along with a small admixture of (desaturated) bronchial venous blood. The LA is dorsal and extends slightly caudal to the left ventricle (LV) through which it communicates across the left AV or mitral valve. The left atrial pres-sure is closely tied to that of the pulmonary circulation, and at resting heart rates, the pulmonary arterial (PA) diastolic pressure is just above those filling the LA and LV.

The 2 atrial chambers communicate in the fetus via the foramen ovale, but are sepa-rated in life by an intact atrial septum. In both premature and full-term foals, a portion of the foramen ovale is visualized echocardiographically as a mobile membrane within the atrial septum projecting into the left side of this structure. Normally, pulmonary venous return increases the LA pressure sufficient to functionally close this interatrial pathway. However, a patent foramen ovale offers a conduit for right-to-left shunting, hypoxemia, and cyanosis when RA pressures are increased, as in severe pulmonary hypertension (PH) or in cases of tricuspid or pulmonary atresia.

The atria have 3 main functions, (1) reservoir during ventricular systole when venous return is collected and the atria achieve maximal size; (2) conduit during early to mid-diastole, when venous return continues across opened AV valves; and (3) presystolic pump function initiated by active contraction of the atrial myocardium. Normally, atrial pressures are relatively low but sufficient to fill the ventricles and establish ventricular preload. However, with extreme exercise, a marked increase in LA pressure occurs that can contribute to pulmonary hemorrhage (see Pulmonary hypertension owing to exercise). The large atrial mass and high resting vagal tone, which shortens atrial cell refractory period, are predispositions to atrial flutter and atrial fibrillation. The loss of the atrial contraction associated with these arrhythmias is recognized clinically by the absence of a distinctive atrial (fourth) heart sound. Ventricular filling become highly dependent on atrial contraction when the heart rate is high (increasing its contribution from approximately 10% to 15% at resting rates to >45% at rates of >200/min). Accordingly, atrial fibrillation is especially likely to cause exercise intolerance in maximally exercised horses.

Ventricles

The RV lies mostly cranial to the LV, and appears crescent shaped on cross-sectional echocardiographic examination. During ventricular systole, the chamber ejects desaturated blood across the pulmonary valve into the pulmonary trunk. Pressures in the pulmonary arteries are relatively lower than in the systemic circulation (about ¼), but these pressures increase markedly during exercise. Anatomically the RV projects an approximate U shape with 3 multiplane components (inlet, apex, and outlet). The tricuspid valve (**Fig. 2**) and proximal inflow tract are situated dorsally and to the right of the midline; the RV apex is located ventrally; and the outflow tract crosses the midline such that the pulmonary valve is oriented dorsally and superficial to the aorta along the anatomic left surface of the heart. The RV is challenging to assess using echocardiography because of the complex geometry that include these 3 main components. Additionally, the major shortening of the RV involves contraction in the apical-to-basilar direction, an assessment limited by the lack of good apical imaging planes.

The LV chamber is a thick, high-pressure pump that also incorporates about two-thirds of the curved septum that separates the ventricles. Internally, the LV is also partitioned into inflow and outflow tracts. These change shape during diastole and systole to facilitate filling and ejection, respectively. The mitral and aortic valves lie in fibrous continuity, and the internal chamber projects a relative V shape from the LV inlet to the apex to the outflow tract. The LV outflow tract is continuous with the ventricular septum cranially and the anterior (septal) mitral leaflet caudally. These relationships are relevant to understanding echocardiographic imaging. The aortic valve and proximal aorta are situated near the center of the cardiac base and just medial to the pulmonary trunk. On cross-sectional imaging across the heart base, the aorta forms the small circle in the center of the picture.

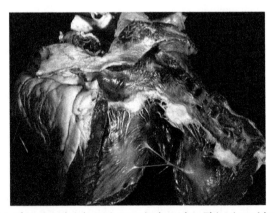

Fig. 2. Appearance of a normal right atrioventricular valve. This tricuspid valve has 3 leaflets with numerous supporting chordae tendineae. Note the absence of a visible pulmonary valve, which is located anatomically to the other side of the thorax. Papillary muscles are less distinctive than for the left side. A specialized conduction bundle (moderator band) is evident spanning the RV and does not attach to the valve cusps.

The components of the LV and related structures are readily evaluated by 2-dimensional (2D) echocardiography (Online Video 1). The LV is roughly conical in appearance when viewed in the long axis and relatively circular in cross-section during short-axis imaging. The ventricular septum is approximately the thickness of the LV free wall, except for the subaortic ventricular septum, which measures somewhat thicker. The greater thickness and the arrangement of myocardial fibers within the LV walls allow this chamber to accommodate the higher pressures and impedance of the systemic arterial circulation. Longitudinal, circumferential, and radial shortening and lengthening of myocardial segments occur during the cardiac cycle. Such movements can be appreciated by advanced echocardiographic imaging (strain or deformation studies) and might represent sensitive methods for evaluating heart function. Additionally, the LV rotates in opposite directions at the apex and base, creating a systolic twisting and diastolic untwisting that contribute to both ejection and to diastolic properties and filling of the LV.

Compared with other species, the equine ventricular myocardium is uncommonly affected by primary cardiomyopathies. However, persistent embryologic openings in the ventricular septum—ventricular septal defects—represent the most common cardiac malformation in horses. Additionally, ventricular chambers can increase in mass in response to exercise training, valvular heart disease (VHD), malformations, and systemic or PH. Multifocal areas of fibrosis (**Fig. 3**A) are observed regularly at autopsy but the etiology of these scars—be it prior inflammation, parasitic insult, toxic injury, or ischemic necrosis—is elusive. Various toxic elements, including

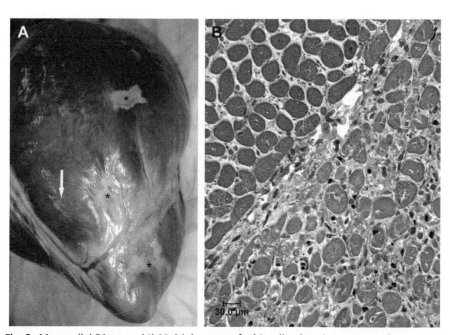

Fig. 3. Myocardial Diseases. (A) Multiple areas of white discoloration representing myocardial fibrosis (*asterisks*). The normal fat surrounding coronary arteries is evident. Small dilated superficial vessels (veins or lymphatics) are also evident (*arrowhead*). (B) Histologic section of myocardium showing extensive myocardial necrosis. Note the degenerative changes and loss of cardiomyocytes and increased cellularity and interstitial change (compared with the normal at upper left).

ionophores, cardiotoxic plants, cantharidin, and snake venom, can induce mild to severe myocardial injury (**Fig. 3**B) with functional consequences that can include fatal arrhythmias. Rarely, a dissection of the ventricular septum or RV wall is observed. A reversible dilated cardiomyopathy phenotype can develop from relentless tachycardias; these are typically ventricular in origin and at heart rates exceeding 120/min.

Cardiac Valves

The cardiac chambers and great vessels are partitioned by the 4 heart valves. These largely collagenous structures are lined by endocardium. The vibrations generating the 4 normal heart sounds of the horse are dictated by abrupt changes in pressure and blood flow, regulated by the function of these valves. Although mitral and aortic valves are in fibrous continuity, the right heart valves are separated, with the tricuspid valve to the right, and pulmonary valve on the left side of the thorax. These locations are relevant to both auscultation and to echocardiography (See John A. Keen's article, "Examination of Horses with Cardiac Disease," and Colin C. Schwarzwald's article, "Equine Echocardiography," in this issue). Valvular diseases are among the most common equine heart diseases. Clinically, valve structure and motion are evaluated by 2D and M-mode echocardiography (See online Videos 1 and 2). Valvular function is assessed by cardiac auscultation and when necessary by color and spectral Doppler echocardiographic techniques.

Atrioventricular valves

The mitral and tricuspid valves close during systole and allow the atria to fill at relatively low pressures. The attendant vibrations generate the first heart sound, and significant AV valvular regurgitation results in a systolic heart murmur over the respective valve area. Both AV valves are anchored by collagenous chordae tendineae, papillary muscles, and, to varying degrees, by annular and atrial tissues. The valve chordae demonstrate arborization with thicker primary chords attaching at the papillary muscles and progressively finer secondary and tertiary chords connecting to the edges and ventricular surfaces of the valves (**Fig. 4**).

The mitral valve is a saddle-shaped structure composed of a large anterior (cranial, septal) leaflet and an expansive posterior (caudal, mural) leaflet that includes several accessory cusps. The anterior leaflet projects deeper into the ventricular cavity, whereas the posterior leaflet has a greater circumference with a scalloped appearance caused by incomplete commissures. Two prominent papillary muscles anchor this valve to the myocardium. The right AV or tricuspid valve encompasses the largest cross-sectional area and in horses consists of 3 well-defined leaflets (septal, anterior, and posterior; nomenclature varies). Papillary to chordal attachments are similar to the mitral valve; however, the number ($\geq$3) and arrangement are less consistent.

Color Doppler examination of the tricuspid valve often demonstrates low-velocity (<3.0–3.5 m/s) regurgitant flow with a prevalence related to the breed, type of work, and veracity of the echocardiographic examination. Tricuspid regurgitation (TR) is often silent to auscultation, and these small regurgitant jets are thought to be physiologic. It is also common to find TR associated with an obvious cardiac murmur in horses subjected to high-level training. The precise etiology of TR in these horses (often Standardbred or National Hunt breeds) is undetermined, and any impact on exercise is unresolved. Similar to the tricuspid valve, color Doppler echocardiography often reveals clinically insignificant mitral valve insufficiency in horses. These jets seem to be more common with age and especially in horses subjected to intense work. The high sensitivity of Doppler echocardiography can create confusion with respect to the

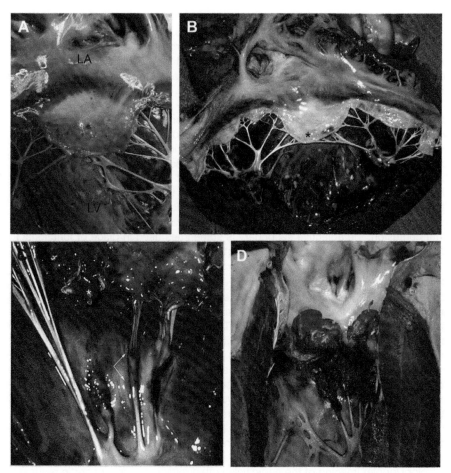

Fig. 4. Pathology of AV valvular disease. (*A*) Mitral valve hamartoma in a young horse with CHF. The anterior leaflet is shown and is shortened and thickened. This was believed to be congenital. (*B*) Myxomatous change of the mitral valve. All leaflets are affected with discoloration and thickening near the free edges of the cusps evident. The left atrium and ventricle are dilated and jet lesions are probably the reason for dense white discoloration in some parts of the atrium. The anterior leaflet is in the center of the image (*asterisk*). Note the different levels of mitral valve chordae tendineae (normal) and the scalloped appearance of the posterior leaflet that extends to either side of the anterior leaflet. (*C*) Noninfective valvulitis of the mitral valve with ruptured chords (*asterisk*). Note the transition of changes within primary chordae tendineae (*arrows*). The mitral leaflets appear distorted and thickened but still glistening. There is scarring of some chordal elements to the myocardium. Etiology was unknown. (*D*) Typical infective endocarditis of the mitral valve. These lesions appear grossly as hemorrhagic thromboses on the leaflets and the chordae tendineae.

clinical significance of mitral regurgitation (MR) or TR. A practical guideline is that clinically relevant AV valvular disease should result in an audible systolic murmur of TR or of MR, this murmur should correlate to 2D and Doppler echocardiographic findings.

The etiology of AV valvular regurgitation can stem from lesions in any portion of the valve apparatus, or from dilation of the cardiac chambers. Most primary valvular disorders are due to congenital malformation, degenerative (myxomatous or fibrotic) tissue change, infective endocarditis,[5] or some poorly characterized lesion such as valvulitis or valvular hamartoma (see **Fig. 4**A). Ruptured mitral chordae tendineae are another reason for valvular regurgitation and the severity usually relates to the location of the tear. Both degenerative changes of the chords and inflammatory lesions affecting the valve such as endocarditis can predispose to chordal rupture.

The term functional valvular regurgitation refers to the MR or TR secondary to cardiac remodeling or papillary muscle dysfunction. For example, PH can induce high-velocity (>3.5 m/s) TR. This is caused by increased PA and RV systolic pressures with secondary ventricular remodeling affecting tricuspid valvular support. When dilated forms of cardiomyopathies do develop in horses, these are often accompanied by functional MR or TR. In these cases, the cause of valvar regurgitation is dilation of the valve annular plane and apical distraction of the leaflets by the papillary muscles (tenting). These murmurs should not be mistaken for normal, physiologic murmurs caused by ejection and filling murmurs that are also called functional murmurs. To prevent confusion, the adjective secondary is sometimes used in place of functional to distinguish normal from pathologic regurgitation.

Aortic and pulmonary valves

Each of these valves is composed of 3 semilunar leaflets anchored by a functional annulus. The leaflets open during systole and close during diastole to prevent regurgitation of blood from the great vessels. This permits the respective ventricle to fill at lower venous and atrial pressures. Semilunar valve closure occurs within the outer edges of the semilunar leaflets, so there is some leaflet redundancy. Central thickenings or excrescences (nodules of Arantius) are normal structures thought to contribute to valve coaptation, and these might occasionally be visualized by 2D echocardiography. Studies have shown that aortic valvular tissue in horses is both passive and active, and contracts in response to a number of adrenergic and vascular agonists, including angiotensin II and endothelin.[6] The left coronary artery and the normally dominant right main coronary artery originate from the aortic valve sinuses (of Valsalva). Extramural coronary disease in horses is exceedingly rare.

Color Doppler imaging of the aortic valve often reveals thin jets of aortic regurgitation (AR) silent to auscultation. Regurgitant flow across the aortic valve is more prominent in horses subjected to aggressive training. When a diastolic murmur is also evident, the valvular insufficiency is more likely to be clinically relevant and warrant further investigation. Pathologic AR with an associated diastolic murmur is quite common in horses more than 10 years of age. The underlying cause is progressive degeneration of the valvular connective tissues,[7] and the associated echocardiographic findings are diastolic prolapse of 1 or more leaflets and, less often, a torn cusp. Another cause of AR is a ventricular septal defect (See Brian A. Scansen's article, "Equine Congenital Heart Disease," in this issue). Many of these lesions are sited immediately below the right or noncoronary aortic cusps. Loss of aortic root support can lead to valvular prolapse into the defect. Infective endocarditis (see **Fig. 4**D; **Fig. 5**) is a rare etiology of AR or valvar stenosis. As discussed in Annelies Decloedt's article, "Pericardial Disease, Myocardial Disease, and Great Vessel Abnormalities in Horses," in this issue, the aortic sinuses can rupture leading to an acquired left-to-right shunt into the ventricular septum, RV, RA, or PA. Of note is the rare occurrence of aortic or subvalvular aortic stenosis in horses, especially when compared with dogs and humans. This difference is clinically relevant because most ejection murmurs detected over the aortic valve area in the horse are physiologic in origin, and aortic stenosis is rarely a tenable diagnostic consideration.

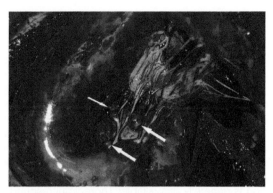

Fig. 5. Infective endocarditis of tricuspid valve. Note the vegetative lesions on the chordae tendineae (*arrows*). This was associated with a ruptured chorda tendinea. (*Courtesy of* Dr Colin Schwarzwald, Zurich, Switzerland.)

The pulmonic (pulmonary) valve guards the RV outflow tract. Similar to the tricuspid valve, color Doppler imaging often shows trivial low velocity (<2.2 m/s) regurgitant diastolic flow that is silent to auscultation. Pulmonary regurgitation (PR) is generally inaudible owing to the relatively low PA pressures and flow volumes involved. However, in severe PR, or when there is PH, the murmur can become audible.

CLINICAL PATHOPHYSIOLOGY

An appreciation of both normal and pathologic cardiovascular physiology is fundamental to an understanding of cardiac disease in the horse. Some key aspects have been noted and others are considered within the context of pathologic physiology.

Congestive Heart Failure

CHF is a pathophysiologic state and clinical syndrome, not a specific disease. It is the consequence of cardiac dysfunction and compensations chronically activated to maintain systemic BP in the setting of a failing heart. BP relates to the product of CO and systemic vascular resistance. When the BP decreases owing to cardiac pump limitations, a series of vascular, hormonal, neural, and renal adaptations occur to maintain arterial filling and BP. Presumably, the pathophysiology of CHF in horses is similar to that of humans.[8] Chronically activated, these compensations are considered maladaptive, and include (1) remodeling of the heart, (2) activation of the sympathetic nervous system, (3) release of vasoconstricting, sodium-retaining hormones (renin–angiotensin–aldosterone; vasopressin), (4) increased activity of endothelial vasoconstrictors (endothelin), and (5) kidney retention of sodium and water owing to changes in intrarenal blood flow and stimulation of adrenergic, mineralocorticoid, vasopressin 1, and endothelin receptors. These systems overwhelm natriuretic peptides despite their increased release by the heart. Fluid retention, combined with a failing cardiac pump, increases venous and capillary hydrostatic pressures, overwhelming lymphatic reserves, and creating the edematous state characteristic of CHF. Neurohormonal activation is also responsible for increasing afterload on the ventricles by causing vasoconstriction. Further injuries include microscopic changes and damage to myocardial and vascular tissues, including cellular hypertrophy, necrosis, apoptosis, and fibrosis. The fundamental paradigm is CHF is characterized by vasoconstriction, renal sodium retention, and abnormal tissue growth (including hypertrophy and fibrosis).

Epidemiologically, CHF is relatively uncommon in horses and most often is associated with the combination of structural heart disease (valvular or congenital) and AF. Possible causes have been summarized in the prior sections and are covered in other articles. Mares in the late stages of gestation can develop CHF because the hemodynamic burden of pregnancy is greatest then. Clinical signs of CHF are known to most veterinarians and are summarized in **Box 3**. Of note is that horses with acute left-sided CHF are often misdiagnosed with pneumonia, and that chronic left heart disease often progress to biventricular CHF related to PH or superimposition of atrial fibrillation.

The diagnosis of right-sided CHF is straightforward and based mainly on observation (**Fig. 6**), physical examination, and ultrasound evaluation. Isolated left-sided CHF is a challenging diagnosis because clinical signs are similar to those of pneumonia. Thoracic radiography can reveal perihilar interstitial to alveolar densities (**Fig. 7**); however, this examination is generally unavailable. Thoracic ultrasound examination can reveal pleural effusion or multiple B-lines suggesting an air–fluid interface within the lung parenchyma. Echocardiography is particularly useful in identifying cardiac lesions that might include pericardial effusion, cardiac chamber dilation, valvular lesions, or cardiac malformation.[9] Enlargement of the LA and LV in the horse often results in rounding of the affected chamber along with measurable enlargement. Ventricular

---

Box 3
Congestive heart failure: findings and diagnosis

Historical and observational signs
  Exercise intolerance
  Altered behavior (depression)
  Weight loss and muscle wasting (cardiac cachexia)
  Respiratory signs: tachypnea or coughing
  Subcutaneous edema
  Colic-like signs

Cardiovascular abnormalities
  Resting tachycardia (examination, electrocardiography)
  Altered arterial pulse (eg, hypokinetic, arrhythmic, paradoxicus)
  Superficial (jugular) venous distension
  Abnormal heart sounds (possible causes)
    Soft first sound (decreased contractility or effusion)
    Tympanic second heart sound (pulmonary hypertension)
    Absent atrial sound (atrial fibrillation)
    Premature beats (premature atrial/ventricular complexes)
    Arrhythmia (atrial fibrillation/ectopic ventricular rhythm)
  Cardiac murmur(s)
  Evidence of structural heart disease (echocardiography)

Abnormal extravascular fluid (association/diagnosis)
  Pulmonary edema (left-sided CHF/auscultation of loud bronchial sounds or crackles, radiography, thoracic ultrasound)
  Pleural effusion (left- or right-sided CHF/muffled breath sounds; thoracic ultrasound examination)
  Subcutaneous, ventral edema (right-sided or biventricular CHF)
  Ascites (right-sided CHF/abdominal ultrasound examination)

Clinical laboratory tests (comments)
  Azotemia (nonspecific)
  Elevated blood cardiac troponin-I or -T (myocardial injury, nonspecific)
  Elevated blood natriuretic peptides (myocardial stretch, poorly defined in horses)

Abbreviation: CHF, congestive heart failure.

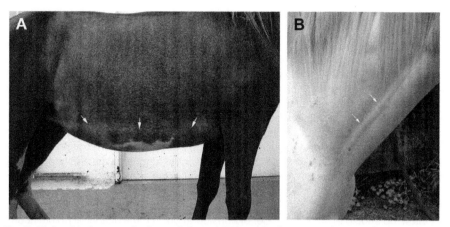

Fig. 6. Right-sided congestive heart failure. (*A*) Ventral edema is evident in a horse with cardiomyopathy. Note the sharp demarcation in the tissue edema (*arrows*). (*B*) Jugular venous distension in a horse with pericarditis and right heart failure.

systolic function is variable, and can be hyperdynamic in primary mitral or aortic valve diseases. Dilated pulmonary arteries with left-sided cardiomegaly suggest postcapillary PH. Routine laboratory tests are not diagnostic, but mild azotemia is often observed and markers of cell injury or natriuretic peptide release might be identified.

The prognosis for horses with CHF is always guarded, unless a potentially reversible etiology such as pericardial effusion or tachycardia-induced cardiomyopathy is identified. The horse should never be ridden or driven, and there is a risk of collapse or sudden death from arrhythmia or rupture of the pulmonary artery. Some horses can be maintained as companions or for reproduction. With catastrophic lesions, such as flail

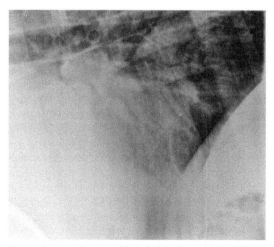

Fig. 7. Thoracic radiographs in a horse with left sided congestive heart failure because of severe mitral regurgitation. Note the cardiomegaly with bulging and rounding of the left atrium, prominent pulmonary vascular markings, and increased interstitial lung density. Bronchial markings are also prominent that might indicate concurrent disease or peribronchial fluid collection.

mitral valve or severe vegetative endocarditis, animals are unlikely to survive long term.

The medical therapy for CHF owing to valvular or myocardial diseases includes furosemide and digoxin. Digoxin is especially indicated when accompanied by atrial fibrillation, although the drug is (relatively) contraindicated in horses with ventricular ectopy. Chronic administration should include monitoring of blood concentrations. Digoxin has been safely administered in the final trimester of pregnancy. Initial intravenous doses are often administered every 12 hours, and this is followed by chronic oral administration every 12 to 24 hours, if feasible. Parenteral furosemide is a mainstay for CHF and initially used intravenously. Chronic intramuscular administration is sometimes possible. Pimobendan and angiotensin-converting enzyme inhibitors have been prescribed. Evidence for these drugs and usual dosages are summarized in Adam Redpath and Mark Bowen's article, "Cardiac Therapeutics in Horses," in this issue.

Follow-up should include a number of considerations: (1) the historical points noted in **Box 3**, (2) resting heart rate and rhythm (motivated clients can record smartphone-based electrocardiograms for transmission), (3) respiratory signs (resting respiratory rate, cough), (4) body condition and weight if available (marked gains can indicate fluid retention), and (5) jugular venous distension and pulsation. Physical and ultrasound examinations are usually focused on the identification of edema and effusions. Pertinent clinical laboratory tests (renal function, electrolytes, and serum digoxin concentration) can be obtained. It might be helpful to consult with a cardiac specialist regarding prognosis and management. Unfortunately, the majority of horses released to the farm will not survive for more than 6 months, with most euthanatized or suffering an unwitnessed death.

Pulmonary Hypertension

PH indicates an increased BP in the pulmonary arteries and implies an increase in CO, pulmonary vascular resistance, or both determinants of PA pressure. Although this pressure elevation is assumed to occur at rest, severe exercise can induce PH both physiologically and accentuate an underlying cause for this pathophysiologic state. PH in humans is classified in a number of ways, but mainly by etiology. Within this classification, some of the causes potentially relevant to horses are listed in **Box 4**. PA hypertension (PAH) is characterized by "cellular fibrosis and proliferation and fibrosis of small pulmonary arteries" that leads to a "progressive rise in pulmonary vascular resistance."[10] This designation of PAH is especially relevant to people owing to the substantial number of patients with idiopathic (primary) PH. However, in horses, it might be more practical to use a functional or pathophysiologic classification for PH, such as (1) exercise-induced PH, (2) postcapillary PH, (3) PH owing to advanced pulmonary disease, and (4) precapillary PAH. This grouping is simply one of convenience; there are no veterinary consensus statements about this disorder.

The pressure in the PA depends on flow (CO) and pulmonary vascular resistance. The equine heart carries tremendous heart rate and SV reserves such that CO can increase to extraordinary levels with maximal exercise (more than five-fold) taxing the vascular compliance of the lungs and the left heart. As noted, vascular resistance in the lungs is not solely related to arterial resistance, but is also influenced significantly by pulmonary capillary density and compression, and by left heart function and pressures. As such, left heart failure, widespread pulmonary disease, or arterial constriction or narrowing can increases pulmonary vascular resistance and PA pressures.

Box 4
Potential etiologies of pulmonary hypertension

Exercise-related PH
  High cardiac output–related PH

PAH
  Congenital heart disease (Eisenmenger's pathophysiology)
  Pulmonary venoocclusive disease
  Drug or toxin induced
  Persistent PH of the newborn
  Pulmonary arteriopathy
  Idiopathic PAH (?)

PH owing to left heart disease
  Left ventricular dysfunction
  Valvular heart disease
  Congenital disease

PH owing to lung disease or hypoxia
  Chronic reactive (obstructive) pulmonary disease (asthma)
  Interstitial lung disease
  Pleuropneumonia (?)
  Chronic exposure to high altitude (?)

Chronic thromboembolic PH (?)

Abbreviations: ?, uncertain relevancy to horses; PAH, pulmonary arterial hypertension; PH, pulmonary hypertension.

Modified from Classification of European Society of Cardiology & European Respiratory Society. Eur Respir J 2015;46:903–75; with permission.

Pulmonary hypertension owing to exercise

Exercised-induced pulmonary hemorrhage (EIPH) is a well-known disorder affecting performance horses and likely stems from the combination of normal and pathologic airway mechanics, augmented CO, and elevations in postcapillary vascular resistance and pressure in what might be viewed as an overfilling of the left heart. Although increased pulmonary blood flow can increase PA pressures in other disorders, as with ventricular septal defect, exercise-induced PH in horses is unique. As the heart rate increases to about 240/min, the CO soars, the LV end-diastolic pressure exceeds 40 mm Hg, and the mean LA pressures can exceed 60 mm Hg. These hemodynamic changes, along with other pulmonary and physical factors, result in stress rupture of pulmonary capillaries into the alveolar space. The consequences are pulmonary hemorrhage and airway bleeding, along with pathologic lung remodeling (noted in recurrent cases). PA pressure can be reduced by the preexercise administration of furosemide (where permitted). The prevention of EIPH is also approached by other treatments that focus on airway dynamics (such as nasal strips). The disorder of EIPH is predisposed by high-intensity exercise, associated with PH, is clinically extensive, and presents an expansive topic beyond the scope this article. The reader is referred to reviews of EIPH[11] and to the American College of Veterinary Internal Medicine Consensus Statement on this subject.[12]

Postcapillary pulmonary hypertension

Postcapillary pulmonary hypertension is either left heart disease or the recently reported pulmonary venoocclusive disease.[13] PH can be caused by severe MR, left heart failure, or increased resistance to flow caused by remodeling of pulmonary veins. Acute left heart failure, as with infective endocarditis or flail mitral leaflet, is more likely to result in pulmonary edema owing to elevated venous pressures. However, PA arterial pressures must also increase proportionally to overcome the hydrostatic resistance to venous return. Consequently, most horses with left-sided CHF are likely to have some degree of postcapillary PH. Chronically, left heart failure can lead to progressive PH with RV enlargement and potentially to biventricular CHF. This finding is especially common if there is a superimposed reactive pulmonary arteriopathy (poorly characterized in horses) or if atrial fibrillation supervenes, because this markedly reduces CO.

Pulmonary hypertension owing to lung disease

Chronic, severe lung disease—especially diffuse interstitial lung diseases—increase the pulmonary vascular resistance by destroying a large cross-sectional area of lung, including capillaries and small vessels. Although PH is poorly characterized in chronic lung diseases of horses,[14] it is likely that it is underrecognized, and most severe in disorders such as multinodular pulmonary fibrosis. Dixon[15] measured invasive PA pressures in a number of horses with recurrent airway obstruction and overall found mild to moderate increases in PA pressures at rest, with mean PA pressure approximately doubling in affected cases. It is likely that PH becomes more severe in these horses during exercise.

Precapillary pulmonary hypertension

This category is similar to human PAH inasmuch as the level of increased resistance resides largely within the medium and small pulmonary arteries. Potential causes include idiopathic PAH and pulmonary thromboembolism (see **Box 4**); however, these disorders are largely unrecognized in horses. Aside from the rare causes of pulmonary arteriopathy, this category is probably unimportant in horses. It is likely that a precapillary component of reactive pulmonary vasoconstriction occurs in any cause of significant alveolar hypoxia, including equine asthma and left-sided CHF.

Cor pulmonale

The development of RV enlargement or hypertrophy secondary to acute or chronic pulmonary disease is termed cor (Latin for heart) pulmonale. In terms of defining this condition, right heart changes secondary to left heart failure are excluded from this designation (**Fig. 8**). In nearly every case, the pathophysiologic basis of cor pulmonale is underlying PH, generally from increased resistance to PA blood flow or from extensive loss of alveolar–capillary units. Acute pulmonary disease, such as an exacerbation of equine asthma, can lead to reversible dilation of the right heart and PA. Chronic or recurrent pulmonary diseases such as multinodular pulmonary fibrosis are more likely to result in persistent RV hypertrophy.

Clinical signs

Clinically, significant PH leads to right heart dysfunction. It is likely that the most common clinical sign is exercise intolerance related to diminished CO. However, the precise etiology can be challenging to pin down because most horses with symptomatic PH have other excuses for poor performance, such as bronchopulmonary disease or left heart dysfunction. Exercise intolerance in this disorder is fundamentally a type of heart failure; however, only in extreme cases of PH do clinical signs of right-sided CHF develop. History and physical examination might indicate evidence of pulmonary disease, including tachypnea, cough, pulmonary crackles, and wheezes.

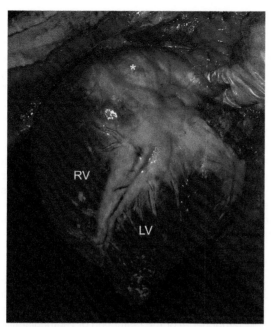

Fig. 8. Cor pulmonale. Note the right heart enlargement (compared with the left side) and dilated pulmonary artery (*asterisk*).

Diagnostic tests

Imaging studies can be helpful. Although thoracic radiography is not widely available, thoracic ultrasound examination and echocardiography can identify pulmonary disease or features of cor pulmonale. Dilation of the pulmonary trunk and branch pulmonary arteries are the typical echocardiographic features of PH. Ultrasound examination can also identify supravalvular pulmonary stenosis owing to a lung mass (a differential diagnosis). The pattern of RV enlargement is variable and more often "mixed" inasmuch as the wall thickness increases modestly along with dilation of the RV and the RA. Chamber dilation is especially likely if there is concurrent CHF or significant TR or PR (secondary to PH). If PR or TR is evident by Doppler imaging, the peak regurgitant velocity will be increased. As rough guidelines, in resting horses, a TR velocity exceeding 3.5 m/s or a PR velocity of greater than 2.5 m/s on continuous wave Doppler echocardiography are quite suggestive of increased PA pressures.

Other diagnostic tests are focused toward identification of underlying respiratory pathology. These studies often involve a complete blood count/fibrinogen, airway endoscopy, and bronchoalveolar lavage with cytology and culture (adding special microbiological tests as indicated). More invasive testing in PH includes lung biopsy and right heart catheterization. Catheterization is the definitive method to document PH, and a pulmonary capillary wedge pressure can help to exclude underlying or occult left heart dysfunction.[16] In left heart failure, the pulmonary capillary wedge pressure—an estimate of LA pressure—increases, approximating the level of the PA diastolic pressure at normal heart rates. When the pulmonary capillary wedge pressure is substantially lower than the diastolic PA pressure, the cause of PH is likely anatomic or reactive pulmonary vascular disease, advanced lung disease, or both.

Management

The treatment of postcapillary PH generally involves treating underlying left heart failure with diuretics, digoxin, and angiotensin-converting enzyme inhibitors (See Adam Redpath and Mark Bowen's article, "Cardiac Therapeutics in Horses," in this issue). The management of PH owing to pulmonary disease involves identifying and treating the underlying bronchopulmonary disorder, as with antimicrobials, airway dilators and antiinflammatory drugs. Precapillary PH in other species is often successfully treated with phosphodiesterase V inhibitors such as sildenafil. These agents maintain the activity of cyclic GMP, the second messenger of nitric oxide, a potent PA vasodilator. However, sildenafil was ineffective in preventing exercise-induced PH in 1 equine study; nevertheless, this class of drug has not been suitably evaluated in PAH or PH owing to spontaneous lung disease. Inhaled nitric oxide has been used to treat foals with neonatal PH, but this therapy is expensive and impractical. In 1 study, inhaled nitric oxide decreased exercise-induced PH, but did not protect the lung from EIPH. Drugs used to treat PAH in humans, including endothelin receptor blockers, have not been sufficiently studied in horses.

Pericardial Diseases

The clinical signs of heart failure in pericardial disease are attributed to diastolic ventricular dysfunction, altered ventricular interdependence, the development of CHF, and the underlying etiology (see **Fig. 1**). Cardiac dysfunction stems from external compression (cardiac tamponade) or the restriction of ventricular filling. Cardiac tamponade is characterized by increased (positive) intrapericardial pressure and reduced cardiac filling despite increases in ventricular filling pressures. With tamponade, the total cardiac volume within the 4 chambers is fixed such that inspiratory augmentation of right heart filling shifts the ventricular septum leftward, reducing LV preload; this reverses during expiration. Acutely, rapid intrapericardial fluid collection can lead to hypotension or sudden death, as with intrapericardial rupture of the aorta. Chronically, pericardial constraint impairs CO, leading to predictable compensations previously noted for CHF. These changes are recognized clinically as right-sided CHF. Some cases of pericarditis progress to constrictive pericardial disease, in which the effusion is reabsorbed and the pericardial layers and inflammatory debris organize causing the epicardium and parietal pericardium to adhere. A transition stage is termed constrictive–effusive disease. In addition to signs of cardiac failure, systemic and constitutional signs related to inflammation or infection might be evident in affected horses, depending on the underlying etiology.

The resting arterial pulse rate is increased from sinus tachycardia, and pulse character can be hypokinetic from reduced SV or vary markedly with phases of ventilation. A pronounced inspiratory decrease in the BP (*pulsus paradoxicus*) should be sought by palpation of the facial arterial pulse or measurement of Doppler flow BP with a protracted and deliberate release of pressure in the tail cuff. With pulsus paradoxicus, Doppler flow sounds are eventually lost during inspiration, but reemerge during expiration. This finding is related to exaggerated ventricular interdependence with swings in left and right heart filling. The systemic BP in chronic disease is likely to be normal, owing to fluid retention, elevated venous pressures, arterial vasoconstriction, and increased heart rate.

The initial therapy for cardiac tamponade is logically pericardiocentesis, because this procedure relieves the initiating pathophysiology of the disease. The value of intravenous fluid therapy to increase cardiac filling is more controversial, although small infusion volumes might improve CO and BP in some cases. Therapy for constrictive disease is highly problematic unless there is a substantial effusive component. Clinical findings, diagnostic studies, and management of pericardial diseases in horses are discussed in more detail in Annelies Decloedt's article, "Pericardial Disease, Myocardial Disease, and Great Vessel Abnormalities in Horses," in this issue.

Myocardial Diseases

Cardiomyocytes can hypertrophy (increase in mass) as a response to exercise, increased work owing to structural cardiac disease, or secondary to a noncardiac disorder. Volume overloads, if significant, are recognized echocardiographically (or at postmortem examination) as eccentric hypertrophy with dilation and often apical rounding of the affected chamber. The uncommon causes of systolic pressure overload (pulmonary stenosis; PH; systemic arterial hypertension) can lead to wall thickening or a concentric form of ventricular hypertrophy on the affected side of the heart.

The clinical manifestations of myocardial disease, regardless of the underlying injury, can be attributed to 4 pathophysiologic processes: (1) systolic dysfunction with reduced myocardial contractility and ventricular ejection fraction, (2) diastolic dysfunction with impaired ventricular filling, (3) secondary AV (mitral or tricuspid) valve incompetency caused by cardiac dilation or papillary muscle dysfunction, or (4) the development of heart rhythm disturbances. Persistent premature ventricular complexes or ventricular tachycardias are common features of myocardial disease. Although atrial arrhythmias such as atrial fibrillation are more often a primary electrical disturbance in horses, these arrhythmias can also develop with cardiomyopathies (**Fig. 9**). Although it is tempting to diagnose myocardial disease in the setting of any heart rhythm disturbance, it should be appreciated that rhythm abnormalities can be primary electrical disturbances, without a gross anatomic substrate. This point is especially relevant to horses suffering from electrolyte or other metabolic imbalances, adrenergic excess, sepsis or toxemia, hypoxemia, or hypotension–ischemia–reperfusion. For example, in horses examined for sudden death at a racetrack, gross or

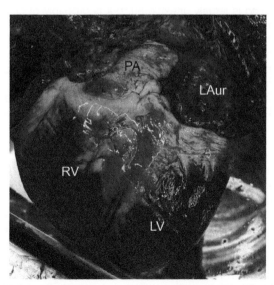

Fig. 9. Autopsy of left lateral perspective of a heart affected with dilated cardiomyopathy. Note the dilated left atrium/auricle (LAur) and rounding of the left ventricular (LV) apex. The right ventricle (RV) is also enlarged. Compare this heart to **Fig. 8**.

microscopic myocardial lesions are a relatively uncommon finding and nearly one-fourth of cases are unexplained.[17]

The overall cardiac disability engendered by myocardial disease varies greatly. Some horses have no detectable clinical signs other than perhaps an increase in a circulating biomarker test such as cardiac troponin-I or troponin-T. Others demonstrate exercise intolerance, life-threatening arrhythmias, signs of CHF, or sudden death. Clinical findings, diagnostic studies, and management of myocardial diseases in horses are discussed in more detail in Annelies Decloedt's article, "Pericardial Disease, Myocardial Disease, and Great Vessel Abnormalities," in this issue.

Valvular Heart Disease

Progressive, hemodynamically significant valvular regurgitation induces cardiac remodeling. MR is characterized by LA dilation, eccentric LV hypertrophy, and alterations of the intercellular matrix that are largely beyond the view of conventional echocardiography. Acute and chronic AR place a volume (and to some degree a pressure load) on the LV, leading to eccentric or mixed hypertrophy with increased LV mass. These changes are especially likely once regurgitation becomes moderate to severe. The LA in chronic AR can also enlarge consequent to mitral valve disease or to LV diastolic or systolic failure. For equal regurgitant volumes, the load on the LV is greater with AR because with MR much of the ventricular SV is ejected into the lower pressure LA before the opening of the aortic valve. This allows the LV to both decrease in volume and increase in wall thickness before actual ejection of blood, decreasing wall stress. Conversely, in chronic AR, the additional end-diastolic volume must be ejected into the high-pressure systemic arterial system. This factor probably explains the greater degree of LV mass that often develops with severe AR, as well as the greater likelihood of heart failure and possibly ventricular arrhythmias when AR is present. In cases of TR, the changes found in MR are mirrored on the right side of the heart. When TR is caused by PH, the degree of RV hypertrophy is likely to be greater.

The role of neurohormonal activation in the pathogenesis of valvular disease and ventricular remodeling is largely unexplored, but is probably of clinical relevance in some horses. Limited biomarker studies have shown some trends for increased values of natriuretic peptides and cardiac troponins, but the sensitivity of these for predicting outcomes in primary valvular disease is likely to be low. Ultimately, such pathophysiology becomes relevant to clinicians once studies demonstrate a meaningful reduction in disease progression, clinical signs, or mortality associated with treatment. Some treatments used in management of equine valve disease today, such as inhibitors of the renin–angiotensin–aldosterone system, have a reasonable theoretic basis for their use, but also lack sufficient evidence to dogmatically advance (see Adam Redpath and Mark Bowen's article, "Cardiac Therapeutics in Horses," in this issue).

Clinically relevant VHD is recognized by the presence of a cardiac murmur, usually localized over the affected valve area. The source of the murmur can be refined by comparing the results of auscultation to those of echocardiography and especially Doppler imaging. The consequences of a valvular lesion depends largely on the severity of regurgitation (or stenosis) across the valve and the secondary responses that develop within the cardiac chambers and pulmonary vasculature.[18] These are best seen by echocardiography. As noted, many horses adapt to trivial, mild, or even moderate VHD with no apparent consequence on performance. This also depends on the disease severity relative to the level of work. Some practical considerations for assessing the severity of valvular disease are: (1) the etiology and lesion severity responsible for VHD; (2) the severity of the regurgitation as assessed by

Doppler imaging; (3) the degree of cardiac remodeling; (4) ventricular function; (5) the pulmonary vascular response if any; (5) the heart rhythm; and (7) clinical effects of VHD on exercise performance. These issues, along with management approaches and prognostic considerations, are described in more detail in Celia M. Marr's article, "Equine Acquired Valvular Disease," in this issue.

Disease of the Impulse-Forming and Conduction Systems

Disorders of the cardiac rhythm are discussed elsewhere in this issue, and page space limits a detailed discussion of the mechanisms of arrhythmogenesis aside from listing these as (1) enhanced (normal) automaticity, (2) triggered (pacemaker) activity, and (3) various forms of microreentry and macroreentry that include many ventricular tachycardias as well as myocardial flutter and fibrillation. Clinical associations of cardiac arrhythmias stem from 1 of 5 categories: (1) primary structural or electrical heart disease, (2) autonomic influences, (3) metabolic (electrolyte) or endocrine disorders, (4) drugs, anesthetics, and toxins, and (5) noncardiac disorders, notably hypotension/reperfusion, severe gastrointestinal disease, hypoxia, or systemic inflammation.

The pathophysiology of arrhythmias in terms of hemodynamics relate largely to their impact on ventricular filling and pumping. CO (L/min) is the product of (ventricular SV [mL/beat] × heart rate [beats/min]). The SV is strongly affected by filling or preload along with myocardial inotropy and impedance to ejection (wall stress, afterload). Additionally, the sequence of ventricular contraction (synchrony) and influence of myocardial oxygen delivery (relative to demand) affect ventricular performance. Severe bradyarrhythmias, relatively rare in horses, reduce CO by virtue of the low heart rate. Conversely, tachyarrhythmias can encroach on the diastolic filling and coronary perfusion periods of the ventricle, while increasing demands for myocardial oxygen. As such, tachyarrhythmias can reduce preload and induce demand ischemia of the heart muscle. Tachyarrhythmias associated with irregular ventricular rhythms (such as atrial fibrillation), further encroach on filling during short cardiac cycles. Some arrhythmias reduce AV synchrony, negatively affecting ventricular filling. For example, atrial fibrillation eliminates the effective atrial contraction so necessary for filling at higher heart rates, and ventricular tachycardias often cause AV dissociation in which atrial and ventricular activations are no longer synchronized. Ventricular ectopy is also likely to result in uncoordinated ventricular contractions, or dyssynchrony, which further limits SV.

Ultimately, cardiac arrhythmias become clinically relevant for 2 reasons. The first is their effect on BP and tissue perfusion, most evident as signs of low CO causing exercise intolerance, azotemia, or colic. More serious is the potential to induce a severe or fatal rhythm disturbance that causes syncope or sudden death. Recognition and management of arrhythmias are the focus of Katharyn J. Mitchell's article, "Equine Electrocardiography," and Gunther van Loon's article, "Cardiac Arrhythmias in Horses," in this issue.

SUPPLEMENTARY DATA

Supplementary data related to this article can be found online at https://doi.org/10.1016/j.cveq.2019.01.001.

REFERENCES

1. Schwarzwald CC. The cardiovascular system. In: Reed SM, Bayly WM, Sellon DC, editors. Equine internal medicine. 4th edition. Philadelphia: Saunders Elsevier; 2017. p. 387–541.

2. Else RW, Holmes JR. Cardiac pathology in the horse. 1. Gross pathology. Equine Vet J 1972;4:1–8.
3. Reef VB, Bonagura J, Buhl R, et al. Recommendations for management of equine athletes with cardiovascular abnormalities. J Vet Intern Med 2014;28:749–61.
4. Worth LT, Reef VB. Pericarditis in horses: 18 cases (1986-1995). J Am Vet Med Assoc 1998;212:248–53.
5. Maxson AD, Reef VB. Bacterial endocarditis in horses: ten cases (1984-1995). Equine Vet J 1997;29:394–9.
6. Bowen IM, Marr CM, Chester AH, et al. In-vitro contraction of the equine aortic valve. J Heart Valve Dis 2004;13:593–9.
7. Bishop SP, Cole CR, Smetzer DL. Functional and morphologic pathology of equine aortic insufficiency. Pathol Vet 1966;3:137–58.
8. Tanai E, Frantz S. Pathophysiology of heart failure. Compr Physiol 2015;6:187–214.
9. Reef VB. Advances in echocardiography. Vet Clin North Am Equine Pract 1991;7:435–50.
10. Lau EMT, Giannoulatou E, Celermajer DS, et al. Epidemiology and treatment of pulmonary arterial hypertension. Nat Rev Cardiol 2017;14:603–14.
11. Poole DC, Erickson HH. Exercise-induced pulmonary hemorrhage: where are we now? Vet Med (Auckl) 2016;7:133–48.
12. Hinchcliff KW, Couetil LL, Knight PK, et al. Exercise induced pulmonary hemorrhage in horses: American College of Veterinary Internal Medicine consensus statement. J Vet Intern Med 2015;29:743–58.
13. Williams KJ, Derksen FJ, de Feijter-Rupp H, et al. Regional pulmonary veno-occlusion: a newly identified lesion of equine exercise-induced pulmonary hemorrhage. Vet Pathol 2008;45:316–26.
14. Schwarzwald CC, Stewart AJ, Morrison CD, et al. Cor pulmonale in a horse with granulomatous pneumonia. Equine Vet Educ 2006;18:182–7.
15. Dixon PM. Pulmonary artery pressures in normal horses and in horses affected with chronic obstructive pulmonary disease. Equine Vet J 1978;10:195–8.
16. Gehlen H, Bubeck K, Stadler P. Pulmonary artery wedge pressure measurement in healthy warmblood horses and in warmblood horses with mitral valve insufficiencies of various degrees during standardised treadmill exercise. Res Vet Sci 2004;77:257–64.
17. Lyle CH, Uzal FA, McGorum BC, et al. Sudden death in racing Thoroughbred horses: an international multicentre study of post mortem findings. Equine Vet J 2011;43:324–31.
18. Reef VB, Bain FT, Spencer PA. Severe mitral regurgitation in horses: clinical, echocardiographic and pathological findings. Equine Vet J 1998;30:18–27.

Examination of Horses with Cardiac Disease

John A. Keen, BVetMed, PhD, Cert EM (Int Med), MRCVS

KEYWORDS

- Equine • Clinical evaluation • Auscultation • Blood pressure • Cardiac biomarkers

KEY POINTS

- Despite advances, increased convenience, and availability of echocardiography and other diagnostic techniques, a comprehensive clinical examination still forms the essential first step in any cardiac evaluation.
- Signalment and historical findings provide important perspective on the case, whether abnormalities are detected during routine examination or when there are specific presenting signs that may be attributable to cardiac disease.
- Good auscultation skills are imperative and this skill improves with thought and practice.
- Ancillary tests, such as blood pressure measurement and blood analysis, may provide useful additional information, particularly in specific cases.

 Video content accompanies this article at http://www.vetequine.theclinics.com.

INTRODUCTION

A thorough medical history and clinical examination at rest forms the cornerstone of any cardiac evaluation. This article describes an approach based on the assumption that cardiac disease is suspected and highlights some ancillary techniques that complement the initial examination of such a case. Clinicians may be alerted to potential cardiac disease following routine examinations, such as those at scheduled vaccinations or during prepurchase evaluation. Conversely, clinicians may be prompted to examine a horse for cardiac disease because of a specific presenting complaint (**Box 1**). Consideration of the presenting signs, or lack of, is an important first step in considering whether clinically relevant cardiac disease is likely and for reflecting on the potential differential diagnoses. Cardiac disease is rare in the horse in comparison with other domestic species and, because of the large cardiac reserve of the

Disclosure Statement: None.
The Royal (Dick) School of Veterinary Studies, Easter Bush Campus, Roslin, Midlothian EH25 9RG, UK
E-mail address: john.keen@ed.ac.uk

Vet Clin Equine 35 (2019) 23–42
https://doi.org/10.1016/j.cveq.2018.12.006   vetequine.theclinics.com

> **Box 1**
> **Presenting signs that may prompt specific evaluation for cardiac disease**
>
> Detection of a murmur/arrhythmia during routine examination
>
> Altered demeanor
>
> Poor performance/exercise intolerance
>
> Dyspnea/cough
>
> Weakness
>
> Collapse
>
> Colic
>
> Distended peripheral veins/ventral edema
>
> Epistaxis
>
> Persistent tachycardia of unexplained origin
>
> Fever of unknown origin

horse, overt clinical signs are often only noted when severe dysfunction is present or during vigorous exercise testing. Although murmurs and arrhythmias are commonly detected in horses, these are often physiologic in origin and may well be of no pathologic significance.

SIGNALMENT AND HISTORY

Considering the signalment of the case that is presented for evaluation is a crucial first step in any evaluation because there are some conditions that are more likely, or have more importance in certain breeds, ages, and sexes of horse and pony. For example, the detection of aortic regurgitation is potentially more relevant in a young horse,[1] ventricular septal defects (VSD) occur with increased frequency in Welsh Section A ponies,[2] Arabian horses may have predisposition to congenital lesions,[3] and Friesian horses have a predisposition to aortopulmonary fistulae.[4,5] Similarly, stallions are more prone to the development of fistulae in the aortic root[6,7]; large athletic horses commonly have atrioventricular (AV) valve regurgitation,[8–10] not always clinically relevant but nonetheless important; and the suspicion of tricuspid regurgitation has different implications in a small pony versus a Thoroughbred horse.

Many horses presented for further cardiac evaluation may have no or minimal relevant history. Even under these circumstances, however, it is important to collect key information that should include background facts and specific questions about the presenting signs. In the case of a recent detection of a murmur or rhythm abnormality, determining when the heart was last auscultated and whether this was apparently normal or abnormal is an important question that provides key context to the ensuing examination. Asking specifically about the presence of other presenting signs (see **Box 1**) may be useful because the client may not have recognized their clinical relevance.

CLINICAL EVALUATION

The clinical evaluation should be thorough and comprehensive, and although in the case of a cardiac patient this naturally focuses on the cardiovascular system, other body systems should also be considered. For example, dyspnea may be noted in cases with mitral regurgitation and atrial fibrillation leading to a suspicion of left-sided heart failure, but one must question whether the type of dyspnea is consistent with pulmonary congestion (typically rapid shallow breaths caused by decreased lung compliance; Video 1, cardiac dyspnea) or more consistent with concurrent primary respiratory disease, such as equine asthma (Video 2, increased expiratory effort). Conversely synovial distention is common and often of minimal significance in older horses, but in tandem with intermittent pyrexia of unknown origin and the sudden appearance of a cardiac murmur, this finding may be consistent with the synovitis frequently noted in endocarditis cases.[11,12] Furthermore, the presence of even subtle ventral edema (**Fig. 1**) is an important finding in the context of cardiac disease, potentially suggesting right-sided or biventricular congestive heart failure.

Pro forma sheets (**Fig. 2**) are useful for ensuring that clinical recording is consistent between examinations and are a useful *aide memoire* when revisiting cases. The following discussion picks up on key points of the clinical examination.

Evaluation of the Peripheral Circulation

Mucous membranes should be assessed in good ambient light. With clinically relevant cardiac disease, sympathetic activity is enhanced, the peripheral perfusion is poor, and membranes may display pallor or even cyanosis in severe cases. Impaired tissue oxygenation, such as may occur with right-to-left cardiac shunts in complex congenital heart disease where the lungs are bypassed to varying degrees, may also impart a blue tinge to the membranes. The oral mucosa is the most convenient to assess but ocular, vulval, and rectal mucosa can also be evaluated. Although rare in the horse, a patent ductus arteriosus may present with differential oxygenation of the cranial versus caudal vasculature.[13]

A pulse is easily palpable as the facial artery crosses the ramus of the mandible, whereas the transverse facial artery is an alternative site on the head for assessing pulses. Other sites that are used include the palmar digital artery, the dorsal metatarsal artery (foals), and the median artery; the latter is useful to palpate while auscultating as an aid to differentiating between systole and diastole. Palpation of the pulse provides an appreciation of rhythm and rate but also provides a subjective assessment of pulse pressure. For example, pulse pressures may be weak with low-output heart failure. In contrast bounding pulses may be present in cases of moderate-to-marked aortic

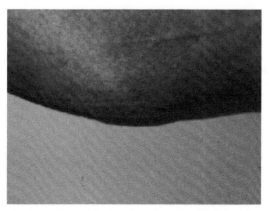

Fig. 1. Subtle ventral edema in a horse in acute-onset heart failure; such findings may be missed if not specifically looked for, especially in horses with full winter coats.

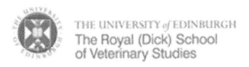

THE UNIVERSITY of EDINBURGH
The Royal (Dick) School
of Veterinary Studies

The Equine Hospital

AFFIX STICKER

Equine Cardiac Examination

Presenting signs: ....
Pulse (rate/quality/ rhythm): ....
Mucous membranes: ....
Heart rate and rhythm: ....
Respiration rate: ....
Other (e.g. jugular vein/ oedema): ....
BLOOD PRESSURE ....

LEFT SIDE AUSCULTATION

S1   S2   S1   S2

1. PMI: _____ GRADE: _____ QUALITY: _____ DIAGNOSIS: _____
2. PMI: _____ GRADE: _____ QUALITY: _____ DIAGNOSIS: _____

RIGHT SIDE AUSCULTATION

S1   S2   S1   S2

1. PMI: _____ GRADE: _____ QUALITY: _____ DIAGNOSIS: _____
2. PMI: _____ GRADE: _____ QUALITY: _____ DIAGNOSIS: _____

Fig. 2. Pro forma sheet for cardiac examination. (*Courtesy of* University of Edinburgh, Edinburgh, UK.)

regurgitation, where diastolic pressures fall (because of diastolic backward flow from the aorta into the left ventricle) and systolic pressures rise (because of left ventricular volume overload resulting in increased stroke volume) creating an increased pulse pressure. Increased pulse pressure indicates significant left ventricular enlargement and should be regarded as a negative prognostic finding in aortic regurgitation.[1]

Evaluation of Central Venous Pressures

A useful clinical proxy for central venous pressure assessment involves examination of the jugular furrow to assess the jugular vein filling and pulsation. When the head is in a resting position, the normal blood pressure in the right atrium (0–5 mm Hg) causes filling to a level approximately one-third of the way up the horse's jugular furrow. When right atrial pressure is elevated, such as with right-sided or biventricular congestive heart failure, then this column of blood extends up the furrow (increased jugular filling, **Fig. 3** and Video 3) and pulsation may become more evident. Pulsation in the jugular vein is caused by changes in atrial filling pressure that occur through the cardiac cycle and the underlying pulsations from the carotid artery; in the face of elevated right atrial pressure and jugular filling, this pulsation becomes more obvious. Central venous pressure is assessed by invasive means using intracardiac catheters (See Andre Shih's article, "Cardiac Monitoring in Horses", in this issue.), but this is rarely necessary.

Cardiac Auscultation

Cardiac auscultation is a crucial part of the cardiac examination and usually enables the formulation of a differential diagnosis list if not the actual diagnosis to be made.

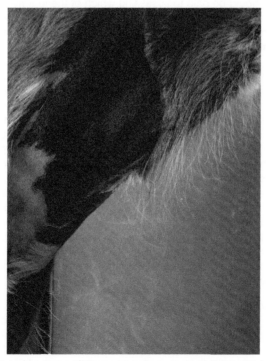

Fig. 3. Abnormal jugular venous filling suggesting elevated right atrial pressure in a foal with cardiac disease.

More advanced diagnostic tests described later in this text confirm the diagnosis and assess its clinical relevance.

Effective cardiac auscultation is well described and the reader is directed elsewhere for a more comprehensive review.[14–16] In general, most cardiac problems do not require sophisticated or expensive stethoscopes to reach a diagnosis. The more expensive stethoscopes are better, however, for more subtle abnormalities and are more comfortable to use. Several models of electronic stethoscopes are now available that allow the recording of sounds, which is useful in some cases for repeated re-evaluation and for sharing with others; the quality of the playback can, however, be variable. A quiet environment is crucial to block out extraneous sounds, and sufficient thought to the process and time are especially important to the novice clinician. Palpating the apex beat is a useful part of the examination and landmark providing the starting point for auscultation.

Heart rate

Measuring heart rate is a crucial first step that is often forgotten in the face of interesting auscultation abnormalities. The heart rate at rest (reference interval 28–40 beats/min) gives an important indication of cardiac function. It is often worth assessing this variable at the start and the end of the examination, because the rate can change as the horse relaxes during an examination. Measuring the heart rate should ideally be 30 seconds with normal rhythm and longer when an arrhythmia is present. Note that smaller ponies may have a slightly higher heart rate at rest compared with larger horses.[17]

Normal heart sounds and rhythm

Specific attention should be paid to assessing which of the four normal heart sounds are audible, because this helps with ascertaining the timing of murmurs and rhythm assessment. Sounds 1 and 2 (S1 and S2) (**Table 2**, Audio 1A) are high-frequency sounds that almost invariably are audible unless obscured by a loud murmur. Sounds S3 and S4 (**Table 2**; Audios 1B, 1C) are lower frequency sounds and are therefore harder to hear; they are often close in timing to S2 and S1, respectively, and some people may find it difficult to distinguish between sounds that are close together; this is a skill that improves with practice. With good auscultation skills, splitting of the S2 sound, caused by the slight difference between aortic valve and pulmonic valve closure, is heard cranially on the left side in thin-chested horses. If it is obvious, then this could indicate pulmonary disease associated with pulmonary hypertension. Splitting of the S1 sound is rarely detected but occasionally noted in arrhythmias, such as atrial fibrillation. Normal heart sounds may sound quiet or muffled in cases of pericarditis or where there is a large mass in the pleural cavity. Sound S3 may increase in intensity with significant mitral regurgitation and marked volume overload.

The rhythm should be assessed as regular or irregular and, if it is irregular, whether it is regularly or irregularly irregular. Many arrhythmias are suspected based on auscultation, although an electrocardiogram (ECG) provides the definitive diagnosis (See Katharyn J. Mitchell's article, "Equine Electrocardiography"; Gunther van Loon's article, "Cardiac Arrhythmias in Horses," in this issue).

Auscultating arrhythmias

The human ear is good at detecting arrhythmias and these are frequently identified during auscultation. The most common arrhythmia detected is a regular irregularity that usually represents second degree AV block. This is confirmed if the S4 sound is clearly audible because this is heard on its own within the block. In the absence of an audible S4, AV block cannot be distinguished from the less common sinoatrial block. Sinus arrhythmia is less common than in small animals but does occur, perhaps more commonly in donkeys.[18] It is rarely synchronized with respiration unless there is markedly increased respiratory effort because of severe lung disease. Early beats may represent supraventricular or ventricular ectopic activity; it is frequently difficult to distinguish between these two options on auscultation and ECG is definitive. Early beats from both sites may occur occasionally in normal horses, hence the determination of "normal" is the subject of considerable discussion (See Gunther van Loon's article, "Cardiac Arrhythmias in Horses," in this issue). The detection of an irregular irregularity usually signifies atrial fibrillation (see **Table 2**, Audio 6); again ECG confirmation is required. Exercise is useful if there is any doubt distinguishing between physiologic and pathologic arrhythmias and for assessing the clinical relevance of ectopic rhythms. The decrease in parasympathetic and increase in sympathetic input with exercise should be associated with abolition of the arrhythmia when the arrhythmia is physiologic or where the sinus rate "overdrives" an ectopic rhythm. In contrast, the persistence of an arrhythmia during exercise is of increasing concern and suggests further evaluation is warranted.

Understanding and assessing murmurs

Murmurs are sounds that occur between the normal heart sounds. Most of these are characteristic and commonly heard with ease. Murmurs are usually categorized according to five key criteria (**Table 1**) and fit into specific groups (**Fig. 4**). Less commonly detected are brief clicking sounds that may be heard in midsystole with careful auscultation over the cardiac apex and may be similar to systolic clicks heard in humans, thought to be associated with mitral valve prolapse (**Table 2**, Audio 3). Equally rarely detected in the horse are the friction rubs associated with pericarditis, which are typically triphasic (one systolic and two diastolic components relating to cardiac movement) and are characteristically squeaky or scratchy in nature (see **Table 2**, Audio 4). Murmurs are either caused by normal physiologic flow of blood or pathologic abnormalities (see **Fig. 4**).

Physiologic murmurs

These are caused by the normal flow of blood into and out of the horse's heart and their presence is explained with a basic appreciation of flow dynamics, which describes the flow of fluid in tubes; the heart is essentially a series of specialized tubes. When flow is high, fluid turbulence is likely and this may be manifest as a murmur during auscultation of the heart; high flow only occurs briefly and at specific points in the cardiac cycle. Physiologic murmurs are therefore typically short, are rarely loud and often have a characteristic quality. Physiologic systolic murmurs are also known as "ejection murmurs" and are caused by blood accelerating out of the great vessels, usually the aorta; they are typically crescendo-decrescendo in character and are only in the early part of systole, never reaching the S2 (**Table 3**, Audios 7A, 7B). Physiologic diastolic murmurs are also known as "filling murmurs" and may occur at either the beginning or the end of diastole. In early diastole, the active relaxation of the ventricle causes a sudden influx of blood into the ventricle and this may be audible as an early diastolic murmur; typically these may be high pitched (squeak) or low pitched (rubbing) (see **Table 3**, Audios 9A, 9B). In late diastole, the atrial contraction may lead to a short murmur between S4 and S1 (see **Table 3**, Audios 10A, 10B). Diastasis, the middle of diastole where blood flow is minimal, should be silent under normal circumstances.

Special consideration should be given to systemic diseases that may alter the rheologic properties of blood. In the context of diseases, such as anemia,

Table 1	
Criteria for describing and categorizing murmurs	
Criterion	**Comment/Options**
Timing	With respect to the cardiac cycle Systolic vs diastolic vs continuous Early/mid/late Holosystolic/holodiastolic (whole of systole/diastole but S1/S2 clearly audible) Pansystolic/pandiastolic (whole of systole/diastole encompassing S1 and S2)
Point of maximal intensity	Where is the murmur loudest? Left vs right side of chest Base vs apex of heart According to valve position: mitral, aortic, pulmonic, tricuspid valve
Grade	Intensity/loudness of the murmur Note that this grade does not necessarily relate to the severity of the regurgitation 1: Very quiet and localized, often labile 2: Quiet, localized but easily detected 3: Moderate murmur less loud than S1/S2 4: Moderate murmur louder than S1/S2 5: Palpable thrill detected on chest wall 6: Audible with stethoscope off the chest wall
Radiation	Degree broadly relates to intensity, but not necessarily Dorsal/ventral/concentric
Character and shape	Descriptive terms; typical terminology includes Character Soft Harsh Whooping Musical Vibrant Buzzing Squeak Shape Band/plateau (even through the murmur) Crescendo (increase in intensity) Decrescendo (decrease in intensity)

hypoproteinemia, and colic, murmurs may be evident that are not normally present. These so called "hemic murmurs" are confusing and the horse is best reassessed when the systemic disease is resolved.

Pathologic murmurs

Pathologic murmurs are caused by abnormalities in the flow of blood caused by changes to cardiac structures. These may be split into three categories: (1) valve regurgitation (or leakage), (2) valvular stenosis (or narrowing), and (3) abnormal communications between chambers and/or vessels.

Valve regurgitation Backflow though leaky valves is the most common nonphysiologic cause for a cardiac murmur. In this case, the regurgitating blood mixes with the normal flow into that chamber, creating turbulence and hence a murmur. Valve regurgitation is common, especially in athletic breeds of horse.[8] Unfortunately for the diagnosing clinician, not all regurgitation is necessarily of great clinical

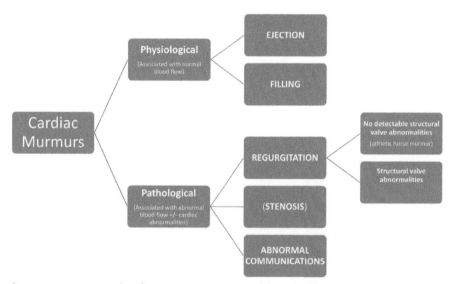

Fig. 4. Basic murmur classification into physiologic versus pathologic processes, and the possible causes for each (see text for details). Note that in situations where rheologic properties of blood are altered (extracardiac pathology), murmurs caused by normal flow of blood may be more likely.

consequence. A large number of normal athletic horses have some degree of regurgitation, especially from the AV valves, and this regurgitation does not necessarily affect performance.[9,10] Distinguishing between this athletic horse regurgitation and more significant regurgitation is tricky for even the most experienced clinicians and relies heavily on echocardiographic evidence, which may detect structural valve abnormalities (See Colin C. Schwarzwald's article, "Equine Echocardiography"; Celia M. Marr's article, "Equine Acquired Valvular Disease," in this issue).

Valve stenosis Unlike in dogs, where isolated valve stenosis is a common diagnosis, this finding is rare in horses and usually only suspected in cases with complex congenital abnormalities. Although stenosis should not be completely discounted, it is not a common differential for a murmur in the horse. A potentially confusing diagnosis is the murmur of relative pulmonic stenosis, which is frequently encountered alongside a VSD, when there is increased flow from the left to right ventricle during systole. This murmur is caused by increased flow across a normal pulmonary artery, making turbulence more likely and hence creating a systolic murmur over the pulmonic valve area: a less confusing and more accurate term may be a pulmonic ejection murmur.

Abnormal communications between chambers and vessels These conduits may either be congenital or acquired. Because the chambers and great vessels of the heart are pressurized to varying degrees, a communication leads to passage of blood down the pressure gradient leading to blood mixing, turbulence, and therefore a murmur. All variants of congenital disease may occur in the horse,[19] but the most common finding are VSD. These are frequently in the paramembranous part of the interventricular septum below the noncoronary and right coronary cusps of the aortic valve on the left and the septal leaflet of the tricuspid valve on the right side (See Brian A Scansen's article, "Equine Congenital Heart Disease," in this issue).[20] This leads to a characteristic murmur that is loudest on the right-hand side and radiates toward the sternum.

Table 2
Normal and abnormal heart sounds in the horse

Sounds	Comments	Phonocardiogram (and Description of Sounds)	Audio File
Normal heart sounds	S1 and S2 are high intensity sounds and are invariably present in all horses; where there is a loud murmur, this may block the ability to hear them.		Audio 1A
	S4 may be heard in normal horses immediately before S1, and represents sounds associated with atrial contraction.	S1 S2 clearly audible. In this recording the heart rate is regular, 30 beats/min.	Audio 1B
	S3 may be heard in normal horses immediately after the S2 sounds and this signifies the end of rapid ventricular filling.	Note the clearly audible S4 S1 S2 pattern in the recording.	Audio 1C
		Note the S1 S2 S3 rhythm in the recording. The S3 is easiest to hear after the "blocked" beats because it is more separated from S2. Note that a soft MR murmur is also audible in this recording (sound supplied by Dr Karen Blissitt and Professor Lesley Young).	
Split S2	May be heard in normal TB far forward over the pulmonary valve. If more obvious, may be caused by pulmonary hypertension.	Note the 2 sounds at S2 very close together.	Audio 2

Midsystolic click	Very brief sound midsystole; perhaps caused by movement of mitral valve apparatus.	Audio 3
	Very brief snapping sound midsystole.	
Pericardial friction rubs	Triphasic squeaking/creaking quality, associated with pericarditis. Sounds reflect movement of heart within inflamed pericardial sac.	Audio 4
	3 regular and repeating squeaky noises.	
Physiologic arrhythmia: atrioventricular block	A common finding in normal relaxed horses.	Audio 5
	This recording has a clear S4 sound and this is heard on its own during the blocks (sound supplied by Dr Karen Blissitt and Professor Lesley Young).	
Pathologic arrhythmia: atrial fibrillation	Irregularly irregular. Common cardiac cause of poor performance in the horse.	Audio 6
	Note the irregularly irregular rhythm.	

Abbreviation: MR, mitral regurgitation.

Table 3
Auscultation findings with common heart murmurs in the horse

Side of Horse	Position in Cardiac Cycle	Murmur	Common Characteristics	Phonocardiogram (and Description of Murmur)	Audio File
Left	Systolic	Aortic ejection/flow	PMI AoV early to midsystolic; crescendo decrescendo; rarely > grade 3/6	S4 S1 S2 pattern with short murmur after S1	Audio 7A / Audio 7B
		Mitral regurgitation	PMI MV; holosystolic (not always); often band-shaped or crescendo. Late crescendo murmurs are often deemed to be consistent with MV prolapse	S1 S2 pattern with short crescendo-decrescendo murmur after S1; MR plateau shaped, even sound through systole (early diastolic filling murmur also audible); MR crescendo, increasing toward end of systole	Audio 8A / Audio 8B
	Diastolic	Early diastolic filling	PMI MV; short murmur in early diastole; squeak or rubbing quality; rarely > grade 3/6	Squeak sound after S2; Soft/rubbing sound after S2	Audio 9A / Audio 9B

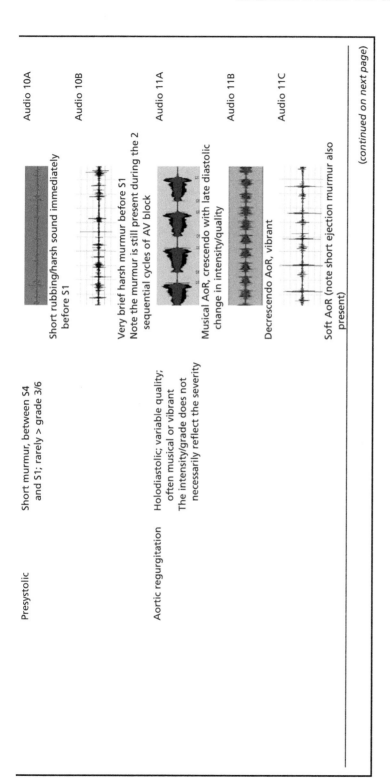

Presystolic	Short murmur, between S4 and S1; rarely > grade 3/6	Short rubbing/harsh sound immediately before S1 — Audio 10A
		Very brief harsh murmur before S1. Note the murmur is still present during the 2 sequential cycles of AV block — Audio 10B
Aortic regurgitation	Holodiastolic; variable quality; often musical or vibrant. The intensity/grade does not necessarily reflect the severity	Musical AoR, crescendo with late diastolic change in intensity/quality — Audio 11A
		Decrescendo AoR, vibrant — Audio 11B
		Soft AoR (note short ejection murmur also present) — Audio 11C

(continued on next page)

Table 3
(continued)

Side of Horse	Position in Cardiac Cycle	Murmur	Common Characteristics	Phonocardiogram (and Description of Murmur)	Audio File
Right	Systolic	Tricuspid regurgitation	PMI TV; holosystolic (not always); band shaped	Holosystolic TR, quality soft	Audio 12
				Early diastolic filling murmur also present in this recording and note the irregularly irregular rhythm (atrial fibrillation)	
		VSD (paramembranous)	PMI TV; radiates cranioventral The intensity/grade does not necessarily reflect the severity		Audio 13A
				Harsh murmur, blocking out S1 and S2 sounds	Audio 13B
	Diastolic	Presystolic	Short, between S4 and S1; rarely > grade 3/6	As above; the rate is high in this recording As above for left side	Audios 10A, 10B
	Diastolic	Aortic regurgitation	PMI TV; character as above; usually one grade less than on left side	As above for left side	Audios 11A–11C

Abbreviations: AoR, aortic regurgitation; AoV, aortic valve; MR, mitral regurgitation; MV, mitral valve; PMI, point of maximal intensity; S1-4, heart sounds 1-4; TV, tricuspid valve.

Acquired communications often involve the aortic root and proximal aorta, leading to communication between the aorta and the right atrium, ventricle, or the pulmonary artery (See Annelies Decloedt's article, "Pericardial Disease, Myocardial Disease, and Great Vessel Abnormalities in Horses," in this issue).[5,7]

Distinguishing Between Physiologic and Pathologic Murmurs

Table 3 shows the common differentials for murmurs with the point of maximum intensity on the right and left side of the chest in systole and diastole, along with their typical characteristics. Differentiating between these common murmurs in horses is described in more detail elsewhere, but in essence the two key aspects for determining physiology versus pathology using a stethoscope are the length of the murmur in relation to the point in the cardiac cycle (ie, systole vs diastole) and the intensity or loudness. Short murmurs are less likely to indicate significant pathology and are usually caused by changes in normal flow or insignificant regurgitation, whereas long murmurs are more likely to be associated with significant pathology. Although all loud murmurs are not necessarily clinically relevant, they usually need to be assessed in case they are; equally although quiet murmurs are not always innocuous, there are usually other indicators of significant dysfunction (eg, elevated resting heart rate) that would suggest further cardiac evaluation is warranted.

Pathologic Murmurs: Distinguishing Between Significant and Nonsignificant Murmurs

The suspicion of aortic valve regurgitation should almost always trigger further re-evaluation using echocardiography, resting and exercising ECG[1]; this is particularly important in the presence of a hyperkinetic pulse (discussed previously). For AV valve regurgitation, the situation is less clear, given that many athletic horses have AV valve regurgitation that is apparently of minimal or no consequence to performance.[9,10] By and large, athletic horse murmurs occur in ostensibly normal horses that are of an athletic type, with a normal resting heart rate and with normal heart rate responses to exercise. If these criteria do not hold true (eg, suspicion of AV valve regurgitation in a pony) or if in doubt, then further evaluation including echocardiography is warranted. For the AV valve murmurs in athletic horses, there are minimal follow-up data to corroborate the clinical impression that these usually do not progress, but this would be most clinicians' experience in the absence of significant valvular changes on echocardiography.

EVALUATION OF BLOOD PRESSURE IN THE HORSE

Blood pressure measurement is not commonplace in general equine practice, although more and more clinicians, including those with a specific interest in cardiology, are starting to assess this variable, especially in the hospital setting. Blood pressure may be measured by either direct (invasive) or indirect (noninvasive) methods. Invasive measurement is perhaps more applicable to anesthetized horses or for specific purposes, where continuous beat-to-beat blood pressure measurement is required. Indirect methods are more suited to the general clinical setting with standing unsedated horses, but are more subject to variability and less accurate.[21]

Direct assessment of blood pressure involves placing a cannula within a suitable artery and connecting the blood within the vessel, via a constant column of fluid (heparinized saline), to a pressure transducer. The pressure transducer is zeroed to atmospheric pressure and leveled at a height that equates to the base of the heart, thus representing right atrial pressure. Measured pressures are then relative to this zero point. Invasive monitoring is regarded as the gold standard, providing a constant assessment of systolic and diastolic and hence, by calculation, mean arterial pressure (MAP = [SBP + 2 (DBP)]/3). This technique is done in the standing horse usually using a facial artery, or in the anesthetized horse using a facial or distal limb artery. In recumbent foals the dorsal metatarsal artery is a common site for invasive monitoring.[22]

Indirect assessment of blood pressure involves the use of either oscillometric or Doppler-based devices for assessing blood pressure during the deflation of an air-filled cuff. Although the Doppler-based (auscultation/sound) devices were used for early work in horses, determining normal reference values for the horse,[23,24] more recent studies have evaluated the more convenient fully automated oscillometric devices in anesthetized horses, standing horses, and neonatal foals.[21,22,25] The fully automated oscillometric devices inflate an air-filled cuff and use an electronic sensor to measure oscillations in pressure around the vessel that change as the cuff deflates. The point of maximal oscillation corresponds to the mean arterial pressure, and algorithms based around the oscillometric envelope are used to determine systolic and diastolic blood pressure.[26] The precise determinants of these algorithms are contentious[27] and because the algorithms are specific to each machine/manufacturer, the precise manufacturer's instructions including cuff width to tail ratio should be adhered to.

In general, studies suggest that indirect methods are less accurate than direct methods and more subject to variability.[21] This is especially the case in the standing horse, with low heart rates or AV blocks, and with very high or low blood pressures. The devices in clinical use generally also detect the heart rate and accuracy of the heart rate provides some confidence in the result obtained. With uniform use, these devices can provide convenient assessment of equine blood pressure.

Pulse Pressure

Pulse pressure is the difference between systolic and diastolic blood pressure. This is assessed subjectively by palpation of a peripheral pulse, but blood pressure measurement provides an objective figure for this variable, despite the limitations noted previously. Pulse pressure can change with disease states and in particular it may be useful for assessment of aortic regurgitation and for monitoring potential progression objectively. With significant aortic regurgitation, diastolic pressure decreases and systolic pressure increases, creating an increased pulse pressure that is detected clinically as a bounding pulse. Pulse pressures greater than 60 mm Hg have been suggested to indicate a poorer prognosis in aortic regurgitation (See Celia M. Marr's article, "Equine Acquired Valvular Disease," in this issue).[1,28] Pulse pressures may also increase in the presence of fistulae around the aortic root/proximal aorta.

LABORATORY EXAMINATION OF THE HORSE WITH CARDIAC DISEASE
Standard Hematology and Biochemistry

Many horses with even significant cardiac pathology have minimal alterations in standard hematologic and biochemical variables. Nevertheless, hematology and biochemistry are useful as part of the examination of cardiovascular disease. Although it rarely provides specific diagnostic information over and above that obtained by other means, it often helps determine the severity of signs and aids in determining prognosis. Standard biochemical profiles should include: hepatocellular enzymes, such as glutamate dehydrogenase and aspartate aminotransferase, which may be raised in congestive heart failure; the markers of muscle damage aspartate aminotransferase and creatine kinase, which may be raised with significant myocardial disease; creatinine for assessing urinary function in congestive heart failure; markers of inflammation, such as serum amyloid A and fibrinogen; and electrolytes, derangements in which can predispose to cardiac arrhythmias. Sequential hematologic analysis may be useful, particularly in cases of infective endocarditis.

Specific Markers of Myocardial Damage and Cardiac Dysfunction

Several proteins that are known to be cardiac specific in other species have also been investigated in the horse, to increase diagnostic information. Early work in this area suffered from the fact that many assays were crude or poorly sensitive or specific in nature, coupled with the fact that horses do not suffer from myocardial infarction and arthrosclerosis, common conditions that drive the research interest into these biomarkers in humans. Early studies in horses showed that lactate dehydrogenase isoenzymes 1 and 2 were more predominant in cardiac muscle, whereas for creatine kinase (CK) the MB isoenzyme predominates with smaller amounts of the MM isoenzyme.[29,30] There were few indications for the use of these assays in clinical practice.

Much of the recent interest in biomarkers in equine cardiology has centered on the cardiac-specific form of troponin (cTn). The Tn complex is made up of three proteins (TnC, TnT, and TnI) and these are integral to skeletal and cardiac muscle contraction. The cardiac-specific proteins cTnI and cTnT are regarded as specific and sensitive indicators of myocardial injury with specific application to myocardial infarction in humans.[31] They have been studied in many veterinary species for various cardiac applications and, because these proteins are conserved, human assays are potentially applicable providing appropriate validation studies are carried out.[32] Reference ranges have been determined using various assays (including those with high sensitivity) for cTnI and cTnT[33–36] and case reports have shown elevations in cTnI in myocardial necrosis, ionophore toxicity, and atypical myopathy.[36–39] In all of the clinical cases described thus far, severe pathology was evident so whether these assays can detect more subtle pathologic changes is less clear. Certainly, however, in the research setting, subtle alterations in cTnI have been noted following exercise in race and endurance horses.[40–42]

The stretch-induced compound atrial natriuretic peptide, which could potentially signify hemodynamic load in the heart, has also been evaluated.[43–47] Preliminary findings suggest that this may be a useful marker of atrial dilatation and stretch in horses with AV valvular disease, but it may have poor sensitivity and further studies are necessary.[44,47–49]

The use of biomarkers in horses currently is as an additional interesting tool in the diagnostic armory, or in research studies, rather than as a sensitive and specific predictor of disease. They may offer an exciting insight into cardiac disease, however, with perhaps the biggest potential applicability in the detection of early myocardial dysfunction, such as in athletic horses where such dysfunction associated with cardiac fatigue could lead to impaired performance.

SUPPLEMENTAL DATA

Supplementary data related to this article can be found online at https://doi.org/10.1016/j.cveq.2018.12.006.

REFERENCES

1. Reef VB, Bonagura J, Buhl R, et al. Recommendations for management of equine athletes with cardiovascular abnormalities. J Vet Intern Med 2014;28(3):749–61.

2. Marr CM. Cardiac murmurs: congenital heart disease. In: Marr CM, Bowen IM, editors. Cardiology of the horse. 2nd edition. London: Saunders Elsevier; 2010. p. 193–205.
3. Hall TL, Magdesian KG, Kittleson MD. Congenital cardiac defects in neonatal foals: 18 cases (1992-2007). J Vet Intern Med 2010;24(1):206–12.
4. Ploeg M, Saey V, van Loon G, et al. Thoracic aortic rupture in horses. Equine Vet J 2017;49(3):269–74.
5. Ploeg M, Saey V, de Bruijn CM, et al. Aortic rupture and aorto-pulmonary fistulation in the Friesian horse: characterisation of the clinical and gross post mortem findings in 24 cases. Equine Vet J 2013;45(1):101–6.
6. Sleeper MM, Durando MM, Miller M, et al. Aortic root disease in four horses. J Am Vet Med Assoc 2001;219(4):491–6, 459.
7. Marr CM, Reef VB, Brazil TJ, et al. Aorto-cardiac fistulas in seven horses. Vet Radiol Ultrasound 1998;39(1):22–31.
8. Patteson MW, Cripps PJ. A survey of cardiac auscultatory findings in horses. Equine Vet J 1993;25(5):409–15.
9. Young LE, Rogers K, Wood JL. Heart murmurs and valvular regurgitation in thoroughbred racehorses: epidemiology and associations with athletic performance. J Vet Intern Med 2008;22(2):418–26.
10. Buhl R, Ersboll AK, Eriksen L, et al. Use of color Doppler echocardiography to assess the development of valvular regurgitation in Standardbred trotters. J Am Vet Med Assoc 2005;227(10):1630–5.
11. Porter SR, Saegerman C, van Galen G, et al. Vegetative endocarditis in equids (1994-2006). J Vet Intern Med 2008;22(6):1411–6.
12. Maxson AD, Reef VB. Bacterial endocarditis in horses: ten cases (1984-1995). Equine Vet J 1997;29(5):394–9.
13. Dufourni A, Decloedt A, De Clercq D, et al. Reversed patent ductus arteriosus and multiple congenital malformations in an 8-day-old Arabo-Friesian foal. Equine Vet Educ 2018;30(6):315–21.
14. Blissitt KJ. Auscultation. In: Marr CM, Bowen IM, editors. Cardiology of the horse. 2nd edition. London: Saunders Elsevier; 2010. p. 91–104.
15. Schwarzwald CC. Disorders of the cardiovascular system. In: Reed SM, Bayly WM, Sellon D, editors. Equine internal medicine. 4th edition. St. Louis (MO): Saunders; 2010. p. 387–541.
16. Jago R, Keen J. Identification of common equine cardiac murmurs. Practice 2017;39(5):222–31.
17. Schwarzwald CC, Kedo M, Birkmann K, et al. Relationship of heart rate and electrocardiographic time intervals to body mass in horses and ponies. J Vet Cardiol 2012;14(2):343–50.
18. Little C, Hansen S, Geering R, et al. Insights into the autonomic control of heart rate. In Proceedings of the Veterinary Cardiovascular Society, November 2011. p. 61–78.
19. Keen JA. Complex cardiac defects: a challenge for the clinician and cardiologist. Equine Vet Educ 2018;30(6):322–5.
20. Reef VB. Evaluation of ventricular septal defects in horses using two-dimensional and Doppler echocardiography. Equine Vet J Suppl 1995;(19):86–95.
21. Heliczer N, Lorello O, Casoni D, et al. Accuracy and precision of noninvasive blood pressure in normo-, hyper-, and hypotensive standing and anesthetized adult horses. J Vet Intern Med 2016;30(3):866–72.
22. Giguere S, Knowles HA Jr, Valverde A, et al. Accuracy of indirect measurement of blood pressure in neonatal foals. J Vet Intern Med 2005;19(4):571–6.

23. Parry BW, McCarthy MA, Anderson GA. Survey of resting blood pressure values in clinically normal horses. Equine Vet J 1984;16(1):53–8.

24. Parry BW, Anderson GA. Importance of uniform cuff application for equine blood pressure measurement. Equine Vet J 1984;16(6):529–31.

25. Nout YS, Corley KTT, Donaldson LL, et al. Indirect oscillometric and direct blood pressure measurements in anesthetized and conscious neonatal foals. J Vet Emerg Crit Car 2002;12(2):75–80.

26. Geddes LA, Voelz M, Combs C, et al. Characterization of the oscillometric method for measuring indirect blood pressure. Ann Biomed Eng 1982;10(6): 271–80.

27. Babbs CF. Oscillometric measurement of systolic and diastolic blood pressures validated in a physiologic mathematical model. Biomed Eng Online 2012;11:56.

28. Horn J. Sympathetic nervous control of cardiac function and its role in equine heart disease. London: Royal Veterinary College, University of London; 2002.

29. Thornton JR, Lohni MD. Tissue and plasma activity of lactic dehydrogenase and creatine kinase in the horse. Equine Vet J 1979;11(4):235–8.

30. Argiroudis SA, Kent JE, Blackmore DJ. Observations on the isoenzymes of creatine kinase in equine serum and tissues. Equine Vet J 1982;14(4):317–21.

31. Morrow DA, Cannon CP, Jesse RL, et al. National academy of clinical biochemistry laboratory medicine practice guidelines: clinical characteristics and utilization of biochemical markers in acute coronary syndromes. Circulation 2007; 115(13):e356–75.

32. Serra M, Papakonstantinou S, Adamcova M, et al. Veterinary and toxicological applications for the detection of cardiac injury using cardiac troponin. Vet J 2010;185(1):50–7.

33. Rossi TM, Kavsak PA, Maxie MG, et al. Analytical validation of cardiac troponin I assays in horses. J Vet Diagn Invest 2018;30(2):226–32.

34. Rossi TM, Pyle WG, Maxie MG, et al. Troponin assays in the assessment of the equine myocardium. Equine Vet J 2014;46(3):270–5.

35. Shields E, Seiden-Long I, Massie S, et al. Analytical validation and establishment of reference intervals for a 'high-sensitivity' cardiac troponin-T assay in horses. BMC Vet Res 2016;12(1):104.

36. Van Der Vekens N, Decloedt A, Ven S, et al. Cardiac troponin I as compared to troponin T for the detection of myocardial damage in horses. J Vet Intern Med 2015;29(1):348–54.

37. Cornelisse CJ, Schott HC 2nd, Olivier NB, et al. Concentration of cardiac troponin I in a horse with a ruptured aortic regurgitation jet lesion and ventricular tachycardia. J Am Vet Med Assoc 2000;217(2):231–5.

38. Schwarzwald CC, Hardy J, Buccellato M. High cardiac troponin I serum concentration in a horse with multiform ventricular tachycardia and myocardial necrosis. J Vet Intern Med 2003;17(3):364–8.

39. Van Der Vekens N, Decloedt A, Sys S, et al. Evaluation of assays for troponin I in healthy horses and horses with cardiac disease. Vet J 2015;203(1):97–102.

40. Rossi TM, Kavsak PA, Maxie MG, et al. Post-exercise cardiac troponin I release and clearance in normal Standardbred racehorses. Equine Vet J 2019;51(1): 97–101.

41. Holbrook TC, Birks EK, Sleeper MM, et al. Endurance exercise is associated with increased plasma cardiac troponin I in horses. Equine Vet J Suppl 2006;(36): 27–31.

42. Shileds E, Seiden-Long I, Massie S, et al. 24-hour kinetics of cardiac troponin-T using a 'high-sensitivity' assay in thoroughbred chuckwagon racing geldings

after race and associated clinical sampling guidelines. J Vet Intern Med 2018; 32(1):433–40.

43. Trachsel DS, Grenacher B, Weishaupt MA, et al. Plasma atrial natriuretic peptide concentrations in horses with heart disease: a pilot study. Vet J 2012;192(2): 166–70.

44. Trachsel DS, Schwarzwald CC, Bitschnau C, et al. Atrial natriuretic peptide and cardiac troponin I concentrations in healthy Warmblood horses and in Warmblood horses with mitral regurgitation at rest and after exercise. J Vet Cardiol 2013;15(2):105–21.

45. Trachsel DS, Schwarzwald CC, Grenacher B, et al. Analytic validation and comparison of three commercial immunoassays for measurement of plasma atrial/A-type natriuretic peptide concentration in horses. Res Vet Sci 2014;96(1):180–6.

46. van der Vekens N, Decloedt A, de Clercq D, et al. Atrial natriuretic peptide vs. N-terminal-pro-atrial natriuretic peptide for the detection of left atrial dilatation in horses. Equine Vet J 2016;48(1):15–20.

47. Leroux AA, Al Haidar A, Remy B, et al. Atrial natriuretic peptide as an indicator of the severity of valvular regurgitation and heart failure in horses. J Equine Vet Sci 2014;34(10):1226–33.

48. Trachsel DS, Grenacher B, Schwarzwald CC. Plasma atrial/A-type natriuretic peptide (ANP) concentration in horses with various heart diseases. J Vet Cardiol 2015;17(3):216–28.

49. Van Der Vekens N, Hunter I, Timm A, et al. Total plasma proANP increases with atrial dilatation in horses. Vet Rec 2015;177(24):624.

Equine Echocardiography

Colin C. Schwarzwald, Prof Dr med vet, PhD

KEYWORDS

- Ultrasound • Heart • Cardiac • Horse • Measurements • Cardiac structures
- Chamber dimensions • Myocardial function

KEY POINTS

- Echocardiographic assessment of cardiac structures, chamber dimensions, and myocardial function is challenging and limited by a variety of technical, anatomic, and physiologic factors that need to be considered.
- An echocardiographic study should address morphologic lesions, motion abnormalities, cardiac chamber and great vessel size, cardiac valve function, blood flow disturbances, ventricular systolic and diastolic function, and hemodynamic variables, including pressure gradients and filling pressures.
- This requires a systematic approach and application of at least 2-dimensional, motion mode, and flow Doppler modalities. In selected cases, tissue Doppler imaging should be used for assessment of left ventricular diastolic function.
- Assessment of severity of valvular regurgitation should not be limited to evaluation of the regurgitant jet as visualized by color flow mapping but should also include measures of chamber size and geometry.
- Independent of the methods used, the findings obtained during echocardiography should be critically assessed in the light of clinical findings. Also, despite the availability of quantitative echocardiographic measurements, subjective assessment remains crucial and must not be neglected.

 Video content accompanies this article at http://www.vetequine.theclinics.com.

INTRODUCTION

Echocardiography is part of every comprehensive cardiac examination in horses. However, the echocardiographic assessment of cardiac structures, chamber dimensions, and myocardial function is challenging and limited by a variety of technical, anatomic, and physiologic factors that need to be considered.[1–3] In recent years,

Disclosure Statement: No disclosures. The author does not have any relationship with a commercial company that has a direct financial interest in subject matter or materials discussed in article or with a company making a competing product.

Clinic for Equine Internal Medicine, Equine Department, Swiss Equine Cardiology Consulting, Vetsuisse Faculty, University of Zurich, Winterthurerstrasse 260, Zurich 8057, Switzerland
E-mail address: cschwarzwald@vetclinics.uzh.ch

Vet Clin Equine 35 (2019) 43–64
https://doi.org/10.1016/j.cveq.2018.12.008
0749-0739/19/© 2019 Elsevier Inc. All rights reserved.

novel echocardiographic methods, such as tissue Doppler imaging (TDI), 2-dimensional (2D) speckle tracking (2DST), and 3-dimensional (3D) echocardiography, have been investigated in horses to complement the traditional 2D, motion mode (M-mode), and Doppler echocardiographic methods, and to overcome some of their limitations. This article mainly focuses on the traditional echocardiographic techniques and provides some information on the more advanced techniques as far as they are considered clinically relevant. More details on echocardiographic findings in various equine heart diseases have been described elsewhere.[4,5]

INDICATIONS FOR ECHOCARDIOGRAPHY

Echocardiography is used to identify (or rule out) cardiac disease, make the correct anatomic diagnosis, assess hemodynamic and structural consequences of disease (chamber enlargement, remodeling, quantification of pressure gradients), provide important prognostic data, monitor response to treatment and progression of the disease, and identify complications of a known diagnosis. The medical history and the results of the physical examination, including the cardiac rhythm and the findings of auscultation, should all be taken into consideration before interpreting the echocardiogram. **Table 1** lists the most important indications for echocardiography in horses.

A complete echocardiographic study should address morphologic lesions, motion abnormalities, cardiac chamber and great vessel size, cardiac valve function, blood flow disturbances, global and regional ventricular systolic function, estimates of hemodynamic variables (including pressure gradients and volumetric flow), and ventricular diastolic function and filling pressures (realizing that these latter two are challenging to measure in mature horses).[6] A comprehensive assessment requires the application of at least 2D, M-mode, and flow Doppler modalities, if possible complemented by TDI for assessment of left ventricular (LV) diastolic function.

EQUIPMENT AND TECHNICAL CONSIDERATIONS

The ultrasonographic equipment for echocardiography in large-size adult horses should include a phased-array sector transducer working at frequencies between 1.3 and 3.5 MHz. Tissue harmonic imaging often improves the image quality, particularly in the far field and in large horses, by providing a higher signal-to-noise ratio, better contrast, and higher spatial resolution. The depth of penetration should reach at least 25 to 30 cm. When such transducers are not available, low-frequency (noncardiac) curvilinear transducers can often produce images of sufficient quality for 2D imaging. Simultaneous recording of a surface electrocardiogram is required and allows exact timing of flow events and measurements. Contemporary echocardiography systems offer digital raw data storage of still frames and cine loop recordings. This is extremely useful because it reduces the contact time with the patient and allows postprocessing and off-line analysis of the stored data.

Two imaging modalities, 2D echocardiography (2DE; brightness mode) and M-mode echocardiography and are commonly used (**Figs. 1–3**). When Doppler studies or contrast echocardiography is added, blood flow can be detected relative to the 2D and M-mode images (**Fig. 4**).

Two-dimensional (B-Mode) Echocardiography

The 2DE generates a tomographic image by sweeping an ultrasound beam across the heart (**Fig. 1**A, B; **Figs. 2** and **3**). Different image planes must be used to fully interrogate the 3-dimensional heart. These imaging planes are designated long-axis, short-axis, apical (when the transducer is near the left apex), and angled (hybrid) views.

Table 1 Indications for an echocardiogram in horses	
Indication	**Clinical Use and Relevance of Echocardiography**
Evaluation of heart murmurs	Differentiation between physiologic flow murmurs and pathologic murmurs (eg, valvular regurgitation), assessment of clinical relevance of pathologic murmurs Note: Due to the high prevalence of heart murmurs in healthy horses, an echocardiographic examination is not strictly recommended in all horses with murmurs.[6] The consensus is that echocardiography is indicated in the presence of the following: 1. Previously diagnosed functional murmurs that are louder on serial examinations 2. Grade 3–6/6 left-sided murmurs compatible with mitral regurgitation or aortic regurgitation (AR) 3. Grade 4–6/6 right-sided systolic murmurs compatible with tricuspid regurgitation 4. Suspected ventricular septal defect or other congenital heart lesions 5. Continuous or combined systolic-diastolic murmurs 6. Murmurs associated with poor performance 7. Murmurs detected on prepurchase examinations. Note that the current recommendations are based on murmur grades, on the assumption that murmurs of grade 1–2/6 are less likely to be clinically relevant. However, murmur grade might not be directly related to clinical relevance or severity of disease. Therefore, in case of doubt, an echocardiogram is always indicated in horses with murmurs.
Clinically important arrhythmias (whether murmur is present or not)	Detection of underlying cardiac disease (eg, mitral regurgitation and left atrial dilatation with atrial fibrillation)
Suspected congenital defects	Evaluation of heart murmurs, unexplained cyanosis, arrhythmias, or signs of heart failure in neonates
Suspected myocardial disease	With unexplained tachycardia, supraventricular or ventricular ectopy, increased plasma cardiac troponin concentrations
Exercise intolerance, poor performance, collapse, or episodic weakness	Detection or rule-out of cardiac disease
Muffled heart sounds	Detection or rule-out of pericardial disease
Fever of unknown origin or specific suspicion for infectious or inflammatory cardiac disease	Detection or rule-out of endocarditis or pericarditis
Clinical signs of congestive heart failure	Cause of heart failure, assessment of severity, monitoring of progression, and response to treatment
Severe respiratory disease	Detection of pulmonary hypertension, detection of patent foramen ovale in foals with respiratory disease

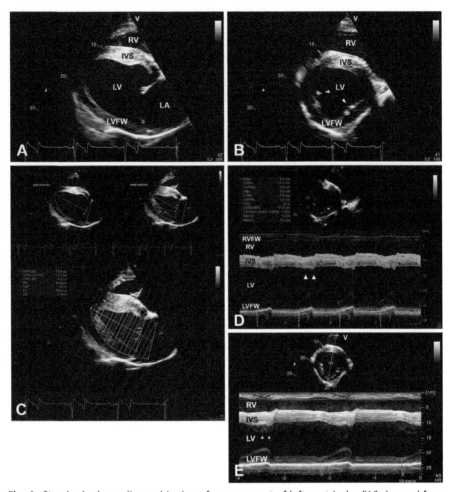

Fig. 1. Standard echocardiographic views for assessment of left ventricular (LV) size and function. (*A*) Right parasternal long-axis 4-chamber view centered on the LV (Video 1). The transducer is positioned in the right fourth intercostal space at a level slightly above the olecranon, angled caudally, and rotated clockwise to the 1 o'clock position. Slight changes in transducer placement (including moving to another intercostal space) may be necessary to optimize the image plane. The operator must ensure that the mitral valve annulus and the LV apex remain within the image plane throughout the cardiac cycle to avoid artificial foreshortening of the ventricle during systole. This view is best suited to assess the structures, dimensions, and mechanical function of the LV. Because this image is centered on the LV, the left atrium (LA) may not be imaged in its entirety throughout the cardiac cycle. Assessment of the right heart is limited due to its anatomic position, its complex geometry, and its visualization in the narrow near field of the imaging sector. IVS, interventricular septum; LVFW, left ventricular free wall; RV, right ventricle. (*B*) Right parasternal short-axis view of the LV at the level of the chordae tendineae (*arrowheads*) (Video 2). This view is obtained by rotating the transducer 90° clockwise from a 4-chamber view. It is commonly used for measurement of the diameter and the area, respectively, of the LV and evaluation of LV systolic function. (*C*) Same image plane as in *A*, showing tracings (*green dotted lines*) of the LV internal area and longitudinal axis at end-diastole (*top left*), and peak-systole (*top right*). The bottom image shows the end-diastolic area tracing superimposed to the peak-systolic area tracing (*green dotted lines*). Applying a geometric model, such as the modified (single-plane) Simpson's model of discs, allows calculation of the estimated LV

Because of anatomic restrictions, apical images are difficult or impossible to obtain except in foals. By convention, in long-axis and short-axis recordings, the dorsal regions of the heart (atria, heart base) and the cranial regions of the heart (right ventricular [RV] outflow tract), respectively, are displayed to the right of the screen. The real-time 2DE is typically done at sampling rates (frame rates) of 20 to 40 frames per second, with the frame rate inversely related to penetration depth and sector width. Fully digital echocardiographs can display much faster frame rates, often exceeding 60 per second. Newer applications, such as 2DE-based anatomic M-mode (AMM)[7] or 2DST[8] demand a frame rate between 40 and 90 Hz to achieve sufficient temporal resolution. 2DE allows assessment of cardiac anatomy, detection of macroscopic structural lesions, subjective evaluation, and measurement of chamber and vessel dimensions, and evaluation of left atrial (LA) and LV function.

M-Mode Echocardiography

In an M-mode echocardiogram (**Fig. 1**D, E), the movement of the cardiac structures (vertical axis) is displayed over time (horizontal axis). Visualization of the characteristic movements of cardiac structures permits the experienced viewer to evaluate and quantify cardiac anatomy and myocardial function. The high sampling rate of the M-mode study makes it excellent for visualizing rapidly vibrating structures, such as the oscillating mitral leaflet in aortic (Ao) regurgitation.

Contrast Echocardiography

Contrast echocardiography, whereby agitated saline is used to delineate the path of blood flow, is useful for the detection of right-to-left shunts in foals, including patent

---

volume at end-diastole (LVIVd) and LV volume at peak-systole (LVIVs), ejection fraction (EF) (%EF = [LVIVd − LVIVs] / LVIVd × 100), stroke volume (SV) (SV = LVIVd − LVIVs), and cardiac output (CO) (CO = SV × HR). HR, heart rate; LVIVd (S) (500), LVIVd estimated by Simpson's model and allometrically scaled to a BWT of 500 kg. (D) Right parasternal short-axis view (top) and corresponding M-mode recording (bottom) of the LV at the chordal level. The motion of the IVS and the LVFW are displayed over time. Care must be taken that the LV is bisected by the cursor line into 2 symmetric parts throughout the cardiac cycle. The RV and the RV free wall are (RVFW) displayed in the near field. A small amount of spontaneous echo contrast is frequently seen in the ventricular lumen (arrowheads). Measurement of LV wall thickness and internal dimensions, evaluation of septal motion, and calculation of LV fractional shortening (FS) allow assessment of LV size and systolic function. The blue dotted lines indicate measurement of the IVS thickness, the LV internal diameter (LVID) and the LVFW thickness at end-diastole (defined as the onset of the electrocardiographic QRS complex) and at peak systole (defined as the time at which the LV internal lumen is narrowest). These measurements allow calculation of the FS (%FS = [LVIDd − LVIDs] / LVIDd × 100), mean wall thickness at end-diastole (MWTd) (MWTd = [IVSd + LVFWd] / 2), and relative wall thickness at end-diastole (RWTd) (RWTd = [IVSd + LVFWd] / LVIDd). LVIDd (500), LV internal diameter allometrically scaled to a BWT of 500 kg; LA diameter (max)/LVIDd, ratio of maximum LA diameter to LVIDd; d, measurements at end-diastole; s, measurements at peak systole. (E) Anatomical M-mode (AMM) image of the LV (bottom), reconstructed from a digitally stored 2D cineloop recording obtained from a right parasternal short-axis view at the chordal level (top). Notice that the AMM cursor (green line) can be freely positioned on the 2D image, independent of the sector apex, to bisect the IVS, the LV cavity, and the LVFW into 2 equal parts throughout the cardiac cycle. (From [A, B, and E] Schwarzwald CC. Ultrasonography of the heart. In: Kidd JA, Lu KG, Frazer ML, et al, editors. Atlas of equine ultrasonography. Oxford (United Kingdom): Wiley; 2014; p. 380; with permission.)

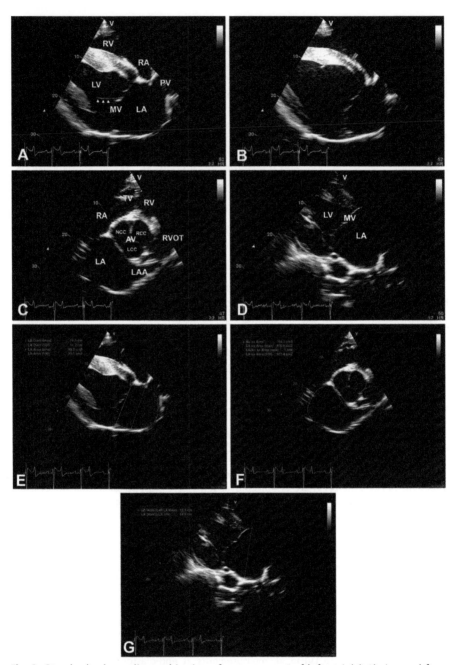

Fig. 2. Standard echocardiographic views for assessment of left atrial (LA) size and function. (*A, B*) Right parasternal 4-chamber view centered on the LA, to image the LA in its entirety throughout the cardiac cycle (Video 3). At an imaging depth of 30 cm, this view is best suited to assess the mitral valve (MV) apparatus, LA dimensions, and LA mechanical function. Only in rare cases (eg, large draft breeds, horses with severe cardiomegaly), the LA cannot be displayed in its entirety from this window. (*A*) Image recorded at the end of ventricular systole, 1 frame before opening of the MV, when the LA is at its

foramen ovale. Saline contrast echocardiography does not require specific equipment and can be done with any ultrasound machine and transducer.

Doppler Echocardiography

Doppler echocardiography relies on the Doppler principle to measure the direction and velocity of red blood cells moving through the heart (**Fig. 4**A–D). The information is displayed as a spectral tracing, showing time along the horizontal axis, the flow direction as above (toward the transducer) or below (away from the transducer) a zero baseline, and blood flow velocity along the vertical axis. With all Doppler modalities, parallel alignment with the direction of movement of the target is crucial because excessive angle of interrogation (ie, >20°) will lead to an underestimation of velocities. Therefore, technically, velocities can only be accurately measured for blood flowing parallel to the ultrasound beam (ie, toward or away from the transducer) but not for blood moving perpendicular to the beam. Digital angle correction should not be applied for Doppler measurements of intracardiac blood flow because true direction of flow in the cardiac chambers is unknown and cannot be derived from the Doppler signals.

◄──

maximum dimensions. Chordae tendineae are seen in the left ventricular (LV) cavity (*arrowheads*). PV, pulmonary vein ostium; RA, right atrium; RV, right ventricle. (*B*) Image recorded at the end of diastole, immediately after closure of the MV, when the LA is at its minimum dimensions. Note the obvious change in LA dimensions within a single cardiac cycle (ie, between *A* and *B*), indicating that timing of measurements of LA dimensions is critical. Generally, LA dimensions should be assessed at the end of ventricular systole (*A*). (*C*) Right parasternal short-axis view at the level of the aortic valve (AV) (Video 4). This view is obtained by rotating the transducer 90° clockwise from a right parasternal LV outflow tract view (see **Fig. 3**A). In this view, the AV with its 3 cusps is visible in the center of the image. The surrounding structures include RA, tricuspid valve (TV), RV, RV outflow tract (RVOT), LA, and LA appendage (LAA). The apparent triangular separation (at the 12 o'clock position) evident between the noncoronary cusp (NCC) and the right coronary cusp (RCC) is a normal finding and does not represent an anomaly. LCC, left coronary cusp of the AV. (*D*) Left parasternal long-axis view of the LA, MV, and LV (Video 5). The transducer is positioned in the fifth or fourth intercostal space slightly above the olecranon, oriented perpendicular to the chest wall, and angled dorsally. This view has traditionally been used for assessment of LA dimensions. However, as opposed to the right parasternal views (*A*, *B*), this view often does not allow imaging of the LA in its entirety due to interference with the ventral lung border. Nonetheless, imaging LA and MV from a left thoracic window provides additional information and should complement the right parasternal views. (*E*) Same image plane as in *A*, showing tracings (*blue dotted lines*) of the maximum LA internal area (LA area [max]) and the maximum LA diameter parallel to the MV annulus (LA diameter [max]) at the end of ventricular systole, 1 frame before MV opening. LA diameter (500) and LA area (500), maximum LA diameter and area, respectively, allometrically scaled to a BWT of 500 kg. (*F*) Same image plane as in *C*, showing tracings (*blue dotted lines*) of the aortic short-axis area (Ao sx area) and the short-axis area of the LA (ie, the LA body and LAA) (LA sx Area [max]) at the end of ventricular systole, 1 frame after AV closure. The size of the LA can be directly compared with the Ao area (LA/Ao sx Area [max] ratio). LA sx Area (500), short-axis area of the LA allometrically scaled to a BWT of 500 kg. (*G*) Same image plane as in *D*, showing measurement of the maximum LA diameter in left long-axis view (LA diameter [left LX view]) at the end of ventricular systole, 1 frame before MV opening. Note that the maximum diameter often cannot be measured parallel to the MV annulus in this image plane. LA diameter (LLX 500), LA diameter in left long-axis view allometrically scaled to a BWT of 500 kg. (*From* [A–D] Schwarzwald CC. Ultrasonography of the heart. In: Kidd JA, Lu KG, Frazer ML, et al, editors. Atlas of equine ultrasonography. Oxford (United Kingdom): Wiley; 2014. p. 381; with permission.)

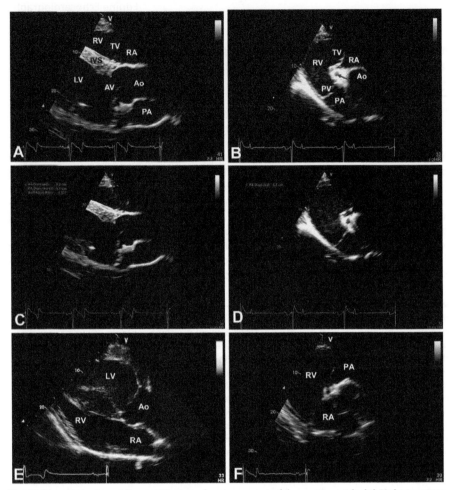

Fig. 3. Standard echocardiographic views for assessment of the great vessels. (*A*) Right parasternal long-axis view of the left ventricular outflow tract (LVOT) (Video 6). Starting from a 4-chamber view (see **Fig. 1**A), the transducer is angled more cranially, tilted dorsally, and rotated to the 2-o-clock position to obtain this view. It is best suited to assess the structures, dimensions, and function of the aortic valve (AV), the sinus of Valsalva, the ascending aorta (Ao) and the pulmonary artery (PA). The size of the PA should be smaller than the diameter of the Ao. IVS, interventricular septum; LV, left ventricle; RA, right atrium; RV, right ventricle; TV, tricuspid valve. (*B*) Right parasternal long-axis view of the right ventricular outflow tract (RVOT) (Video 7). Starting from an LVOT view (*A*), the transducer is angled more cranially to obtain this view; occasionally the transducer has to be moved 1 intercostal space cranially. The RA, the TV, the RV, the RVOT, the pulmonic valve (PV), the PA, and cross section of the Ao and the right coronary artery (*arrow*) can be visualized. (*C*) Same image plane as in *A*, showing measurements (*blue dotted lines*) of the Ao diameter at the level of the sinus of Valsalva (Ao diameter [ed]) and PA diameter (PA diameter [ed-sx]) at the end of diastole. The ratio of the Ao sinus diameter to the cross-sectional PA diameter can be calculated (Ao/PA [sx] ratio) and should always be greater than 1.0. (*D*) Same image plane as in *B*, showing measurement (*blue dotted line*) of the PA diameter at the level of the sinus at the end of diastole (PA diameter [ed]). (*E*) Left parasternal long-axis view of the LVOT. The transducer is positioned in the fifth or fourth intercostal space at a level slightly above the olecranon and angled slightly cranially. (*F*) Left parasternal long-axis view of the RVOT. Starting from the LVOT view (*E*), the transducer is moved 1 intercostal space more cranially to obtain this image. (*From* [*E* and *F*] Schwarzwald CC. Ultrasonography of the heart. In: Kidd JA, Lu KG, Frazer ML, et al, editors. Atlas of equine ultrasonography. Oxford (United Kingdom): Wiley; 2014; p. 382; with permission.)

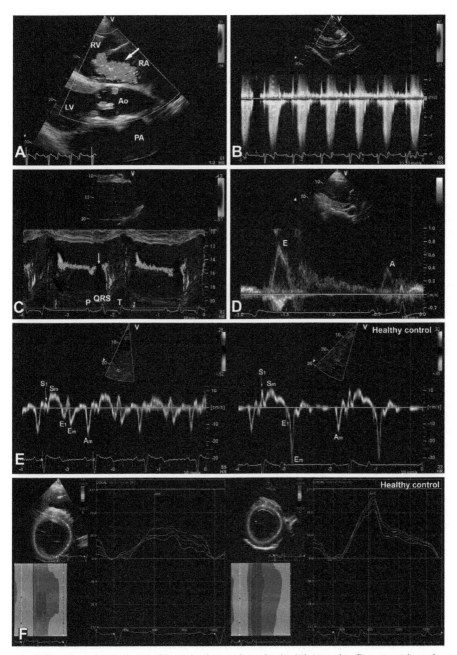

Fig. 4. Doppler echocardiography and advanced methods. (*A*) 2D color flow Doppler echocardiogram demonstrating marked tricuspid regurgitation (TR) (*arrow*). The right atrium (RA), the right ventricle (RV) and the pulmonary artery (PA) appear enlarged when compared with the left ventricle (LV) and the aorta (Ao). Blood flow directed toward the transducer is color-coded in red and yellow, flow directed away from the transducer is coded in blue, and turbulent flow (variance) is coded in green. The color seen in the Ao is caused by normal systolic flow. (*B*) Continuous-wave (CW) Doppler recording of the TR jet shown in *A*. The maximum jet velocity is 4.8 m/s, corresponding to an RV-to-RA pressure gradient

Pulsed-wave (PW) Doppler methods measure direction and velocity of red blood cells within a discrete area of the heart, determined by the observer when placing the sample volume within the cardiac chambers or great vessels (see **Fig. 4**D). Color-coded Doppler imaging, which is also called color flow mapping (CFM), is a more refined variant of PW Doppler imaging that is superimposed on 2D or M-mode images. Flow toward the transducer is coded in red and flow away is represented in blue. Velocity is displayed in relative shades of these colors, and green or yellow are often added to the color map to identify turbulent blood flow (variance) (see **Fig. 4**A, C). Color Doppler imaging is useful because large areas of the heart can be screened

---

of 92 mm Hg (modified Bernoulli equation: $dp = 4 \times v_{max}^2$). In the absence of RV outflow obstruction, the high-velocity TR jet indicates severe pulmonary hypertension. TR jet velocities associated with normal RV pressures are typically less than 3.2 m/s. (*C*) Color M-mode echocardiogram in a right parasternal long-axis view obtained from a horse with Ao regurgitation. The cursor line is placed immediately below the aortic valve (*top*). This imaging mode is particularly useful for timing of flow events and identifying brief regurgitant signals or normal valve closure noise. In this case, an Ao regurgitant jet is visible as a turbulent flow pattern, starting at the beginning of diastole (ie, after the T wave) and ending at the onset of systole (ie, immediately after the QRS complex). Notice the absence of turbulent flow during the PQ interval (*arrow*). This can be explained by a change in LV pressure occurring after atrial contraction or a reorientation of the regurgitant jet relative to the cursor owing to translational movement of the heart. (*D*) Transmitral flow velocity profile from a healthy horse recorded from a left parasternal long-axis echocardiographic view with the pulsed-wave Doppler cursor positioned between the open tips of the mitral valve leaflets. Note that the cursor line could not be aligned with the presumed direction of transmitral blood flow, leading to an underestimation of measured flow velocities. The early-diastolic transmitral flow velocity (E wave) is larger than the late-diastolic transmitral flow velocity (A wave, caused by active atrial contraction), indicating a normal filling pattern. (*E*) Pulsed-wave tissue Doppler imaging (PW TDI) analysis of the LV free wall recorded at the level of the chordae tendineae in a right parasternal short-axis view obtained in a horse suffering from masseter myopathy and nutritional myocardial damage (plasma cardiac troponin I concentration 11.6 ng/mL; normal <0.06 ng/mL). E_m depicts the peak radial wall motion velocity during early diastole and A_m depicts the peak radial wall motion velocity during late diastole. The E_m/A_m inversion (*left*) indicates diastolic dysfunction and impaired ventricular relaxation. Notice the normal E_m/A_m ratio (with E_m being markedly larger than A_m) in the healthy control (*right*) for comparison. S_1, peak radial wall motion velocity during isovolumic contraction; S_m, peak radial wall motion velocity during ejection; E_1, peak radial wall motion velocity during isovolumic relaxation. (*F*) Two-dimensional speckle tracking (2DST) analyses of an LV short-axis recording from the same horse shown in *E*. Trace screens of the 2DST software are shown, containing the following information: *Top left*: 2D image with the segmented region of interest (ROI) and parametric color coding. *Bottom left*: M-mode with parametric color coding. *Right*: Trace display for radial strain (ie, percent myocardial deformation). The colors of the traces correspond to the colors of the segmented ROI. The start and the end of the cycle (onset of the QRS complex) are marked on the electrocardiogram with yellow dots. The time of aortic valve closure (AVC) is indicated by a green vertical line, dividing the cycle in its systolic and diastolic component. Note that peak radial strain (*left*) in this case is markedly reduced compared with the healthy control (*right*), indicating depressed LV systolic function. (*From* [*C*] Schwarzwald CC. Ultrasonography of the heart. In: Kidd JA, Lu KG, Frazer ML, et al, editors. Atlas of equine ultrasonography. Oxford (United Kingdom): Wiley; 2014; p. 392; and [*E* and *F*] Schefer KD, Hagen R, Ringer SK, et al. Laboratory, electrocardiographic, and echocardiographic detection of myocardial damage and dysfunction in an Arabian mare with nutritional masseter myodegeneration. J Vet Intern Med 2011;25:1171–80; with permission.)

for flow disturbances. A pivotal limitation of color Doppler is temporal resolution, particularly when using ultrasound systems that are not specifically designed for cardiovascular imaging. With low frame rates, it may become necessary to time flow events using either spectral Doppler (see **Fig. 4**B) or color-M-mode echocardiography (see **Fig. 4**C), which both provide considerably higher temporal resolution. Correct timing of blood flow prevents the clinician from misinterpreting normal backflow signals related to valve closure or diagnosing a diastolic flow event as systolic. PW spectral and color Doppler techniques can provide accurate information about the location of flow disturbances but cannot measure high-velocity flow accurately. High-velocity flow is encountered as blood is ejected from high to low pressure zones across incompetent valves, stenotic valves (rare in horses), and intracardiac and extracardiac shunts. In general, when velocities exceed about 2.5 m/s (the exact velocity depends on Doppler frequency and imaging depth), part of the returning Doppler signal is displayed in the opposite direction. This physical phenomenon is called signal aliasing. To quantify high-velocity flow, CW Doppler must be applied (see **Fig. 4**B), which has virtually unlimited ability to record very high blood flow velocity but does not provide the spatial discrimination as found in the PW Doppler modality.

Tissue Doppler Imaging and Two-dimensional Speckle Tracking

In recent years, more advanced echocardiographic methods, such as TDI (**Fig. 4**E)[9–13] and 2DST imaging (**Fig. 4**F)[8,9,12,14–16] (which is based on conventional 2DE cineloop recordings and independent of the Doppler principle) have been investigated in horses to complement the traditional echocardiographic methods and to overcome some of their limitations. These modalities allow quantitative assessment of myocardial motion velocity, deformation (strain), deformation rate (strain rate), displacement, and rotation in longitudinal, radial, and circumferential imaging planes, and they may provide more sensitive methods for assessing regional or global myocardial function in horses. TDI is a promising tool for detection of LV diastolic dysfunction.[16–18] 2DST may be helpful for detection and quantification of LA stunning after treatment of atrial fibrillation (AF) and LV systolic dysfunction in horses with myocardial disease[12,16,17,19]; however, clinical applications and the added value compared with traditional echocardiographic methods still need further definition.

STANDARD EXAMINATION

A systematic approach should be used to perform a complete echocardiographic examination. The author uses the approach outlined in **Box 1**. Note that certain lesions cannot be detected in standard views and require nonstandard angled, tilted, or rotated views to be explored.

Some horses do not tolerate the echocardiographic procedure and require sedation to allow conducting the examination safely and with sufficient quality. Many of the echocardiographic changes seen with sedation are small and, in the light of marked variability, the clinical relevance of the effects of sedation may be minor. Nonetheless, sedation should be avoided if possible because cardiac function will be altered due to drug effects on contractility, preload, afterload, rate, and rhythm. Generally, alpha-2 agonists tend to reduce LV systolic performance and worsen regurgitation because of an increase in afterload and myocardial depression, whereas acepromazine may improve LV systolic performance and reduce regurgitation due to a decrease in afterload.[20–23]

Currently, no generally accepted consensus has been reached by experts on how to quantify chamber size and function in horses and other species. In the following sections, the author's approach is summarized. Reference intervals for individual

---

Box 1
Systematic approach for a complete echocardiographic examination.

1. Right parasternal views
   a. Long-axis: 2D echocardiography
      i. RV outflow tract, pulmonic valve, pulmonary artery (**Fig. 3**B and Video 7)
      ii. LV outflow tract, aortic valve, aorta (**Fig. 3**A and Video 6)
      iii. 4-chamber view angled dorsally, optimized to display entire LA (**Fig. 2**A and Video 3)
      iv. 4-chamber view angled ventrally, optimized to display entire LV (**Fig. 1**A and Video 1)
   b. Short-axis: 2D echocardiography
      i. LV at apical and papillary muscle level (if searching for muscular lesions)
      ii. LV at chordal level (**Fig. 1**B and Video 2)
      iii. LV at mitral valve level
      iv. Aorta, LA and LA appendage (**Fig. 2**C and Video 4)
   c. Short-axis: M-mode echocardiography
      i. Aortic valve, LA appendage
      ii. Mitral valve
      iii. LV at chordal level (**Fig. 1**D, E)
   d. Short-axis: Pulsed-wave tissue Doppler imaging
      i. LV free wall at chordal level (**Fig. 4**E)
   e. Long-axis and short-axis: Flow Doppler and saline contrast studies
      i. Color flow mapping: All 4 valves, shunts (if applicable) (**Fig. 4**A)
      ii. Color M-mode as necessary for timing of flow events (**Fig. 4**C)
      iii. PW or CW Doppler as necessary (always for tricuspid and pulmonic insufficiencies and ventricular septal defects to calculate pressure gradients) (**Fig. 4**B, D)
      iv. Saline contrast as necessary (particularly to detect right-to-left shunts)

2. Left parasternal views
   a. Long-axis: 2D echocardiography, Color flow mapping
      i. LV, mitral valve, LA (**Fig. 2**D and Video 5)
      ii. LV, aortic valve (**Fig. 3**E)
      iii. Pulmonary artery, pulmonic valve, RV, RA (**Fig. 3**F)
   b. Long-axis and short-axis: 2D echocardiography, color flow mapping, Doppler studies, saline contrast studies
      i. As indicated for specific lesions

---

echocardiographic variables and detailed guidelines for interpretation of abnormal findings are published elsewhere.[5]

CARDIAC ANATOMY AND STRUCTURES

As a first step of every echocardiographic examination, the clinician should obtain an anatomic overview and identify the general situs of the heart and cardiac structures (ie, atria, ventricles, cardiac septa, great vessels, and cardiac valves). With adequate training and experience, this is straightforward in most cases; however, it can be very challenging in patients with complex cardiac malformations that are characterized by an unusual arrangement of the cardiac chambers and great arteries (See Brian A. Scansen's article, "Equine Congenital Heart Disease," in this issue). In such cases, a systematic approach using segmental sequential analysis is strongly advised.[24]

The echocardiographer should watch out for the presence of unanticipated or lack of expected structures, and rule out extrapericardial and pericardial mass lesions and effusion (See Annelies Decloedt's article, "Pericardial Disease, Myocardial Disease, and Great Vessel Abnormalities in Horses," in this issue). Diastolic collapse of the right atrium (RA) or RV indicates cardiac tamponade or a large bilateral pleural effusion. The echo texture of the myocardium can be difficult to assess because it is largely influenced by machine settings, imaging planes, the angle of incidence of the ultrasound beam relative to the course of the myocardial fibers, and the presence of ultrasound artifacts. Heterogeneous or focal hypoechoic or hyperechoic myocardium, displayed in multiple image planes, might suggest myocarditis, ischemia, infiltration, infarction, necrosis, or fibrosis (See Annelies Decloedt's article, "Pericardial Disease, Myocardial Disease, and Great Vessel Abnormalities in Horses," in this issue). The interventricular septum (IVS) is examined in both long-axis and short-axis image planes for echo dropout or discontinuity suggesting ventricular septal defects (See Brian A. Scansen's article, "Equine Congenital Heart Disease," in this issue). The valves are inspected for the number and morphology (eg, increased echogenicity, thickening) of the leaflets and cusps, the integrity of the support apparatus (ie, the annulus; for the atrioventricular valves also the chordae tendineae and papillary muscles), and the motion during the cardiac cycle (including valve prolapse and flail leaflets) (See Celia M. Marr's article, "Equine Acquired Valvular Disease," in this issue).

ASSESSMENT OF CHAMBER AND GREAT VESSEL DIMENSIONS

One of the main goals of echocardiography is the detection of cardiac chamber dilation or hypertrophy and the grading of the enlargement, if present, as mild, moderate, or severe. The internal dimensions of all cardiac chambers, their wall thickness, and the size of the great vessels must be subjectively assessed. Subsequently, they can be quantified using linear, area, and volumetric methods that are based on 2D and M-mode echocardiography, considering that all of them are limited by a variety of issues.[2] The core measurements most relevant for the equine practitioner are shown in **Figs. 1–3** (see later discussion).

Left Ventricle

LV enlargement is a common consequence of valvular regurgitation, left-to-right shunt, cardiomyopathy, myocarditis, or persistent tachyarrhythmia. LV hypertrophy, characterized by thickening of the LV wall at the expense of its lumen, can be seen with volume depletion or endotoxemia (pseudohypertrophy), acute myocarditis, chronic systemic hypertension (eg, because of chronic kidney disease, metabolic syndrome, laminitis, chronic pain, pheochromocytoma), chronic digitalis poisoning (eg, foxglove, oleander, yew), overuse of anabolic steroids or clenbuterol, or (in rare cases) of hypertrophic cardiomyopathy, infiltrative cardiomyopathy (eg, amyloidosis, lymphoma, other neoplasia), or outflow tract obstruction.

Assessment of LV dimensions is a crucial part of every echocardiographic examination and provides important information on hemodynamics, LV remodeling, and severity of cardiac disease. LV internal dimensions and LV wall thickness, respectively, are usually measured from a right parasternal short-axis view or from a right parasternal 4-chamber view using 2DE or M-mode recordings (see **Fig. 1**).[3] Sole linear measurements of the LV minor dimension (see **Fig. 1**D) may not well describe true LV size and geometry because asymmetric LV dilation and dimensional changes along the major axis of the ventricle are neglected. Similarly, linear measurements of wall thickness at a single location may not be accurate estimates of LV mass, particularly if asymmetric thickening is present or if the M-mode cursor crosses a papillary muscle or fails to sample the thickest part of the free wall or septum. Furthermore, standardized placement of the M-mode cursor is difficult to verify in all 3 dimensions. This limitation can be partially overcome by use of AMM technology, which allows free orientation of the cursor line within the imaging plane independent of the apex of the imaging sector (**Fig. 1**E).[7]

Measures that consider the long-axis and short-axis area (instead of diameter) of the LV (ie, various area-length models and the Simpson's method of discs, see

Fig. 1C) may be more accurate estimates of internal LV dimensions and LV mass.[2,25,26] The accuracy of these methods, on the other hand, is limited because the true LV long-axis may be difficult to measure by 2DE due to the LV shape, translational motion of the LV during contraction and relaxation, and artificial foreshortening of the ventricle. Furthermore, all conventional volumetric indices are calculated based on several geometric assumptions and may, therefore, be prone to error. Nonetheless, in addition to conventional linear measurements, one should consider using area measurements and volume estimates for quantification of chamber dimensions, particularly in cases in which the subjective evaluation and conventional measurements provide equivocal results. In the future, real-time 3D echocardiography may be applied to horses, eliminating the need for model-based estimation of chamber dimensions and minimizing measurement errors caused by suboptimal imaging planes.

Left Atrium

The magnitude of LA enlargement is used to assess the severity of mitral valve disease, left-to-right shunts, cardiomyopathies, or other diseases causing systolic or diastolic LV dysfunction. In horses, assessment of LA size has traditionally been limited to subjective evaluation and measurement of the LA diameter in a 2DE in a left parasternal long-axis view (**Fig. 2**D, G). However, this view often does not allow imaging of the LA in its entirety owing to interference with the ventral lung border; this often results in measurements of the LA diameter that are not parallel to the mitral valve annulus or that are made too close to the annulus and thereby underestimate the true maximum atrial diameter. Also, the exact timing of LA measurements is often not specified in the older equine literature, leading to uncertainties when comparing results from different studies.

With contemporary echocardiographic systems, the LA can usually be displayed in its entirety from a right parasternal window in long-axis and short-axis views (**Fig. 2**A–C,E,F), which provide sufficient anatomic landmarks (ie, mitral valve anulus, pulmonary vein ostia) for consistent and reliable measurement of LA dimensions.[27,28] In addition to LA diameter, assessment of LA area should be considered because enlargement may not occur in a uniform fashion and LA geometry may change over time. The LA size is best measured at the end of the ventricular systole, 1 frame before mitral valve opening, when the LA chamber is at its greatest dimension. Methods and reliability of 2DE measurements of LA size and function in horses have been described.[27]

Right Atrium and Right Ventricle

Causes of RA and RV dilation include severe tricuspid valve disease (regurgitation, rarely atresia), pulmonary hypertension, atrial septal defect, large ventricular septal defect, right heart failure, and biventricular heart failure. Subjective assessment of the right heart chambers in multiple image planes is important. Objective quantification of the RA and RV dimensions has recently been described in horses[29] but is difficult because the geometric shape of the right heart is complex and the apparent internal dimensions of the RA and the RV cavity largely depend on transducer placement and imaging plane. When measured in M-mode from a right parasternal short-axis window (see **Fig. 1**D, E), the internal diameter of the RV should be markedly smaller than the diameter of the LV.

Great Vessels

Great vessel dimensions should be assessed in absolute terms and in relation to each other. Generally, the Ao dimensions should always exceed the pulmonary artery (PA) dimensions.[5] The Ao diameter can be decreased with low cardiac output (CO) and systemic hypotension. Ao dilation is seen in horses with chronic severe aortic regurgitation (AR), with Ao sinus of Valsalva aneurysm, and in a variety of congenital malformations (eg, tetralogy of Fallot, persistent common arterial trunk, patent ductus arteriosus). Decrease in PA diameter or absence of the PA usually suggest malformation (eg, pulmonary atresia, PA hypoplasia), whereas PA dilation results from pulmonary hypertension, left-to-right shunt, or (rarely) poststenotic dilation resulting from pulmonic stenosis.

The semilunar valves and great vessels can be imaged in right parasternal long-axis (**Fig. 3**A–D) and short-axis (see **Fig. 2**C, F) views and in left parasternal long-axis views (**Fig. 3**E, F). As for all cardiac structures, timing and anatomic location of the measurement are crucial. The minimal dataset should include measurements of the Ao and PA sinus diameter, and the PA short-axis diameter at end-diastole (ie, at the onset of the electrocardiographic QRS complex) in right parasternal long-axis views of the RV and LV outflow tracts (see **Fig. 3**C, D).

Allometric Scaling of Measurements

Cardiac size and function in horses is influenced by body size, breed, and athletic condition.[5,30–34] The influence of body size on cardiac dimensions can be corrected for by using the principles of allometric scaling.[35–37] Among the different approaches that have been described, the author prefers a practical and intuitive approach, in which measurements are normalized to a body weight (BWT) of 500 kg using the following equations: diameter (500) = measured diameter / $BWT^{1/3} \times 500^{1/3}$; area (500) = measured area / $BWT^{2/3} \times 500^{2/3}$; volume (500) = measured volume / $BWT \times 500$. This approach is advised to correct chamber dimensions for differences in BWT among Warmblood horses,[36,38] but has not been validated in other breeds or for use across different breeds. Theoretically, the use of the ideal BWT, as opposed to the actual BWT, should be preferred but would introduce an additional source of error. In situations in which an accurate BWT cannot be obtained, the size of the Ao can serve as an internal reference for body size (except in cases with severe Ao valve or great vessel disease).[27,36]

ASSESSMENT OF SYSTOLIC VENTRICULAR FUNCTION

The echocardiographic detection of myocardial failure and deterioration of systolic function has great prognostic implications. However, the functional characteristics of the cardiac chambers have been incompletely studied in horses, and most of the indices used in clinical practice serve to evaluate global systolic LV function, whereas diastolic LV function, LA function, right heart function, regional myocardial function, and myocardial synchrony are rarely considered. Also, it is important to realize that the echocardiographic indices of systolic ventricular function generally do not reflect contractility per se but are (to a variable extent) influenced by preload, afterload, heart rate, and rhythm. Generally, it is advised to use a variety of echocardiographic variables to assess LV systolic function and to interpret them in the context of the clinical findings.[1–3]

Two-Dimensional Ejection Phase Indices

The 2D ejection phase indices are based on measurements of LV dimensions, and the same limitations as previously discussed apply to these indices. LV ejection fraction (EF) (%EF = SV / LVIVd × 100; where SV is stroke volume and LVIVd is LV end-diastolic volume) has traditionally been the standard index of LV systolic function. The LV fractional shortening (FS) (%FS = [LVIDd−LVIDs]/LVIDd × 100; where LVIDd and LVIDs are the LV internal diameter at end-diastole and peak systole, respectively) approximates the

%EF and is the most commonly used index of LV systolic function in horses. In fact, often it is the only one used in routine echocardiography because it can be easily calculated from M-mode recordings (see **Fig. 1**D, E). However, reliance on this index as a single measurement of LV function may be problematic.[19] The %FS represents the relative shortening of the LV short-axis in only a single dimension, disregarding that the LV contracts in all 3 dimensions. Also, it may lack accuracy when the IVS and the LV free wall do not contract synchronously, or when the cursor line is not placed optimally.

Area-based measurements, such as the LV fractional area change, are less sensitive to asynchronous wall motion and allow assessment of shortening in 2 dimensions. Volume-based measurements (%EF, SV, CO) can be calculated based on estimates of LV volume previously described (see **Fig. 1**C) and are preferred by this author.[19] They are generally considered more accurate and less effected by altered chamber geometry. However, there are differences and limitations related to the geometric model used.[1,2,25,26] As previously stated, the use of volume-based measurements of LV systolic function should be considered in cases in which the subjective evaluation and conventional measurements provide equivocal results.

Note that in horses with marked LV volume overload and normal myocardial function, both %EF and %FS can be increased due to the increased preload (ie, because of activation of the Frank-Starling mechanism) and, in case of mitral regurgitation (MR), because of decreased afterload (ie, because of systolic regurgitation of blood into the low-pressure atrial chamber). Conversely, a normal %EF and %FS in the presence of severe LV volume overload may indicate (but do not necessarily prove) myocardial failure.

Doppler-Derived Indices of Stroke Volume and Cardiac Output

Doppler-based estimates of SV and CO are indices of global ventricular function. The SV is calculated by multiplying the velocity time integral of the aortic or the pulmonic flow signal by the cross-sectional area of the respective vessel. There are many limitations of this technique, including the angle-dependency of Doppler-based flow measurements, inaccuracies in the determination of the flow area, and uncertainties as where exactly to measure flow and the cross-sectional area (or diameter) of the vessel.[39] In adult horses, adequate alignment of the Doppler beam with blood flow by transthoracic echocardiography is difficult and Doppler estimates of SV are neither considered very accurate nor reliable.[26] In foals, alignment of the ultrasound beam with blood flow can be achieved using apical imaging planes. Although this may improve the accuracy of CO measurements by Doppler echocardiography, volumetric 2DE measurements using the bullet method have been shown to provide better agreement with CO by lithium dilution than Doppler estimates of CO.[25] In horses with heart disease, myocardial dysfunction generally must be severe for blood flow indices to be affected, because CO is maintained in the failing heart until the compensatory mechanisms are overwhelmed.

Measurement of Systolic Time Intervals

Systolic time intervals (STIs), including LV preejection period (PEP), LV ejection time (ET), and LV PEP-to-ET ratio (PEP/ET), can be measured from M-mode images of Ao valve motion and from Doppler tracings of Ao blood flow, respectively.[3,40] The STIs may serve as complementary indicators of LV function that are independent of ventricular shape and geometry, and that may be superior to the calculation of the %FS. However, they are also variably influenced by heart rate and loading conditions.[3] Accurate time intervals may be difficult to obtain owing to the inability to clearly identify the onset and the end of ejection on M-mode or Doppler tracings.

This limitation may be overcome by use of TDI for measurement of STIs (see later discussion).[8,18] The clinical value of STIs has not been well established in horses with cardiovascular disease.

Tissue Velocity, Strain, and Strain Rate Imaging

TDI allows quantifying myocardial wall motion velocity.[9] The tissue velocity signals can be displayed as spectral tracings (PW TDI; see **Fig. 4**E) or as color-coded maps that are superimposed on a 2D gray-scale image (color TDI). Similar to other Doppler-based methods, velocity measurements by TDI depend on the angle of insonation and can only be performed in a single dimension. Tissue velocity imaging is used in humans and small animals for assessment of global systolic and diastolic LV function, detection of regional wall motion abnormalities, diagnosis of ventricular dyssynchrony, and estimation of ventricular filling pressures.

Echocardiographic strain and strain rate imaging provides additional indices for assessment of regional and global ventricular function.[9] Strain (ε) is a measure of deformation of a myocardial segment, expressed as percentage of change from its original dimension. For normal myocardium, systolic ε is an analog of regional EF. Strain rate (Sr) is the temporal derivative of ε and describes the rate of deformation. Systolic Sr reflects regional contractile function. In people, ε and Sr have been valuable for diagnosing subclinical myocardial disease and coronary artery disease, and for differentiating hypertrophy caused by hypertension or cardiomyopathy. Strain and strain rate imaging may further be useful to detect subclinical systolic dysfunction in valvular heart disease, and it may allow objective assessment of myocardial performance during stress testing to identify stunning, acute ischemia, and myocardial infarction. ε and Sr can be calculated using TDI and 2DST.[9] The latter method is based on conventional 2D recordings. It analyzes the grayscale speckles as they move during contraction and relaxation and allows tracking of myocardial motion throughout the entire cardiac cycle (see **Fig. 4**F). The 2DST method offers a Doppler-independent approach to the measurement of ε and Sr that may overcome some of the limitations of strain measurements by TDI. Importantly, 2DST is independent of the angle of insonation and allows simultaneous measurement of ε and Sr in 2 dimensions. Thus, if complex regional wall motion patterns are to be investigated, 2DST is considered the preferred method.

To current knowledge, horses rarely suffer from clinically relevant coronary artery disease and myocardial infarction, and the prevalence of congestive heart failure is certainly low. The clinical relevance of myocardial ischemia, regional wall motion abnormalities, and ventricular dyssynchrony is still unknown in horses. However, myocardial diseases may be underappreciated in horses, at least in part because of the limitations of the currently used diagnostic methods. Therefore, there is a need to investigate these novel echocardiographic methods to better quantify LV function and to identify echocardiographic indices that may indicate occult myocardial disorders. Over the last few years, several reports on the use of TDI[10,12,16,17,29] and 2DST[8,12,14–17,29] in horses have been published. The results of these studies indicate that radial LV wall motion velocities and STIs measured by TDI as well as ε and Sr measured by 2DST can be reliably used to characterize LV wall motion and to assess LV systolic and diastolic function in healthy horses at rest and after exercise, and in horses with primary myocardial disease (see **Fig. 4**E, F).[12,16,17] Further studies are required to further define the clinical value of these novel echocardiographic methods in horses to assess disease-related alterations in LV systolic function and their relation to severity of disease, exercise capacity, and prognosis.

ASSESSMENT OF DIASTOLIC VENTRICULAR FUNCTION

Diastolic ventricular function is more complex than systolic function. Ventricular filling results from the dynamic interplay of active ventricular relaxation, ventricular compliance, filling pressures, pericardial restraint, ventricular interaction, and atrial function. Afterload and contractility will further influence diastolic function. Therefore, the echocardiographic assessment of diastolic ventricular function and filling pressures (which are commonly assessed together) is difficult. In people, diastolic dysfunction is common to virtually all forms of cardiac failure and associated with impaired ventricular relaxation and increased ventricular stiffness. In horses, diastolic ventricular dysfunction may certainly play a role in pericardial and myocardial disease but the clinical relevance of diastolic dysfunction in other types of cardiac disease is not clear and the prevalence of diastolic heart failure is unknown.

Doppler-derived transmitral flow velocities are commonly used in humans and small animals for assessment of diastolic LV function and filling pressures (see **Fig. 4D**).[1] However, optimal alignment with blood flow and consistent placement of the sample volume relative to the position of the mitral valve is not possible in adult horses and velocity measurements are unreliable.[11,27,41] Nonetheless, if marked decrease or reversion of the ratio between the early diastolic (E wave) and the late-diastolic (A wave) transmitral blood flow velocity (ie, the E/A ratio) is present, diastolic dysfunction must be suspected.[17] TDI may provide additional velocity-based (eg, the ratio between the peak radial wall motion velocities during early diastole (E_m wave) and during late diastole (A_m wave), termed E_m/A_m ratio) and time interval-based (eg, isovolumic relaxation time) indices that are easier to obtain and that can be helpful for assessment of LV diastolic function in horses (see **Fig. 4E**).[10,17,18]

ASSESSMENT OF LEFT ATRIAL FUNCTION

LA function is rarely considered during routine echocardiography in horses. However, LA function is impaired in horses with AF and may also be altered in horses suffering from MR or other cardiac disease. LA size and LA mechanical function can be assessed in horses by use of 2DE, transmitral Doppler flow velocity profiles, and analyses of LA wall motion by TDI and 2DST.[27] Clinically, the use of 2DE variables, including LA area and LA fractional area changes, is straightforward and seems most useful, whereas transmitral flow velocities and TDI variables are more difficult to record and less reliable. LA contractile dysfunction can be detected in horses after conversion from AF to sinus rhythm, likely attributed to AF-induced atrial remodeling, and has prognostic value to predict recurrence of AF.[11,42,43] Additional studies will be required to determine the clinical relevance of LA mechanical dysfunction in the presence of cardiac disease in horses, and to relate the changes in echocardiographic variables to severity of disease, exercise capacity, or prognosis, with appropriate outcome measures.

HEMODYNAMIC ASSESSMENT

The hemodynamic load placed on the heart by cardiac lesions can be estimated by echocardiography, combining information of chamber size, cardiac motion, LV systolic and diastolic function, and intracardiac blood flow. Doppler studies can be used to assess intracardiac pressures and pressure gradients. Normal pressure gradients that generate red blood cell flow range between 0.25 and 1.5 m/s. Abnormally high velocities can be found in many cardiac conditions, including ventricular septal defect and valvular regurgitation, in which a pressure gradient drives blood across a restrictive orifice. The pressure gradients are either reflections of normal intracardiac pressures or consequences of pathologically increased pressures. Pressure gradients can be estimated using Doppler echocardiography by using the simplified Bernoulli equation (dp = $4 \times v_{max}^2$, where dp is the pressure gradient in millimeters of mercury and v_{max} is the peak velocity in meters per second). The main indications to measure pressure gradients in horses are the diagnosis of pulmonary hypertension (by interrogation of regurgitant flow at the tricuspid and pulmonic valves; see **Fig. 4**B) and the assessment of ventricular septal defects (by interrogation of shunt flow).

ASSESSMENT OF VALVULAR REGURGITATION

The Doppler technology of current echocardiographic systems is very sensitive to detect valvular regurgitation and care must be taken not to overinterpret the echo findings (particularly in otherwise healthy animals without abnormal clinical findings and in the absence of heart murmurs). Assessment of valvular regurgitation should be achieved using an integrated qualitative and quantitative approach, combining clinical examination (including auscultation of a typical murmur) and 2D, M-mode, and Doppler echocardiography. Measurement of cardiac chamber dimensions provides information on the hemodynamic relevance of chronic valvular regurgitation. Abnormal timing and direction of transvalvular flow, as well as flow turbulences, can be detected by 2D color Doppler, color M-mode, and spectral Doppler echocardiography (see **Fig. 4**A–D). The regurgitant signal in the receiving chamber can be interrogated and used for assessment of severity of valvular regurgitation.[44] Multiple imaging planes must be used to accurately identify origin, extent, timing, and duration of the regurgitation. It is important to realize that color Doppler echocardiography only describes blood flow direction and velocity but not absolute volumetric flow. Quantification of regurgitation by assessing signal strength of the spectral Doppler regurgitant signal or measuring the area of regurgitation within the receiving chamber is, therefore, problematic. The Doppler-derived regurgitant signal is largely influenced by color gain settings, direction of flow, orifice size and shape, driving pressure, flow, and characteristics of the receiving chamber. Therefore, receiving chamber analysis of the regurgitant jet should not be used as a sole measure of severity.

Recently, a scoring system was introduced for staging mild, moderate, and severe AR, based on 3 different criteria.[45] These included LV size and geometry assessed subjectively from a 4-chamber view, LV short-axis diameter measured at end-diastole, and the size and area of the regurgitant jet as visualized by CFM. A similar scoring system could well be applied to cases with MR, including measures of LA size and regurgitant jet area. However, although such scoring systems certainly provide a more comprehensive assessment of AR and MR severity compared with assessment of jet size only, they will need to be validated independently and their prognostic value (eg, with respect to risk of arrhythmia or likelihood of progression of disease) will have to be determined before they can be widely used in clinical practice.

SUMMARY

Echocardiography is well established in horses and recent studies describe the echocardiographic assessment of cardiac size and function in horses by conventional 2DE, M-mode, and Doppler echocardiography, as well as novel TDI, 2DST, and 3D real-time echocardiography. Despite the encouraging findings of some of these studies, one needs to be careful not to be too enthusiastic about the potential diagnostic and prognostic utility of new imaging methods. It is very possible that a few of the novel echocardiographic indices will prove to be of clinical value in future studies. Nonetheless, many or even most of them will probably not withstand the test of time and will not make an entrance into the routine echocardiographic protocols. The conventional techniques will certainly remain the cornerstone of every echocardiographic examination and there are still many open questions, even with respect to these traditional techniques, when it comes to standardization of recordings and measurements, staging of disease, and diagnostic and prognostic value of individual echocardiographic variables. Independent of the methods used, the findings obtained during echocardiography should be critically assessed in the light of clinical findings and should not be overinterpreted or misinterpreted. Also, despite the availability of quantitative echocardiographic measurements, subjective assessment remains crucial and must not be neglected.

SUPPLEMENTARY DATA

Supplementary data related to this article can be found online at https://doi.org/10.1016/j.cveq.2018.12.008.

REFERENCES

1. Otto CM. Textbook of clinical echocardiography. 3rd edition. Philadelphia: Elsevier Saunders; 2004.
2. Lang RM, Badano LP, Mor-Avi V, et al. Recommendations for cardiac chamber quantification by echocardiography in adults: an update from the American Society of Echocardiography and the European Association of Cardiovascular Imaging. J Am Soc Echocardiogr 2015;28:1–39.
3. Boon JA. Veterinary echocardiography. 2nd edition. Oxford: Wiley-Blackwell; 2011.
4. Schwarzwald CC. Ultrasonography of the heart. In: Kidd JA, Lu KG, Frazer ML, editors. Atlas of equine ultrasonography. Chichester (United Kingdom): John Wiley & Sons, Ltd; 2014. p. 379–406.
5. Schwarzwald CC. Disorders of the cardiovascular system. In: Reed SM, Bayly WM, Sellon DC, editors. Equine internal medicine. 4th edition. St. Louis (MO): Saunders Elsevier; 2018. p. 387–541.
6. Reef VB, Bonagura J, Buhl R, et al. Recommendations for management of equine athletes with cardiovascular abnormalities. J Vet Intern Med 2014;28:749–61.
7. Grenacher PA, Schwarzwald CC. Assessment of left ventricular size and function in horses using anatomical M-mode echocardiography. J Vet Cardiol 2010;12:111–21.
8. Schwarzwald CC, Schober KE, Berli ASJ, et al. Left ventricular radial and circumferential wall motion analysis in horses using strain, strain rate, and displacement by 2D speckle tracking. J Vet Intern Med 2009;23:890–900.
9. Stoylen A. Strain rate imaging: cardiac deformation imaging by ultrasound/echocardiography - tissue Doppler and speckle tracking. Available at: http://folk.ntnu.no/stoylen/strainrate/. Accessed December 15, 2018.
10. Schwarzwald CC, Bonagura JD, Schober KE. Methods and reliability of tissue Doppler imaging for assessment of left ventricular radial wall motion in horses. J Vet Intern Med 2009;23:643–52.
11. Schwarzwald CC, Schober KE, Bonagura JD. Echocardiographic Evidence of left atrial mechanical dysfunction after conversion of atrial fibrillation to sinus rhythm in 5 horses. J Vet Intern Med 2007;21:820–7.

12. Decloedt A, Verheyen T, Sys S, et al. Tissue Doppler imaging and 2-dimensional speckle tracking of left ventricular function in horses exposed to lasalocid. J Vet Intern Med 2012;26:1209–16.

13. Decloedt A, Verheyen T, Sys S, et al. Evaluation of tissue Doppler imaging for regional quantification of radial left ventricular wall motion in healthy horses. Am J Vet Res 2013;74:53–61.

14. Decloedt A, Verheyen T, Sys S, et al. Quantification of left ventricular longitudinal strain, strain rate, velocity, and displacement in healthy horses by 2-dimensional speckle tracking. J Vet Intern Med 2011;25:330–8.

15. Decloedt A, Verheyen T, Sys S, et al. Two-dimensional speckle tracking for quantification of left ventricular circumferential and radial wall motion in horses. Equine Vet J 2013;45:47–55.

16. Verheyen T, Decloedt A, De Clercq D, et al. Cardiac changes in horses with atypical myopathy. J Vet Intern Med 2012;26:1019–26.

17. Schefer KD, Hagen R, Ringer SK, et al. Laboratory, electrocardiographic, and echocardiographic detection of myocardial damage and dysfunction in an Arabian mare with nutritional masseter myodegeneration. J Vet Intern Med 2011;25:1171–80.

18. Koenig TR, Mitchell KJ, Schwarzwald CC. Echocardiographic assessment of left ventricular function in healthy horses and in horses with heart disease using pulsed-wave tissue Doppler imaging. J Vet Intern Med 2017;31:556–67.

19. Schefer KD, Bitschnau C, Weishaupt MA, et al. Quantitative analysis of stress echocardiograms in healthy horses with 2-dimensional (2D) echocardiography, anatomical M-mode, tissue Doppler imaging, and 2D speckle tracking. J Vet Intern Med 2010;24:918–31.

20. Patteson MW, Gibbs C, Wotton PR, et al. Effects of sedation with detomidine hydrochloride on echocardiographic measurements of cardiac dimensions and indices of cardiac function in horses. Equine Vet J Suppl 1995;(19):33–7.

21. Gehlen H, Kroker K, Deegen E, et al. Influence of detomidine on cardiac function and hemodynamic in horses with and without heart murmur. Schweiz Arch Tierheilkd 2004;146:119–26 [in German].

22. Buhl R, Ersboll AK, Larsen NH, et al. The effects of detomidine, romifidine or acepromazine on echocardiographic measurements and cardiac function in normal horses. Vet Anaesth Analg 2007;34:1–8.

23. Menzies-Gow NJ. Effects of sedation with acepromazine on echocardiographic measurements in eight healthy thoroughbred horses. Vet Rec 2008;163:21–5.

24. Schwarzwald CC. Sequential segmental analysis - a systematic approach to the diagnosis of congenital cardiac defects. Equine Vet Educ 2008;20:305–9.

25. Giguere S, Bucki E, Adin DB, et al. Cardiac output measurement by partial carbon dioxide rebreathing, 2-dimensional echocardiography, and lithium-dilution method in anesthetized neonatal foals. J Vet Intern Med 2005;19:737–43.

26. McConachie E, Barton MH, Rapoport G, et al. Doppler and volumetric echocardiographic methods for cardiac output measurement in standing adult horses. J Vet Intern Med 2013;27:324–30.

27. Schwarzwald CC, Schober KE, Bonagura JD. Methods and reliability of echocardiographic assessment of left atrial size and mechanical function in horses. Am J Vet Res 2007;68:735–47.

28. Vandecasteele T, Cornillie P, van Steenkiste G, et al. Echocardiographic identification of atrial-related structures and vessels in horses validated by computed tomography of casted hearts. Equine Vet J 2019;51:90–6.

29. Decloedt A, De Clercq D, Ven Sofie S, et al. Echocardiographic measurements of right heart size and function in healthy horses. Equine Vet J 2017;49:58–64.
30. Young LE. Cardiac responses to training in 2-year-old thoroughbreds: an echocardiographic study. Equine Vet J Suppl 1999;30:195–8.
31. Lightfoot G, Jose-Cunilleras E, Rogers K, et al. An echocardiographic and auscultation study of right heart responses to training in young national hunt thoroughbred horses. Equine Vet J Suppl 2006;36:153–8.
32. Buhl R, Ersboll AK, Eriksen L, et al. Changes over time in echocardiographic measurements in young Standardbred racehorses undergoing training and racing and association with racing performance. J Am Vet Med Assoc 2005;226:1881–7.
33. Buhl R, Ersboll AK. Echocardiographic evaluation of changes in left ventricular size and valvular regurgitation associated with physical training during and after maturity in Standardbred trotters. J Am Vet Med Assoc 2012;240:205–12.
34. Flethoj M, Schwarzwald CC, Haugaard MM, et al. Left ventricular function after prolonged exercise in equine endurance athletes. J Vet Intern Med 2016;30:1260–9.
35. Cornell CC, Kittleson MD, Della Torre P, et al. Allometric scaling of M-mode cardiac measurements in normal adult dogs. J Vet Intern Med 2004;18:311–21.
36. Huesler IM, Mitchell KJ, Schwarzwald CC. Echocardiographic assessment of left atrial size and function in Warmblood horses: reference intervals, allometric scaling, and agreement of different echocardiographic variables. J Vet Intern Med 2016;30:1241–52.
37. Brown DJ, Rush JE, MacGregor J, et al. M-mode echocardiographic ratio indices in normal dogs, cats, and horses: a novel quantitative method. J Vet Intern Med 2003;17:653–62.
38. Schwarzwald CC, Berthoud D. Echocardiographic assessment of left ventricular size and systolic function in horses using linear measurements and area-based volume estimates. J Vet Intern Med 2012;26:726.
39. Blissitt KJ, Young LE, Jones RS, et al. Measurement of cardiac output in standing horses by Doppler echocardiography and thermodilution. Equine Vet J 1997;29:18–25.
40. Atkins CE, Snyder PS. Systolic time intervals and their derivatives for evaluation of cardiac function. J Vet Intern Med 1992;6:55–63.
41. Blissitt KJ, Bonagura JD. Pulsed wave Doppler echocardiography in normal horses. Equine Vet J Suppl 1995;(19):38–46.
42. De Clercq D, van Loon G, Tavernier R, et al. Atrial and ventricular electrical and contractile remodeling and reverse remodeling owing to short-term pacing-induced atrial fibrillation in horses. J Vet Intern Med 2008;22:1353–9.
43. Decloedt A, Schwarzwald CC, De Clercq D, et al. Risk factors for recurrence of atrial fibrillation in horses after cardioversion to sinus rhythm. J Vet Intern Med 2015;29:946–53.
44. Young LE, Rogers K, Wood JL. Heart murmurs and valvular regurgitation in thoroughbred racehorses: epidemiology and associations with athletic performance. J Vet Intern Med 2008;22:418–26.
45. Ven S, Decloedt A, Van Der Vekens N, et al. Assessing aortic regurgitation severity from 2D, M-mode and pulsed wave Doppler echocardiographic measurements in horses. Vet J 2016;210:34–8.

Equine Electrocardiography

Katharyn J. Mitchell, BVSc, DVCS, DVM, PhD

KEYWORDS

- Horse • Equine • Electrocardiogram • ECG • Arrhythmia • Heart • Cardiac

KEY POINTS

- A definitive diagnosis of any arrhythmia or investigation of unexplained tachycardia or bradycardia is made with electrocardiography (ECG).
- Resting, exercising, and ambulatory ECGs are important parts of the diagnostic evaluation of many equine patients.
- Recording ECGs in horses is easier than ever with contemporary, digital ECG recorders.
- Good-quality ECG recordings are essential to make an accurate diagnosis.
- A stepwise, logical approach to ECG analysis facilitates recognition and diagnosis of arrhythmias.

INTRODUCTION

Although detection of an abnormal heart rate or rhythm occurs as part of the physical examination, a definitive diagnosis of any arrhythmia or investigation of unexplained tachycardia or bradycardia is made by electrocardiography. The recording of an electrocardiogram (ECG) is an important part of the diagnostic evaluation of many equine patients (**Box 1**).

The type and duration of recording depend on the individual situation, the frequency, and the timing of the arrhythmia. Confirmation of a persistent arrhythmia may be possible with a short duration recording at rest. However, a horse may auscultate normally at rest but have an irregular rhythm in the immediate recovery period after exercise, which would require a telemetric ECG recording before, during, and after exercise to fully evaluate the clinical relevance of the arrhythmia.

Diagnosing and treating arrhythmias in horses first relies on recognition of the normal variation that exists in heart rate, rhythm, and morphology of the P-QRS-T complexes, both at rest and during exercise. Identification of abnormal complexes can be difficult given the horse displays a wide range of "normal" physiologic

Disclosure Statement: No disclosures. The author does not have any relationship with a commercial company that has a direct financial interest in the subject matter or materials discussed in article or with a company making a competing product.

Clinic for Equine Internal Medicine, Equine Department, University of Zurich, Winterthurerstrasse 260, Zurich 8057, Switzerland

E-mail address: kmitchell@vetclinics.uzh.ch

Vet Clin Equine 35 (2019) 65–83
https://doi.org/10.1016/j.cveq.2018.12.007
0749-0739/19/© 2018 Elsevier Inc. All rights reserved.

Box 1
Indications for recording an electrocardiogram

- Horses with an arrhythmia heard on physical examination
- Horses with unexplained tachyarrhythmias or bradyarrhythmias
- Horses with poor performance or exercise intolerance
- Horses with evidence of moderate to severe structural heart disease potentially predisposing to development of arrhythmias
- As part of a prepurchase examination to confirm normal sinus rhythm
- Horses with a history of weakness or collapse
- Monitoring heart rhythm as part of therapy (eg, antiarrhythmic therapy)
- Monitoring heart rate to detect stress or pain (eg, during hospital stay or transport)

---

arrhythmias (eg, sinus pause, sinus arrhythmia, first- and second-degree atrioventricular [AV] blocks) that create variability in the rhythm. Good-quality ECG recordings are essential to allow differentiation of normal from abnormal complexes and artifacts. With the plethora of medical technology available today, recording an ECG in a horse at rest, over prolonged periods of time, or during exercise is becoming easier and more accessible to equine practitioners. Recordings are obtained quickly in a field setting with many handheld or easily attached ECG recording devices that can transmit digitalized data wirelessly. This also enables rapid sharing of data between colleagues for further analysis or second opinion.

INDICATIONS FOR OBTAINING AN ELECTROCARDIOGRAPHIC RECORDING IN HORSES

As indicated in **Box 1**, there are several indications for obtaining an ECG recording in a horse.

Resting Electrocardiograms

Short-duration ECG recordings at rest are quick to obtain and can provide an immediate diagnosis if the abnormal rhythm persists or occurs frequently. Longer-duration (ambulatory or Holter ECG) recordings may be indicated if the problem appears paroxysmal or infrequent. These extended recordings can also be useful when monitoring a response to therapy (eg, antiarrhythmic treatment). Many of the telemetric ECG systems allow for longer-duration recordings with the data being stored locally (eg, on an SD card) or transmitted wirelessly (eg, via Bluetooth or mobile GSM network) to a laptop, computer, smartphone, or a cloud-based server.

Exercising Electrocardiograms

When investigating a horse with a history of exercise intolerance, poor performance, weakness, or collapse, or in a horse with underlying structural heart disease, an exercising ECG is often indicated. In addition, in horses with arrhythmias at rest, it can be informative to know if the arrhythmia is "overdrive-suppressed" by the normal sinus rhythm at higher heart rates or if additional arrhythmias develop (as seen, for example, in with horses in atrial fibrillation [AF] that can develop wide-complex arrhythmias with a rapid ventricular response rate and R-on-T phenomenon during exercise or stress).[1] It is recommended that horses perform at or slightly above their intended level of exercise intensity during an exercising ECG evaluation. Recording with a telemetric device allows continuous assessment of the heart rate and rhythm both during and immediately after exercise, where arrhythmias are most commonly observed.

PRINCIPLES OF ELECTROCARDIOGRAPHY

Cardiac cell depolarization and repolarization result from ions moving across the cell membrane through various pumps, channels, and exchangers, as seen in **Fig. 1**.[2] With simultaneous depolarization and repolarization of a critical mass of cells, the electrical

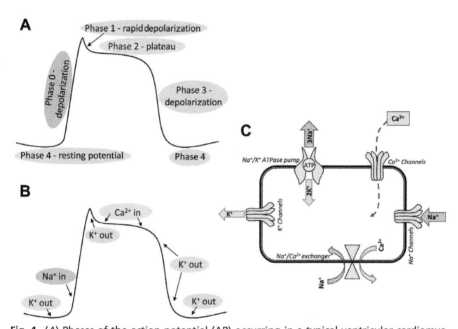

Fig. 1. (A) Phases of the action potential (AP) occurring in a typical ventricular cardiomyo-cyte. There are 4 phases of the AP, with rapid entry of sodium (Na[+]) ions into the cell result-ing in fast depolarization (phase 0) and calcium (Ca[2+]) ions entering more slowly during phase 2, resulting in full depolarization of the cell. Potassium (K[+]) channels open and out-ward movement of K[+] ions account for repolarization of the cell (phases 1 and 3). Phase 4, the maintenance of the resting membrane potential in a state of polarization, results from K[+] diffusing out of the cell following the concentration gradient that is maintained by the Na[+]/K[+]-ATPase (see C). (B) Timing of the movement of ions across the cellular membrane, resulting in the phases of the action potential seen in (A). (C) A stylized cardiomyocyte, de-picting examples of ion pumps, channels, and exchangers that allow the movement of ions across the cell membrane, resulting in depolarization and repolarization of the cell mem-brane. The Na[+]/K[+]-ATPase is primarily responsible for maintaining the resting intracellular concentrations of ions (high intracellular K[+], low intracellular Na[+]). Opening of the Na[+] channels result in rapid influx of Na[+] during early depolarization. Calcium ions enter the cell during the AP through Ca[2+] channels, leading to a Ca[2+]-induced Ca[2+] release from the sarcoendoplasmic reticulum (SER) and subsequent contraction of actin and myosin fila-ments. The excess cytoplasmic Ca[2+] is then either eliminated by reuptake into the SER or removed from the cell via the Na[+]/Ca[2+] exchanger and a Ca[2+] pump (not shown). There are many different K[+] channels that allow K[+] to exit the cell during repolarization and resting state.

potentials are strong enough to be detected on the skin surface. These changes in the electrical field can be recorded using electrodes affixed to the skin. The combination of 2 electrodes (one positive, one negative), placed at points around the heart, measuring the potential difference between them, is called a "lead." When the sum of all electrical potentials aims in the direction of the positive electrode, an upward deflection is seen on the ECG tracing, whereas an electrical vector directed away from the positive electrode results in a downward deflection on the ECG tracing.

Conduction of electrical activity in the heart follows a fairly fixed pathway: From the sinus node, across the atrial myocardium, through the AV node, His bundle, bundle branches, and Purkinje system to the ventricular myocardium. A rhythm originating from the sinus node is called a "sinus rhythm." **Fig. 2**A demonstrates the cardiac conduction system that forms the pathway for depolarization across the myocardium, and **Fig.** 2B depicts the representative segments that are displayed on a surface ECG.

A relatively large amount of myocardial tissue is required for the depolarization or repolarization to be accurately detected on a surface ECG. Therefore, the sinus node depolarizations per se are not visualized, but rather it is the atrial depolarization that creates the P wave seen on the ECG. In horses, the morphology of the P waves is highly variable, with bifid (2 positive peaks), single positive, or biphasic (typically negative/positive) waves commonly observed. As heart rate increases, the P-wave morphology may also change, while some horses also display evidence of a

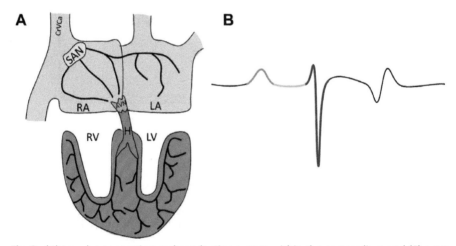

Fig. 2. (A) Impulse generation and conduction system within the myocardium and (B) a surface ECG recording resulting from impulse conduction through the different segments of the conduction system. The impulse is initiated in the sinoatrial node (SAN) and is transmitted across the atrial myocardium, generating the P wave (blue color). Specialized internodal and interatrial (Bachmann bundle) pathways facilitate and direct impulse conduction within the atria. At the atrioventricular node (AVN), impulse conduction is delayed, resulting in the PR interval (yellow color) observed on the surface ECG. Rapid conduction then occurs through the His bundle, bundle branches, and Purkinje fiber network, activating the ventricular myocardium and generating the QRS complex (red color) on the ECG. CrVCa, cranial vena cava; H, His bundle; LA, left atrium; LV, left ventricle; RA, right atrium; RV, right ventricle. (Adapted from van Loon G, Patteson M. Electrophysiology and arrhythmogenesis. In: Marr CM, editor. Cardiology of the horse. 2nd edition. Elsevier; 2010. p. 59–73; and From Schwarzwald CC, Bonagura JD, Muir WW. The cardiovascular system. In: Muir WW, editor. Equine anesthesia. 2nd edition. St Louis (MO): Elsevier; 2009. p. 37–100, with permission.)

wandering pacemaker within the large sinus node, particularly at low heart rates (ie, with high parasympathetic tone), resulting in highly variable P-wave morphology between individual beats. Following atrial depolarization, there is a period of atrial repolarization that can occasionally be seen on a surface ECG as a so-called T_a wave (ie, the atrial T wave).

In a normal horse, the atria and ventricles are electrically separated from each other by nonconducting fibrous tissue, except at the level of AV node. Conduction of the electrical impulse through the AV node is slower than through the other myocardial tissues, resulting in a delay between the atrial and ventricular depolarization. This delay is physiologically important because it allows for the atrial contribution to ventricular filling to occur before the onset of ventricular systole, optimizing preload and therefore cardiac output. Healthy horses commonly have high parasympathetic tone, which can further delay (or even block) AV nodal conduction. Conduction through the AV node does not result in a deflection on the surface ECG, but the conduction delay can be measured through the PR interval.

After leaving the AV node, the electrical impulse travels rapidly through the His bundle and Purkinje system to depolarize the ventricular myocardium. This results in the largest deflection recorded on the surface ECG: the QRS complex. According to international convention, the first downward deflection is the Q wave; the first upward deflection is the R wave, and the next following downward deflection is the S wave. The larger waves are denoted in capital letters; the smaller waves are denoted in lowercase letters. Typically, horses have an rS or S morphology when an ECG is recorded using a base-apex lead configuration (**Fig. 3**). Q waves are rarely identified

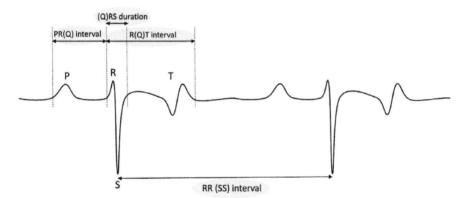

Fig. 3. Typical P-QRS-T complex morphology as recorded with a standard base-apex lead configuration. The important timing intervals are indicated. The equine base-apex lead ECG does not typically have identifiable Q waves. Therefore, the conventional nomenclature of the timing intervals may require modification, the PQ interval becomes the PR interval, the QRS duration is the RS duration, and the QT interval is actually the RT interval. Because the largest deflection of the equine QRS is negative, this is called the S wave, so the interval measured between adjacent QRS intervals is actually the SS interval, rather than the RR interval. However, in most instances, for simplicity and consistency across species, the intervals are still called PQ, QRS, QT, and RR intervals. Note that it can be difficult to accurately define the start and end of the individual deflections. When measuring timing intervals, it can be helpful to increase the paper speed (eg, from 25 mm/s to 50 or 100 mm/s), maintain a standardized approach (eg, always measure from the onset or end of the deflection where it deviates clearly from the baseline), and limit the number of observers (ie, ideally the same person should perform the analysis if repeated measurements over time are required).

on equine surface, base-apex ECG recordings. Despite the largest wave of the typical equine QRS complex being the S wave, rather than the R wave as in the standard human or small animal ECG, for convention, the interval between 2 adjacent QRS complexes is still referred to as the RR interval.

Every depolarization must be followed by repolarization; therefore, *every* QRS complex is *always* followed by a T wave (representing repolarization). Horses have extremely labile T-wave morphology, with variations in polarity and duration highly dependent on parasympathetic tone and heart rate. Although changes in T-wave morphology should not be overinterpreted in the diagnosis of cardiac disease, they can be helpful when determining the presence of abnormal complexes (atrial or ventricular premature complexes [APCs/VPCs]) and detecting artifacts (which do not have T waves).[3]

Recognition of the normal P-QRS-T morphology is critical to assessing an ECG recording, and particular attention should be paid to the polarity of wave forms (particularly the QRS-T) and the timing intervals. As equine ECGs are commonly missing the Q wave, the conventional timing intervals applied from human medicine require modification. The PQ interval becomes the PR interval; the QRS duration becomes the RS duration, and the QT interval becomes the RT interval, although the conventional nomenclature is often referred to for simplicity. These timing intervals are illustrated in **Fig. 3**. It is important to note that because of the extensive Purkinje fiber system within the equine ventricular myocardium (as compared with humans and small animals), the equine QRS complex recorded from a typical base-apex lead configuration provides no reliable information about cardiac chamber size.[4] Twelve-lead ECGs (as opposed to a single-lead base-apex ECG or a traditional limb-lead ECG) provide a larger variety of projections of the heart's electrical activity and have the potential to help determine the origin of premature complexes in horses. However, respective criteria for assessment have not been established so far, and work is currently ongoing in this area (abstract presented by G. Van Steenkiste at ECEIM Congress, November 9, 2018, Ghent, Belgium).

When measuring the time intervals (PR interval, QRS duration, QT interval), the size of the horse should be considered, because body weight is directly correlated with the time intervals (ie, small horses generally have shorter time intervals).[5]

RECORDING ELECTROCARDIOGRAMS IN HORSES
Equipment

The basic equipment required to obtain an ECG recording includes electrodes, a recording device, and a display of the tracing. A large variety of point-of-care medical devices have been brought to the market in recent times, making ECG recording devices easier to use and more affordable for the equine practitioner.

Recording devices

Short-duration recordings can be easily obtained using handheld ECG recording devices (eg, Alivecor Kardia Mobile ECG; Alivecor Inc, Mountain View, CA, USA), any variety of common monitoring devices used for anesthesia, or purpose-built ECG recorders (eg, Televet 100, telemetric ECG system; Engel Engineering Service GmbH, Heusenstamm, Germany). Many of these devices display the ECG tracing on a monitor, smartphone, or tablet computer. It is mandatory for every device to contain some type of storage capability. This storage capability can be a thermoprinter providing hard copies of ECG strips of any length. Preferably, the device should store the data digitally, allowing the ECG to be postprocessed, digitally analyzed, interpreted, or sent to an expert for analysis at a later time.

Longer continuous recordings (eg, longer than 5 minutes) require the use of an ambulatory device, which preferably records both locally (eg, on an SD card) and remotely by sending the signal wirelessly to a storage device with display monitor. The most commonly used veterinary device for this purpose is the Televet recorder, whereas many human or small-animal devices can be adapted for equine use (eg, Lifecard CF; SpaceLab Healthcare, Snoqualmie, WA, USA). It is particularly important that the data from long-term ambulatory recordings be digitalized, stored, and available for further offline processing and analysis. This also allows the easy sharing of ECG recordings between individuals, which can be useful when a second opinion is required.

Several products are currently being developed to improve the ease of ECG recording in horses, particularly during exercise. However, at this time, the Televet recorder is most commonly used, and in the author's opinion, it remains the most reliable and easy-to-use product. It is important to note that the (veterinary) medical technology market has several heart rate monitors currently available, but these should not be confused with an ECG recording device. The heart rate monitors are supposed to detect RR intervals, but an unknown amount of postprocessing occurs with the use of proprietary signal processing algorithms and filters to remove motion artifacts and arrhythmias. Accuracy and reliability of these devices cannot be easily verified by the user, and some of them certainly do not provide accurate results in horses with arrhythmias or with exceptionally high heart rates during exercise.[6] These devices provide no information on P-QRS-T morphology and should not be considered a substitute for an ECG recorder in the diagnosis and management of equine arrhythmias. They can however be useful (acknowledging their limitations), particularly for monitoring heart rates during exercise at home with the owner.

Recently, preliminary investigations in the use of subcutaneous, implantable loop recorders (eg, Reveal; Medtronic, Minneapolis, MN, USA) in horses have shown encouraging results as event recorders for long-term (weeks or months) use. These devices may be useful in patients with paroxysmal arrhythmias that occur infrequently, particularly when investigating horses with collapse. However, these devices are currently cost-prohibitive for most patients and require specific positioning to obtain an optimal ECG signal (research report, R. Buhl, ACVIM forum, Washington DC, June 8, 2017; J. Keen, personal communication, University of Edinburgh, 2017).

Electrodes

Short-term recordings can be obtained using crocodile clips attached on the ends of the ECG cables. However, this is not suitable to obtain longer-term recordings, and some horses will not tolerate these being applied even for a short duration of time. Frequently, the application of water, normal saline, or alcohol to the skin/crocodile clips is required to ensure adequate contact and a good-quality ECG recording.

Self-adhesive gel patch electrodes provide a more comfortable alternative to crocodile clips and frequently remain in place for several hours of recording without issue. For longer duration (overnight) or exercising recordings, the sticky ECG electrodes can be further secured using self-adhesive foam patches or an elastic bandage applied on top (**Fig. 4**A). In most cases, it is not necessary to clip the coat, as long as the gel patch remains moist and the self-adhesive part of the electrode stays dry and provides sufficient adhesive strength. Occasionally, with a thick winter coat, it is necessary to clip the coat to provide better contact with the skin surface. It is essential for the coat to be

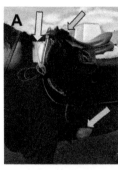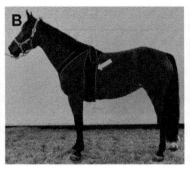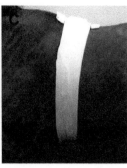

Fig. 4. (*A*) ECG electrodes covered with an adhesive foam patch (*gray arrows*) to secure them during exercise. The ECG cables and the recorder (*green arrow*) are secured out of the way of the rider. (*B*) The use of a commercially available reusable surcingle (Kruuse Tele- vet Electrode support; Jørgen Kruuse A/S, Langeskov, Denmark), which secures the ECG leads and recorder safely in a pocket (*orange arrow*). This system allows longer duration or exer- cising recordings (lunging exercise) to be easily and comfortably performed. (*C*) The use of self-adhesive bandaging material to affix the ECG leads and recorder for an overnight ECG recording. Note the padding over the withers to avoid rubbing and pressure sores.

dry (eg, before exercise) when the sticky electrodes are applied, because they will not stick to a damp or wet surface.

Additional material

For ambulatory recordings, it is necessary to affix the recording/transmitting device to the horse, which can be achieved by a reusable surcingle, purpose built for holding the device and the associated cables safely out of the way of damage, particularly if the horse lies down (eg, Kruuse Televet Electrode support; Jørgen Kruuse A/S, Lange- skov, Denmark; **Fig. 4**B). Alternatively, the device can be affixed using single-use, sticky elastic bandages (**Fig. 4**C). It is important that there is appropriate padding over the withers region, particularly if the device is to be worn overnight or for several days.

Lead Placement

Fig. 5 shows the typical lead placement for a short-duration, resting ECG recording. This is considered a "base-apex" configuration, where either "Lead I" (RA→LA) or "Lead II" (RA→LL) can be chosen on the monitor to display the ECG trace. **Fig. 3** rep- resents the typical P-QRS-T orientation when using this lead placement. **Fig. 6** displays the "modified base-apex" configuration that the author typically uses for long-term ambulatory ECG recordings. With this configuration, "Lead I" will highlight the atrial electrical activity, producing slightly magnified P waves to aid in the differen- tiation of atrial ectopic complexes (**Fig. 7**). "Lead II" will produce the typical ECG seen in **Fig. 3**. "Lead III" (LA→LL) will produce an alternative QRS configuration, which can aid in the detection of ventricular ectopic complexes (**Fig. 8**).

During exercise, the ECG electrodes can remain in the same position as described above (**Fig. 9**A, B) or can be moved to accommodate any equipment necessary (eg, saddle, surcingle, or harness; see **Fig. 4**). **Fig. 9**C is a variation that the author uses particularly for lunging, treadmill, or ridden exercise. The downside of this lead config- uration is that "Lead I" and "Lead II" are very similar (**Fig. 10**), which can make subtle changes in QRS configuration harder to identify but provides a "backup" lead in case one electrode becomes dislodged during exercise.

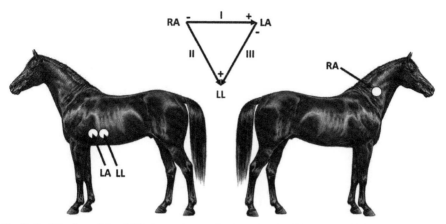

Fig. 5. Positioning of the ECG electrodes to obtain a standard base-apex lead from a resting horse, useful to obtain short-term ECG recordings. The electrode positions described by Eint- hoven triangle are modified and positioned on the body of the horse. The right arm elec- trode (RA) is placed on the right neck of the horse, while the left arm (LA) and left leg (LL) electrodes are placed on the left side of the horse over the apex of the heart. With this electrode configuration, both "Lead I" (RA→LA) and "Lead II" (RA→LL) can be chosen on the ECG recorder to display the base-apex ECG trace. Note that the terminology (LA, RA, LL; lead I, II, III) originates from the Einthoven lead system.

Short-Duration Recordings

Good-quality short-term recordings can be easily obtained from horses well restrained and standing still. Many of the handheld devices require the application of water, normal saline, or alcohol to the skin to facilitate conduction of the signal. Movement

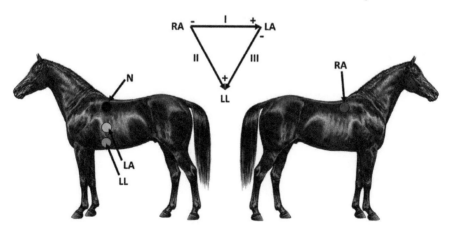

Fig. 6. Positioning of the ECG electrodes to obtain a modified base-apex recording from a resting horse. This electrode configuration allows the 3 leads to each highlight different as- pects of cardiac depolarization/repolarization. This configuration is useful, particularly for telemetric ECG monitoring or long-term (ambulatory, Holter) ECG recordings. LA, left arm electrode; LL, left leg (foot) electrode; N, neutral/ground electrode, RA, right arm electrode. In this example, the electrodes are colored for use with the Televet 100 recording system. Please note that the color system corresponds to the International Electrotechnical Commis- sion (IEC) standard. Other devices might use a different color system (ie, the one defined by the American Heart Association, where RA is white, LA is black, N is green, and LL is red).

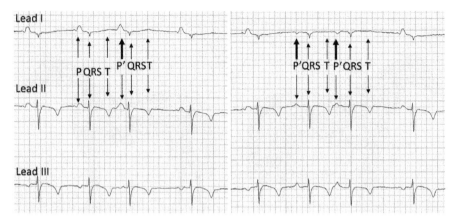

Fig. 7. An example of an ECG, recorded using the modified base-apex lead configuration described in **Fig. 6.** "Lead I" (RA→LA) provides useful information about the morphology of APCs (P', *bold arrows*), because the P and P' waves are more prominent. Two examples of P' morphology are depicted. "Lead II" (RA→LL) will produce the typical ECG. "Lead III" (LA→LL) will produce an alternative QRS configuration, which can also aid in the detection of ectopic complexes as seen in **Fig. 8.** LA, left arm electrode; LL, left leg (foot) electrode; RA, right arm electrode.

artifacts occur frequently and can interfere with the recording quality and subsequent interpretation of the ECG findings (**Fig. 11**), so care must be taken to ensure a good-quality recording is obtained. These recordings are extremely useful if the arrhythmia occurs frequently or continuously (as in a case of chronic AF) but are not useful for paroxysmal or infrequent arrhythmias (eg, paroxysmal AF).

Long-Term Recordings

Ambulatory (Holter) electrocardiographic recordings
Recording an ECG for a longer period of time, particularly overnight or for 24 hours, can be very useful for assessing the type, frequency, and distribution of arrhythmias

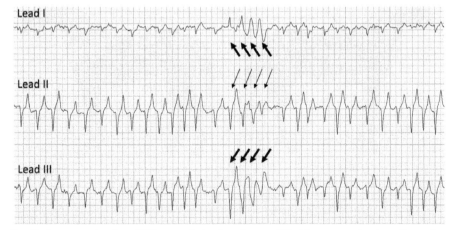

Fig. 8. An example of an ECG, recorded using the modified base-apex lead configuration described in **Fig. 6.** This is an exercising ECG performed in a horse with atrial fibrillation. "Lead I" and "Lead III" provide useful information about the morphology of abnormal QRS-T waves (*bold arrows*) that was not as apparent in the "Lead II" recording (*thin arrows*).

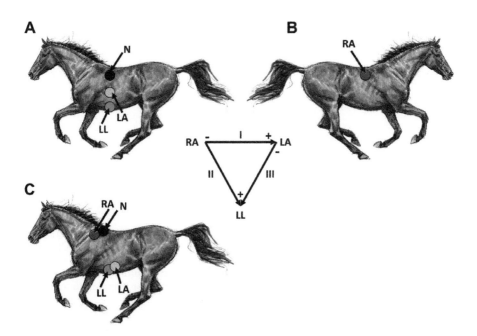

Fig. 9. Positioning of the ECG electrodes to obtain a modified base-apex recording from an exercising horse. (*A-B*) This electrode configuration (same as in **Fig. 6**) allows the three leads to each highlight different aspects of cardiac depolarization/repolarization (see **Figs. 7** and **8**). This may not be practical for some exercise tests, particularly when a rider or equipment interferes the electrode contact, creating artefacts. (*C*) This electrode configuration is useful for ridden exercise or when motion artifacts caused by equipment are present. The drawback of this placement is that both 'Lead I' (RA→LA) and 'Lead II' (RA→LL) are very similar, making abnormal morphology of complexes harder to detect. RA, right arm; LA, left arm; LL, left leg (foot); N, neutral/ground. Please note that the color system displayed here corresponds to the IEC standard (International Electrotechnical Commission) and is the one used by the Televet 100 recording system. Other devices might use a different color system (ie, the one defined by the American Heart Association, where RA is white, LA is black, N is green, and LL is red).

that may be present. Normal horses frequently have vagally mediated arrhythmias at rest.[7] In a recent study, small numbers (on average <3/hour) of premature complexes of atrial origin were present in just under 45% of overnight ECG recordings performed in healthy horses, whereas even smaller numbers (on average <1/3 hours) of VPCs were present in 4.3% of the horses.[8] Horses with clinically relevant arrhythmias often have a much higher frequency of premature complexes, including couplets, triplets, and short runs of tachycardia, that can show multiple P' or QRS-T morphologies or evidence of a short coupling interval with R-on-T phenomenon, particularly at higher heart rates. Bradyarrhythmias can also become apparent in longer recordings, especially overnight when the horse is not stimulated. Details on arrhythmias in horses are discussed in detail by Gunther van Loon's article, "Cardiac Arrhythmias in Horses," in this issue.

In addition, when investigating horses that present for collapse or weakness, longer recordings can be particularly useful, especially when coupled with video monitoring, so that both recordings can be analyzed simultaneously if any events occur during the

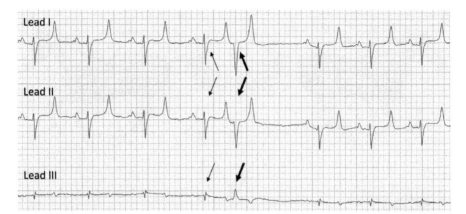

Fig. 10. An example of an ECG, recorded using the modified base-apex lead configuration described in **Fig. 9C**. Both "Lead I" (RA→LA) and "Lead II" (RA→LL) are similar, which provides a backup lead in case one is dislodged during exercise. However, abnormal morphology is not as easy to detect as with the electrode configuration seen in **Fig. 9A, B**. Normal complexes (*thin arrow*) and one premature ventricular complex (*bold arrow*) are shown.

period of observation. Implantable loop recorders for extended event monitoring should be considered in these cases, if budget allows.

Continuous ambulatory ECG monitoring, often combined with telemetric live monitoring of the ECG signal, is frequently used to monitor the effectiveness of anti-arrhythmic or heart failure therapy. Furthermore, it serves to provide diagnostic and prognostic information in humans and small animals with heart disease.[9–12] This approach is also used in equine cardiology, although less supporting evidence for interpretation of any findings is currently available in the equine cardiology literature.

Exercising Electrocardiographic Recordings

The use of ECGs to assess the heart rate and rhythm in horses during exercise is far more widespread, and a larger body of evidence is available in the literature characterizing the normal and abnormal findings in exercising horses. This is covered extensively within the other articles in this issue.

It is important that the type and duration of the exercise test are similar to the horse's typical work (or slightly exceeds it), to fully assess for the presence of clinically relevant exercising arrhythmias. It can be technically challenging to record good-quality exercising ECG recordings, and careful preparation is key, paying particular attention to the placement of the electrodes. Several tested devices include built-in electrodes to avoid the problem of dislodgement during strenuous exercise, although these devices are not readily available.

It is of upmost importance that ECG recording quality is optimized, because the detection of arrhythmias during periods of high heart rate, where motion artifacts are also present, can be very difficult. If necessary, the exercise test should be interrupted and the electrode positioning adjusted, in order to obtain a diagnostic quality ECG recording. In addition, differentiating between normal variation and pathologic arrhythmias can be difficult, although recent studies suggest that there is very little normal beat-to-beat variation present during peak exercise in healthy horses.[13,14]

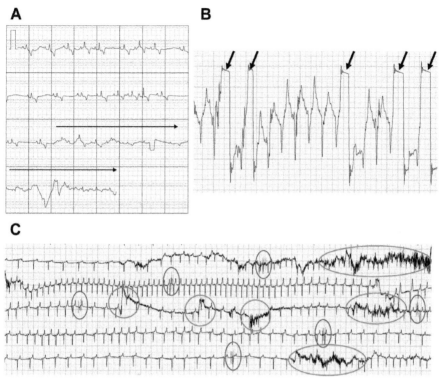

Fig. 11. Examples of artifacts that interfere with ECG interpretation. (*A*) A short duration ECG recorded with a handheld device (Alivecor Kardia Mobile ECG). Note the nondiagnostic section of the ECG (*horizontal arrows*), where P-QRS-T morphology is not clearly differentiated from the motion artifacts. (*B*) An exercising ECG with frequent artifacts (*bold arrows*) caused by a broken lead with exposed wiring. (*C*) Frequent motion artifacts (*green circles*) and poor Bluetooth connectivity (*red hashed lines, orange circles*) causing interruption in the sending of the digitalized ECG recording to the monitor. The first problem might be solved by replacing the ECG electrodes and checking the cables. The latter problem can be avoided by recording the ECG directly (ie, onto an SD card) in addition to transmitting the signal wirelessly and performing any additional analysis on the directly recorded ECG.

Optimization of Recording Quality

Good-quality ECG recordings are essential regardless of whether the ECG is recorded for 2 minutes, 24 hours, or during exercise. Careful attention to the placement of electrodes, ensuring adequate contact with the skin surface to optimally conduct the electrical signal, is critical. The use of additional adhesive material on top of the sticky electrode/lead unit can improve the robustness of the contact, particularly for longer-duration recordings or situations whereby electrode contact may be disrupted (eg, sweating during exercise).

Frequent monitoring of the ECG recording quality is also important, so that any problems (eg, electrodes coming off, batteries exhausted) can be identified and rapidly rectified without interfering with the diagnostic recording duration. If the ECG quality is suboptimal, then steps should be taken to problem solve the issue, checking the placement and contact of the electrodes (and replacing them where necessary), the placement of the surcingle and device, and the connection between the leads and recording device.

ANALYSIS OF ELECTROCARDIOGRAMS IN HORSES
Recognition of a Normal Equine Electrocardiogram

Analyzing any ECG recording should be done in a logical, stepwise manner. It is important to recognize the normal equine ECG morphology (see **Fig. 3**) to detect any abnormal complexes. **Table 1** lists the steps that should be followed to interpret any ECG.

Detection of Abnormal Complexes

Timing and morphology

A detailed description of common equine arrhythmias can be found in Gunther van Loon's article, "Cardiac Arrhythmias In Horses," in this issue. In general, abnormal complexes can be identified by their timing, as those coming earlier than expected based on the underlying rhythm (premature complexes) or those that are slower than expected (as is the case for many bradyarrhythmias and for escape beats). Most premature complexes are followed by a pause, either because of the impulse resetting the sinus node (frequently the case with APCs) or as a result of the abnormal depolarization rending the conduction system or myocardium refractory to transmitting the subsequent normal sinus impulse (seen with many VPCs). There are always possible exceptions to the rule, where a VPC is retrogradely conducted and resets the sinus node tissue or if sinus entry block is present so the sinus node is protected from an APC. Occasionally, a premature complex will not affect the underlying rhythm, resulting in an "interpolated" complex nestled between 2 normal sinus beats. An example is found in Virginia B. Reef's article, "Assessment of the Cardiovascular System in Horses During Prepurchase and Insurance Examinations," in this issue, Fig. 4. "Fusion beats" can occur, when an abnormal impulse is fused with the normal impulse, often resulting in a complex that starts with normal morphology and ends with a different/merged morphology.

The identification of APC and VPCs and other arrhythmias is further discussed in detail by Gunther van Loon's article, "Cardiac Arrhythmias in Horses," in this issue. A basic rule of thumb is that APCs have a P wave (termed P′) associated with the QRS-T and have fairly similar morphology to those of sinus origin (careful evaluation of the ECG is required to identify those P′ buried in the preceding T wave or ST segment). In addition, most APCs reset the sinus node, so that the resulting "noncompensatory pause" (ie, the interval between the premature R wave and the following normal R wave) approximates or is only slightly longer than the normal RR interval. In other words, APCs typically interrupt the underlying sinus rhythm so that the next following normal sinus complex occurs earlier than expected if the rhythm had not been interrupted (See Gunther van Loon's article, "Cardiac Arrhythmias in Horses," in this issue, Fig. 3). If occurring very early during the cardiac cycle, APCs may be blocked in the refractory AV node, so that the P′ wave is not followed by a QRS complex, or the impulse is aberrantly conducted through the partially refractory ventricular conduction system, resulting in an abnormally shaped QRS complex (See Gunther van Loon's article, "Cardiac Arrhythmias in Horses," in this issue, Fig. 4).

VPCs have no associated P wave and frequently show abnormal QRS-T morphology (wide and "bizarre" compared with the normally conducted sinus beat), unless they originate in the interventricular septum, very close to the AV

| Table 1 |
| A stepwise approach to analyze an electrocardiogram |

Step 1	First assess the overall quality of the recording. • The P-QRS-T complexes should be clearly visible and free of obvious artifacts. • Analysis should not be performed if the recording quality is poor, because misdiagnosis of the rhythm is possible.
Step 2	Identify the paper speed (typically 25 or 50 mm/s) and calculate the overall heart rate. • Compare the heart rate with the reference ranges, considering these are body weight dependent.[5] • The heart rate can be divided into 3 broad categories, normal, bradycardic, or tachycardic. • Most digital systems will perform an RR interval analysis and calculate the instantaneous heart rate automatically.
Step 3	Assess if the rhythm is regular or irregular. • If the rhythm is irregular, is there any underlying pattern (regularly irregular) or is there no pattern (irregularly irregular)? • Are there pauses, premature complexes, or both? • If there are pauses, how long are the pauses (shorter than twice the normal RR, twice the normal RR, or longer than twice the normal RR)? • If there are premature complexes, it can be helpful to measure the RR intervals encompassing the abnormal beat (ie, for one abnormal beat, measure 2× the normal RR; for 2 abnormal beats, measure 3× the normal RR, and so forth, and then trace the preceding and the subsequent R waves to determine if the underlying sinus rhythm is disrupted or not). Examples are shown in the Gunther van Loon's article, "Cardiac Arrhythmias in Horses," in this issue, Figs. 3 and 14.
Step 4	Identify the most normal P-QRS-T complexes (if present) and then compare them to the abnormal complexes. • Is there a P for every QRS? • Is there a QRS for every P? • Do they appear related (similar PR intervals) or dissociated (varying PR intervals)? • Is the morphology of all P-QRS-T complexes similar or different? • In particular, are all T waves the same or is there variation in T-wave morphology that could be caused by secondary T-wave changes (ie, if the preceding QRS is abnormal, then likely the following T wave is abnormal as well) or superimposition of other waves (eg, a P′ wave within the preceding T wave)?
Step 5	Measure the PR, QRS, and QT intervals. • Are they similar or varying? • Compare the intervals with the reference ranges, considering these are body weight dependent.[5]
Step 6	Define the rhythm. • Is this a disorder of abnormal impulse formation, abnormal impulse conduction, or both? • Is the rhythm primarily sinus in origin? If no, are the abnormal complexes of atrial, junctional, or ventricular origin? • Is the rhythm sustained or paroxysmal? • What is the timing and frequency of occurrence of abnormal beats?
Step 7	If unsure about the rhythm diagnosis or interpretation of the clinical relevance, seek a second opinion from a person experienced at equine ECG interpretation.

node. Because they usually do not reset the sinus node, they do not interrupt the underlying sinus rhythm, and the next following normal sinus complex occurs at the time expected based on a normal RR interval tracing (the article by Gunther van Loon's article, "Cardiac Arrhythmias in Horses," in this issue, Fig. 14).

Techniques for Detailed Analysis

With longer-duration recordings, additional, more detailed analyses can be performed. Many of these analyses are semiautomated, depending on the ECG software that is supplied with the recording device. Many human ECG systems perform an automated analysis based on morphology, where the normal and abnormal complexes are defined by timing and shape, collated in a library of beats with similar morphology, and then displayed for manual verification by a human operator (eg, Pathfinder SL, Spacelabs Healthcare, Snoqualmie, WA, USA).

Given the wide variety of variation that exists in normal ECG morphology in horses (eg, changing P-waves shape or T-wave inversion with increasing heart rate, body weight-related differences in time intervals, and so forth), many of these automated algorithms are not well suited to analyzing the equine ECG. Usually, a large amount of work is required to "teach" the software, of which complexes are normal or abnormal or to correct the automated analysis using a time-consuming full disclosure mode.

A simpler technique for semiautomated analysis of the equine ECG is to first perform an RR interval analysis, where the software detects RR intervals larger or smaller than a predefined percentage of the previous RR interval and marks these "different" complexes (**Fig. 12**A). Such an algorithm is implemented in the commonly used Televet analysis software. Manual verification can then be performed on any RR intervals that are within or exceed the specified threshold. This does not automatically mean that a marked beat is abnormal, but rather there has been change to the underlying rhythm. The operator must then determine whether this was (a) an artifact, where incorrect RR detection has occurred or RR detection has failed, (b) a normal physiologic variation is present (eg, marked sinus arrhythmia, sinus pause, or second-degree AV block), or (c) an abnormal complex is present that is disturbing the normal sinus rhythm. For (a), the RR detection can be manually overruled and corrected, whereas for (b) and (c), the above algorithm (**Table 1**) should be followed to determine the type of arrhythmia that is present. This method of ECG analysis can speed up the screening of ECGs for rhythm abnormalities, which is particularly helpful for exercising, overnight, or 24-hour recordings. However, this method is not infallible, and manual verification is required for the detection of abnormalities that do not result in a change to the underlying rhythm (eg, abnormal conduction as is seen with bundle branch block). The ability of this method to detect arrhythmias will also depend on the threshold for RR interval variation that is set at the start of the analysis. Typically, the author uses thresholds of 20% beat-to-beat variation at rest and 5% beat-to-beat variation during exercise in horses with predominately sinus rhythm, which is extrapolated from data about the normal beat-to-beat variation seen in healthy horses in sinus rhythm.[13,14] It important to realize that if a premature complex results less than the specified % RR variation, it will not be marked, whereas horses with physiologic arrhythmias like second-degree AV blocks will exceed the 20% threshold and therefore be marked "abnormal." Hence, such RR interval analysis based on timing does not replace the observer's manual analysis and interpretation.

Heart Rate Variability Analysis to Detect and Characterize Arrhythmias

Following RR interval detection and manual verification of appropriate R-wave recognition, the RR interval data can then be exported for advanced statistical and graphical analyses, including heart rate variability analysis (**Figs. 12**B, C). These analyses can be performed on the whole ECG or the ECG can be divided into segments for individual assessment. They provide complementary information, can aid in the detection and

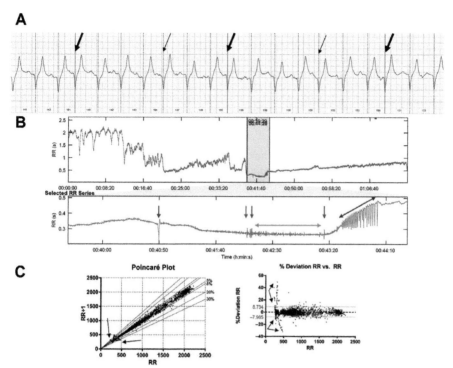

Fig. 12. An example of RR interval detection and subsequent heart rate variability analysis performed on an exercising ECG. This horse presented for poor performance and was found to have frequent arrhythmias during and immediately after exercise. (*A*) A segment of ECG recorded during the immediate recovery period after exercise. The Televet software's RR interval detection has been performed at a threshold of 5%. Several premature complexes have been identified (*red lines, bold arrows*); however, several premature complexes were not identified (*thin arrows*) at this threshold. The instantaneous heart rate is automatically calculated by the software and is displayed in red at the bottom of the tracing. (*B*) The RR interval detection was manually checked, corrected, and then exported to create a graphical RR interval time series plot (RR tachogram) for further analysis. Here the consecutive RR intervals are displayed over time. The upper box displays the entire recording, whereas the lower box displays a section of the recording (*blue box*) in larger detail. This is the section of recording from peak exercise and early recovery. Several areas of abnormality are clearly identified. The red arrow indicates a period of several faster RR intervals in a row, followed by a pause (supraventricular tachycardia based on visualization of the ECG trace). The blue arrows indicate single shorter RR intervals and subsequent pauses (VPCs based on visualization the ECG trace). The purple double-ended arrow indicates a period in early recovery with many short RR intervals and subsequent pauses (a mix of APCs and VPCs based on visualization of the ECG trace). The green double-ended arrow indicates a period of ECG recording where the quality was reduced by motion artifacts, making the identification of any premature complexes more difficult. This example shows how an RR interval time series plot can help assess the number and temporal distribution of abnormal beats. (*C*) The exported RR interval time series is graphically represented as a Poincaré plot and a % RR deviation plot. In the Poincaré plot, every RR interval (x-axis) is plotted against the subsequent RR interval (RR+1, y-axis). In the % RR deviation plot, the % deviation of consecutive RR intervals (y-axis) is plotted against the respective RR interval (x-axis). Both graphs show that at lower heart rates, there is very little beat-to-beat variation, with most beats lying between +5% and −5% beat-to-beat variation. However, at the higher heart rates seen during peak exercise, there is increased variation (more than +30% to −30%; *thin black arrows*), which is the result of the premature complexes and subsequent pauses.

characterization of arrhythmias, and provide additional information on frequency and temporal distribution of rhythm events.[13] Such graphical and statistical analyses are part of the routine ambulatory and stress ECG evaluation in the author's institution. However, further details on how to perform and interpret heart rate variability analysis are beyond the scope of this article, and the reader is directed to other sources if further information is required.[13,15]

SUMMARY

Analyzing equine ECG recordings, making a diagnosis and assessment of any arrhythmias present is an important part of the workup of many equine cases. Accurate analysis requires a good-quality recording, free of as many artifacts as possible, with clear P-QRS-T complex morphology. For sustained arrhythmias, short-term recordings are sufficient to make the appropriate diagnosis before instigating treatment, whereas longer-term recordings are essential for arrhythmias that are paroxysmal, intermittent, or occurring infrequently. A stepwise, logical approach to ECG analysis will help the observer to recognize and correctly diagnose any arrhythmias that may be present.

REFERENCES

1. Verheyen T, Decloedt A, van der Vekens N, et al. Ventricular response during lungeing exercise in horses with lone atrial fibrillation. Equine Vet J 2013;45: 309–14.
2. Opie L. Channels, pumps and exchangers. In: The heart. physiology, from cell to circulation. 3rd edition. Philadelphia: Lippincott-Raven; 1998. p. 71–114.
3. Broux B, De Clercq D, Decloedt A, et al. Atrial premature depolarization-induced changes in QRS and T wave morphology on resting electrocardiograms in horses. J Vet Intern Med 2016;30:1253–9.
4. Hamlin RL, Smith CR. Categorization of common domestic mammals based upon their ventricular activation process. Ann N Y Acad Sci 1965;127:195–203.
5. Schwarzwald CC, Kedo M, Birkmann K, et al. Relationship of heart rate and electrocardiographic time intervals to body mass in horses and ponies. J Vet Cardiol 2012;14:343–50.
6. Lenoir A, Trachsel DS, Younes M, et al. Agreement between electrocardiogram and heart rate meter is low for the measurement of heart rate variability during exercise in young endurance horses. Front Vet Sci 2017;4:170.
7. Eggensperger BH, Schwarzwald CC. Influence of 2nd-degree AV blocks, ECG recording length, and recording time on heart rate variability analyses in horses. J Vet Cardiol 2017;19:160–74.
8. Zuber N, Zuber M, Schwarzwald CC. Assessment of systolic and diastolic function in clinically healthy horses using ambulatory acoustic cardiography. Equine Vet J 2018. https://doi.org/10.1111/evj.13014.
9. Goodwin JK. Holter monitoring and cardiac event recording. Vet Clin North Am Small Anim Pract 1998;28:1391–407, viii.
10. Pedro B, Dukes-McEwan J, Oyama MA, et al. Retrospective evaluation of the effect of heart rate on survival in dogs with atrial fibrillation. J Vet Intern Med 2018; 32:86–92.
11. Pevnick JM, Birkeland K, Zimmer R, et al. Wearable technology for cardiology: an update and framework for the future. Trends Cardiovasc Med 2018;28: 144–50.

12. Motskula PF, Linney C, Palermo V, et al. Prognostic value of 24-hour ambulatory ECG (Holter) monitoring in Boxer dogs. J Vet Intern Med 2013;27: 904–12.
13. Frick L, Schwarzwald CC, Mitchell KJ. The use of heart rate variability analysis to detect arrhythmias in horses undergoing a standard treadmill exercise test. J Vet Intern Med 2018. https://doi.org/10.1111/jvim.15358.
14. Flethoj M, Kanters JK, Pedersen PJ, et al. Appropriate threshold levels of cardiac beat-to-beat variation in semi-automatic analysis of equine ECG recordings. BMC Vet Res 2016;12:266.
15. Task Force of the European Society of Cardiology and the North American Society of Pacing and Electrophysiology. Heart rate variability: standards of measurement, physiological interpretation, and clinical use. Circulation 1996;93: 1043–65.

Cardiac Arrhythmias in Horses

Gunther van Loon, DVM, PhD

KEYWORDS

• Arrhythmia • Diagnosis • Treatment • Atrial fibrillation • Premature depolarizations

KEY POINTS

- Physiologic arrhythmias such as sinus arrhythmia and first- and second-degree atrioventricular block, are common and have no clinical importance as long as they disappear with stress or exercise.
- Atrial premature depolarizations often have no negative impact on performance but, especially in large horses, may predispose to atrial fibrillation.
- Atrial fibrillation is the most common, clinically important arrhythmia that can be treated by quinidine sulfate or transvenous electrical cardioversion.
- Ventricular premature depolarizations, especially when associated with structural heart disease, predispose to ventricular tachycardia or even ventricular fibrillation and may therefore carry a risk for horse and rider.
- Bradyarrhythmias caused by advanced second-degree atrioventricular block or third-degree atrioventricular block may require pacemaker implantation.

INTRODUCTION

Horses often present with cardiac arrhythmias. Although many are physiologic, and usually related to a high vagal tone, others are pathologic and may be a cause of poor performance or may even pose a certain risk to horse and rider. Inducing some kind of stress to the horse will usually abolish the vagally driven arrhythmias, which can be used as a simple trick to make a probable diagnosis of a vagal arrhythmia. For pathologic arrhythmias, one should investigate the presence of underlying cardiac disease (such as acquired valvular disease, congenital deformations, myocardial damage, pericarditis, and endocarditis) or noncardiac disease (such as electrolyte and acid–base disturbances, hypoxemia, endotoxemia, and toxic causes). The importance of an arrhythmia depends on its hemodynamic impact (blood pressure, cardiac output) and the risk of deterioration to a more dangerous rhythm. Ventricular arrhythmias generally carry a bigger risk to become unstable, although atrial fibrillation (AF) can also induce an abnormal ventricular response.

Disclosure Statement: No disclosures.

Department of Large Animal Internal Medicine, Faculty of Veterinary Medicine, Ghent University, Salisburylaan 133, Merelbeke 9820, Belgium

E-mail address: Gunther.vanLoon@UGent.be

There are many ways to subdivide types of arrhythmias. Regarding the duration of arrhythmias, the terms acute versus chronic, and sustained (continuous) versus paroxysmal (intermittently present) are used. Depending on the heart rate, bradyarrhythmias and tachyarrhythmias are described. Arrhythmias can be further categorized in those related to abnormal impulse formation (enhanced automaticity or triggered activity) or abnormal impulse conduction (block, reentry, accessory pathway). Because their impact is related to their site of origin, arrhythmias are very often described based on the anatomic location from which they originate followed by the type of arrhythmia: ventricular (originating in the ventricle) versus supraventricular (any origin except the ventricle) arrhythmias, whereby the latter group is further subdivided into sinus node, atrial, and atrioventricular (AV) node related (junctional) arrhythmias. Per site, the type of arrhythmia is added, such as premature depolarization, tachycardia, fibrillation, and block.

PHYSIOLOGIC ARRHYTHMIAS

Physiologic arrhythmias are mainly arrhythmias related to high vagal tone and usually originate from the sinus node or AV node. They may occur at rest or during a change from sympathetic toward parasympathetic predominance (eg, recovery from exercise). Sinus arrhythmia occurs as a cyclic (over several beats) increase and decrease in the sinus rate whereby the relation between P waves and QRS complexes and QRS morphology remains normal. Slight changes in P wave morphology might be associated with changes in autonomic tone. Sinus arrhythmia often presents after exercise and may start with a sudden PP prolongation, followed by progressive PP shortening after which the cycle repeats itself with a long PP interval (**Fig. 1**). Sinus (exit) block and sinus arrest show a PP interval that is equal to (sinus block) or longer than (sinus arrest) 2 normal PP intervals. PR intervals and QRS morphology remain normal but, owing to the high vagal tone, first- or second-degree AV block often coexist. Sinus bradycardia results from a slow firing rate of the sinus node with long PP intervals, but an otherwise normal ECG.

First-degree AV block shows a prolonged PQ interval that has been shown to depend on body weight.[1] In second-degree AV block, there is intermittent failure of the atrial impulse to be conducted through the AV node toward the ventricle, resulting in a P wave without a QRS complex (**Fig. 2**).

All the arrhythmias described are physiologic and do not require therapy as long as they disappear immediately with stress or exercise and show normal rate response during exercise. When more than 2 consecutive P waves are blocked, especially during stress or exercise, the term high-grade or advanced second-degree AV block is used.[2] These horses are considered less safe to ride and, in rare cases, the arrhythmia may deteriorate into third-degree AV block.

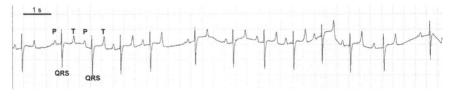

Fig. 1. Sinus arrhythmia after exercise. The electrocardiogram shows a normal P–QRS–T relation, but there is a waxing and waning in the heart rate owing to a progressive change in the PP interval over multiple beats. Slight changes in the P wave morphology occur because of the change in rate, with bifid P waves at slow rates and single P waves at higher rates.

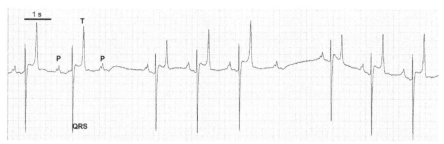

Fig. 2. Second-degree atrioventricular (AV) block is characterized by intermittent failure of the atrial electrical impulse to be conducted through the AV node to the ventricles. The electrocardiogram is characterized by regularly occurring P waves, of which some are not followed by a QRS-T complex. This usually results in a regular irregularity on auscultation, for example, a pause occurring after every third heartbeat.

ATRIAL ARRHYTHMIAS

Classically, atrial (and also ventricular) arrhythmias have been categorized into (isolated) atrial premature depolarizations (APD), atrial tachycardia (AT; >3 consecutive APDs), atrial flutter (AFL; a single macroreentry wave over a fixed pathway) and AF (multiple chaotic reentry waves). However, as in human medicine, the differentiation between AT and AFL cannot always be derived from a surface electrocardiogram (ECG), which leads to confusion. Therefore, the European Society of Cardiology and the North American Society of Pacing and Electrophysiology have suggested to use the general term AT for rapid atrial rhythms, different from AF, irrespective of the underlying mechanism.[3] This general term AT includes both focal AT and macroreentrant AT. Focal AT represents AT that originates from a small area (focus), of which the mechanism is enhanced automaticity, triggered activity, or microreentry. Macroreentrant AT includes different types of AFL and represents a reentry wave turning around a large central obstacle of anatomic or functional origin, usually depending on an area of slow conduction. Elsewhere in this article, the same terminology is used to avoid confusion.

Atrial Premature Depolarizations and Focal Atrial Tachycardia

APDs originate from an ectopic focus in the atrial myocardium. They occur too early (premature), resulting in an early P' wave that may or may not show altered morphology depending on the site of origin within the atrial myocardium (**Fig. 3**). Depending on the prematurity and the sympathetic tone, the P' wave will or will not be followed by a QRS complex. Most commonly, the premature depolarization resets the (timing of the) sinus node, resulting in a noncompensatory pause, which means that the RR interval encompassing the APD is less than 2 times the normal RR interval (see **Fig. 3**). On rare occasions, sinus node resetting does not occur, making the differentiation between supraventricular and ventricular depolarization more difficult, especially at high heart rates when P waves are difficult to identify. The QRS complex after the APD usually has normal morphology, but might show slight differences (mainly in amplitude; **Fig. 4**) especially when associated with short PP' coupling intervals.[4] Such shortly coupled QRS complexes are also associated with T waves that show opposite polarity to the QRS complex (see **Fig. 4**).

Underlying cardiac or systemic disease may be present and, on rare occasions, ultrasound examination may show atrial myocardial lesions. For Standardbred

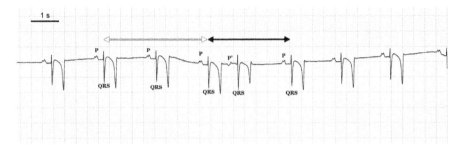

Fig. 3. Atrial premature depolarization characterized by a clearly different P′ morphology. It is followed by a noncompensatory pause, because the premature depolarization resets the sinus node. This means that the RR interval encompassing the premature depolarization (*black double arrow*) is shorter than twice the normal RR interval (*white double arrow*).

racehorses, advancing age has been identified as a risk factor for presence of APDs before racing.[5] Often, APDs disappear during exercise and are not associated with poor performance.[2] One should, however, be aware that such premature depolarizations, even more when they occur with very short coupling intervals, are a potential trigger for AT or AF.[2] This caveat does not apply to small sized animals such as ponies, which are not likely to develop AF because of their small atrial size.

When more than 3 APDs occur in a row, the arrhythmia is called AT. Although impulses may originate from different regions with slightly different P wave morphologies, very often they originate from the same small focus, which is called focal AT. The ECG shows rapid, regularly spaced P′ waves (**Fig. 5**), usually separated by an isoelectric line, although this feature might be absent at high rates. The QRS morphology is normal, but RR intervals are often irregular at rest because of intermittent AV conduction. With decreasing vagal tone and increasing sympathetic tone, more impulses will be conducted to the ventricles, resulting in a more regular 4:1 (4 atrial depolarizations for 1 ventricular depolarization), 3:1, 2:1, or 1:1 atrio-to-ventricular conduction, whereby the ventricular response rate is increased and very quickly equals the atrial rate (**Fig. 6**). The sinus rate may overdrive the focal AT rate during exercise. Focal AT is also a potential trigger for AF, especially at high AT rates. Horses with AF may

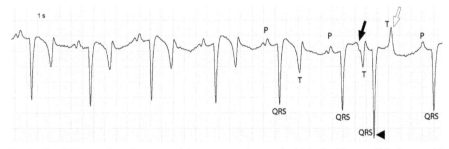

Fig. 4. The QRS complex after an atrial premature beat, of which the P′ wave (*black arrow*) is partially buried in the preceding T wave, shows a larger amplitude (*arrowhead*) and a T wave opposite to the QRS complex (*white arrow*), which is often the case for a short RR interval. Therefore, despite these slight changes in QRS and T morphology, the QRS complex is supraventricular in origin. This example also demonstrates that it is important to carefully inspect the trace to detect superimposed P′ waves.

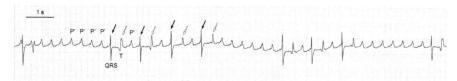

Fig. 5. In this horse with focal atrial tachycardia, the electrocardiogram is characterized by atrial depolarizations (P′) occurring at a rate of 167 bpm. Owing to superimposition of P′ waves, the R (*black arrows*) and T waves (*white arrows*) have altered and varying morphologies. The RR intervals are irregular because of irregular conduction through the atrioventricular node.

develop AT during a medical or electrical cardioversion attempt, which may suggest that these animals initially presented AT. Clinical signs of focal AT include reduced performance, depending on the workload. Compared with AF, the risk for R-on-T during exercise is probably lower.

APDs and focal AT are not life threatening. For APDs, one should consider whether antiarrhythmic therapy is indicated because many antiarrhythmic drugs may induce other (ventricular) arrhythmias. Antiarrhythmic drugs for APDs are mainly indicated in horses that were recently treated for AF to decrease the risk for (early) AF recurrence. Although little hard evidence is currently available, sotalol administered orally at 2 to 3 mg/kg twice a day might be beneficial to decrease the recurrence of AF. Because APDs are thought to originate from diseased or inflammatory myocardium, a resting period or low-level exercise period combined with steroid treatment is often attempted. It is, however, not uncommon for these arrhythmias to persist for a prolonged period of time.

The ECG criteria for differentiation between focal AT and macroreentry AT (AFL) are poorly defined in horses. Electroanatomic mapping, recently described in adult horses,[6] is the only way to differentiate between focal AT and AFL. Similar as for AF, cardioversion can be obtained by means of antiarrhythmic drugs (quinidine sulfate [QS]) or transvenous electrical cardioversion (TVEC), but, at least in human medicine, focal AT is more likely to show early recurrence. Using the mapping technique, successful radiofrequency ablation therapy for focal AT has recently been performed successfully in an adult horse (G. van Loon, personal data, 2018). Such therapy not only terminates the arrhythmia, it also minimizes risk for recurrence.

Macroreentry Atrial Tachycardia or Atrial Flutter

AFL represents a situation where a depolarization wave rotates in the atria over a stable pathway, around a large central obstacle of anatomic or functional origin, usually with an area of slow conduction. This self-perpetuating circling wave produces a

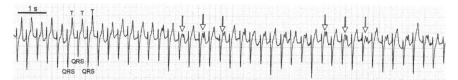

Fig. 6. An electrocardiogram recorded from the same horse as in **Fig. 5**. Already at slow trot, every atrial depolarization is conducted to the ventricles (QRS and T waves), resulting in a regular ventricular rate of 167 bpm. Close inspection allows to identify P′ waves (*white arrows*), but often these are hidden in QRS complex or T waves.

regular saw-tooth pattern of flutter waves on the surface ECG. The differentiation from focal AT (especially at higher rates) can probably not be made with confidence by a standard, bipolar surface ECG recording, and requires sophisticated mapping techniques. Similar as for focal AT, the blocking function of the AV node leads to irregular conduction to the ventricles at rest. However, slight decreases in vagal tone and increases in sympathetic tone allow more impulses to be conducted to the ventricles, resulting in 4:1, 3:1, 2:1, and 1:1 AV conduction,[7] with an increased ventricular rate response during mild exercise and ventricular rates similar (or only slightly higher) to the flutter rate during strenuous exercise. Auscultation may reveal periods of a regular ventricular rhythm. Partially owing to electrical remodeling, AFL is a potential trigger for AF. Clinical signs for AFL are similar as for focal AT. Treatment of AFL is performed similar as for AF, by means of drugs or TVEC (see the section on Atrial Fibrillation).

Atrial Fibrillation

AF is clinically the most important arrhythmia leading to poor performance in horses. The ECG typically shows replacement of P waves by fibrillation (f) waves, irregular RR intervals with normal (supraventricular) QRS morphology (**Fig. 7**). A genetic contribution to the arrhythmia has been identified in Standardbreds.[8] Age has been identified as a significant risk factor for postracing AF.[5] Mitral valve regurgitation, atrial dilation, and atrial electrophysiological characteristics also increase the risk for AF.[9-11] Paroxysmal AF is AF that self-terminates within 5 days and is occasionally seen in racehorses. Most commonly, however, the arrhythmia becomes almost immediately persistent. To sustain, AF needs a trigger to start the arrhythmia and a suitable substrate (the atrial myocardium) to sustain it. APDs, and especially AT or AFL, may induce AF. In human medicine, myocardial sleeves invading the pulmonary veins have been shown to be the most important source of ectopic activity, triggering AF. These myocardial sleeves have been demonstrated in horses and are also a likely source of AF.[12] The perpetuation of AF is facilitated by a large atrial size, structural lesions (fibrosis), and favorable electrophysiological parameters (short refractory period).[13] In small horses and especially ponies, the small atrial size makes it less likely for the arrhythmia to persist.[14,15] Once initiated, AF induces electrical and contractile atrial remodeling that, on their turn, favor perpetuation of the arrhythmia and make it more stable. Especially the shortening of the atrial refractory period allows more reentry wavelets to wander chaotically through the atria and stabilize the arrhythmia. Prompt treatment is therefore indicated, because chronic AF may become more difficult to treat. The high rate of atrial activation (usually around 350 bpm or more), irregular activation pattern, and atrial contractile remodeling result in atrial contractile dysfunction and reduced ventricular filling. Under high vagal tone, the high number

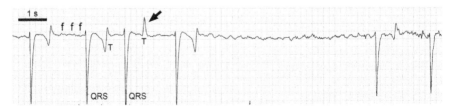

Fig. 7. Atrial fibrillation is characterized by absence of P waves, presence of fibrillation (*f*) waves, and irregular RR intervals with normal (supraventricular) QRS morphology. As always, for short RR intervals, the T wave has opposite polarity to the QRS complex (*arrow*). This pattern should not be misinterpreted as a ventricular ectopic beat.

of atrial impulses is blocked by the AV node. As such, at rest, horses without underlying disease show no clinical signs and have a normal ventricular rate (not rhythm). Stress or exercise decreases the blocking function of the AV node and will suddenly allow a (too) high number of impulses to be conducted to the ventricles. This process results in a disproportionate ventricular response rate at different levels of exercise,[16,17] which may have an impact on performance depending on the hemodynamic demand. More important, some horses present abnormal QRS morphology and R-on-T phenomenon during stress and/or exercise[16,17] (**Fig. 8**). These not only affect performance, but also pose a risk for collapse (**Fig. 9**) or rarely even fatal ventricular arrhythmia during exercise. Finally, some horses have been found to show very pronounced ventricular dyssynchrony at high heart rates, even in the absence of R-on-T phenomenon (G. van Loon, personal data, 2016), which again impairs overall cardiac function and may be a risk factor for collapse.

AF may exist in the absence of detectable underlying disease, called lone AF, or may be a consequence of predisposing cardiac disease, such as valvular dysfunction or congenital heart disease. Horses that gradually develop congestive heart failure will often, as a result of atrial dilation and myocardial fibrosis, suddenly develop AF. Owing to the combination of heart failure and AF, resting heart rates will suddenly increase and lead to overt clinical signs at rest. In horses with severe underlying disease, treatment should be symptomatic and aim to reduce heart rate, increase ventricular contractile function, and improve overall cardiac function (eg, digoxin, diuretics, angiotensin-converting enzyme inhibitors), rather than to try and treat the arrhythmia itself, because AF is very likely to recur quickly.

Most horses, however, present with no underlying heart disease, or only mild valvular regurgitation without cardiac dilation. Horses at rest or used for recreational work often present with no clinical signs, whereas racehorses or eventing horses usually show decreased performance. Depending on the competition level and individual differences, dressage and jumping horses present varying effects on performance. Horses with AF may show epistaxis during exercise.

Racehorses and competition horses, and horses showing high maximal heart rates (>220 bpm) during their regular exercise or horses that present abnormal QRS complexes or R-on-T phenomenon should be treated.[2] For asymptomatic horses, performing at low levels and not presenting an abnormal ventricular response, owners

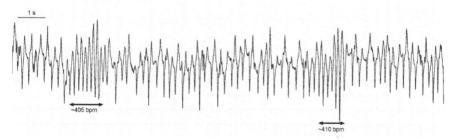

Fig. 8. Lunging exercise test in a Warmblood horse with atrial fibrillation (still being used for show jumping) without underlying heart disease results in 2 episodes with R-on-T phenomenon (*double arrows*), during which the mean heart rate is about 405 bpm. In between both episodes, the mean heart rate is about 270 bpm. The horse showed no clinical signs during this test. However, even in the absence of clinical signs, both R-on-T phenomenon and rapid ventricular response rates exceeding 220 bmp are considered risk factors for collapse or sudden death.

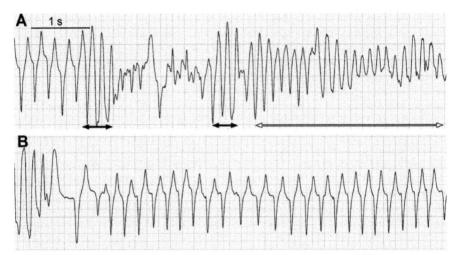

Fig. 9. During a lunging exercise test of a vaulting horse with lone atrial fibrillation, R-on-T (*black double arrows*) occurred after 2 minutes of slow canter (*A*). The rhythm subsequently deteriorated into Torsade de pointes (*white double arrow*). The horse immediately collapsed and remained recumbent for about 30 seconds. Surprisingly, the arrhythmia did not proceed into fatal ventricular fibrillation, but supraventricular tachycardia resumed (*B*) and the horse recovered. (*Courtesy of* Dr. P. A. S. Ivens, DVM, Diplomate, European College of Equine Internal Medicine, Milton Keynes, United Kingdom).

should be well-informed about the small potential risk for riding, treatment options, and recurrence rates. In case no treatment is performed, the AF horse should only be ridden by an adult, informed rider.

Treatment should not be performed in the first few days after AF has developed because the arrhythmia might still be paroxysmal. If so, thorough examinations should be performed, including blood biochemistry and electrolytes, fractional excretion of potassium, echocardiography, and ECG at rest and during exercise to identify predisposing factors. Once AF is sustained, treatment options include medical treatment and TVEC.

Medical treatment
Medical treatment is usually performed with QS via nasogastric tube, although the product becomes increasingly difficult to obtain in many countries. Treatment should be done in a quiet environment under continuous (telemetric) ECG surveillance. Emergency intravenous access should be available. For a maximum of 6 doses a day, 22 mg/kg QS in 3 to 4 L of water is administered via nasogastric tube (left in place) every 2 hours. Horses react very differently to the medication and adverse effects may start to occur after the second dose. In case of toxic adverse effects, the interval between doses is usually prolonged to intervals of 3 to 4 or more hours. Treatment at 6-hour intervals is supposed to maintain steady plasma concentrations, but large individual variations do occur. Unfortunately, most laboratories do not offer rapid measurement of QS plasma concentrations (therapeutic plasma concentrations at 2–5 µg/mL), so that titration of the drug must be done based on clinical signs and the ECG.

Noncardiac adverse effects include nasal edema, depression, colic, diarrhea, and laminitis. Cardiac adverse effects include hypotension, QRS and QT prolongation, supraventricular and ventricular tachycardia (VT), Torsade de pointes, collapse, and death. QRS prolongation should not exceed 25% because of the risk for dangerous ventricular arrhythmia. In case of toxicity, intravenous sodium bicarbonate administration (1 mEq/kg) lowers the free QS plasma concentrations. During QS treatment, some horses may suddenly develop very high ventricular response rates, which are often supraventricular in origin. QS aims at slowing down and organizing an AF rate, whereby gradually f waves change into "P" waves. AT often occurs as an intermediate rhythm before sinus rhythm restores. During such an AT episode, especially at heart rates between about 55 and 80 bpm, every other "P" wave may be perfectly hidden in a T wave with a 2:1 atrio-to-ventricular conduction. In such a situation, the P-QRS-T morphology with the hidden P wave may resemble sinus rhythm while, in fact, cardioversion has not yet occurred (**Fig. 10**). Termination of QS treatment at this stage will lead to a gradual decrease in QS plasma concentrations and a gradual increase in AF rate over the next 24 hours with return of the initial AF.

Intravenous amiodarone treatment is an alternative but generally less efficacious compared with QS.[18–20] The treatment is mainly useful for horses that quickly show QS toxic adverse effects or when oral QS treatment cannot be given. Flecainide administration has been used, but often causes dangerous ventricular arrhythmias in chronic as well as acute AF cases (**Fig. 11**), and sudden deaths have been reported repeatedly after intravenous and oral flecainide treatment.[21–26]

Transvenous electrical cardioversion

TVEC becomes more and more important because of its very high success rate (>95%), even in chronic AF cases and in horses that cannot be converted by QS.[27,28] In addition, it avoids the adverse effects and risks associated with antiarrhythmic drugs. The procedure, however, requires general anesthesia, specialized equipment, and expertise. A defibrillator is needed to deliver a biphasic (truncated exponential or rectilinear) shock through cardioversion catheters, which have a 12-cm-long shock electrode (coil) to achieve a large surface area for safe shock delivery. In addition, a temporary pacing catheter with 2 small electrodes on its tip connected to a temporary pacing unit is used for ventricular pacing in case of temporary complete AV block after shock delivery.[29]

The procedure starts in the standing horse. Alpha-2 adrenergic agonists can be administered as needed. Three introducer sheaths (8.5F or 9F) are placed in the right

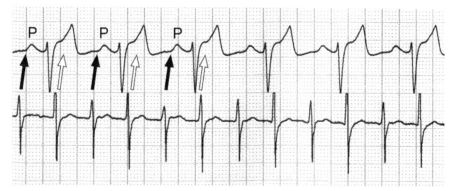

Fig. 10. In this horse with atrial fibrillation, after the fourth dose of quinidine, the surface electrocardiogram (*upper trace*) starts to look like sinus rhythm at 70 bpm with regular RR intervals. The intraatrial electrogram (*lower trace*), however, clearly shows an atrial rate of 140 bpm with atrial depolarizations that produce P' waves (*black arrow*). Every other atrial depolarization produces a P' wave that is buried in a T wave (*white arrow*), mimicking sinus rhythm.

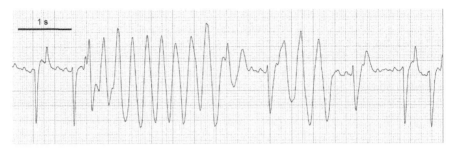

Fig. 11. Wide QRS tachycardia during intravenous flecainide treatment (2 mg/kg) in a horse with chronic lone atrial fibrillation. The horse did not convert to sinus rhythm.

caudal jugular vein. Before insertion, a sterile covering is placed over the catheter so that it remains sterile during the whole TVEC procedure. The first cardioversion catheter is inserted and maneuvered through the right atrium (RA) and right ventricle into the pulmonary artery (PA). Catheter placement is guided by ultrasound imaging from a right parasternal view, ensuring that the tip of the catheter enters the left PA. Subsequently, catheter position is double checked from a left parasternal view in which the catheter tip can be seen to curve around the fourth pulmonary vein ostium. Care must be taken to prevent retroflexion of the catheter tip because this positioning is likely to result in treatment failure.

TVEC catheters with lumen (Gaeltec Devices, Isle of Sky, UK) allow to register blood pressures from the catheter tip, using a fluid-filled line and pressure transducer. The characteristic RA, right ventricle, and PA pressure trace can be identified as the catheter is maneuvered through the heart toward the PA and serves as an additional confirmation of the position of the catheter tip.[27] It does not allow to distinguish catheter position within the PA. Thoracic radiography can also be used to confirm catheter position and the absence of tip retroflexion. It can be done in the standing horse, but is most informative during anesthesia because catheter movement might occur during the induction process. In the standing horse, the PA TVEC catheter is advanced deep into the left PA so that it does not displace during the induction of anesthesia. Total catheter insertion from the caudal jugular vein is usually around 145 cm in an adult 600-kg horse. The same procedure applies to the RA TVEC catheter, which is, at this stage, inserted into the right ventricular apex so that it remains in the right ventricle during the induction of anesthesia.

Finally, the temporary pacing catheter is inserted into the right ventricular apex. Placement of this catheter is guided by ultrasound imaging and facilitated by recording the intracardiac electrogram, which shows no deflections in the jugular vein, rapid deflections in the RA (usually ≥350 per minute), and deflections simultaneous with QRS and T when located in the right ventricle.

Subsequently, general anesthesia is induced. After administration of an alpha-2 adrenergic agonist, anesthesia is induced using ketamine (2.2 mg/kg) and midazolam (0.06 mg/kg) intravenously, and maintained with isoflurane in oxygen. This author prefers to use a sling during induction to get a gentle, controlled left lateral recumbency. The PA TVEC catheter is now slightly withdrawn so that the shock coil is located in the proximal left PA (total catheter insertion of about 135 cm). Next, the RA shock catheter is withdrawn from the right ventricle until the tip of the catheter is located exactly between the closing tricuspid valve so that the shock coil is in the RA. The position of the right ventricular pacing catheter is now optimized to achieve successful right ventricular pacing.

A surface ECG and both cardioversion catheters are connected to the biphasic defibrillator, which is set at synchronous mode. In this mode, the QRS complex is automatically detected and the defibrillator will deliver the shock synchronous with the QRS complex (**Fig. 12**). It is of utmost importance to ensure that only the QRS complex is detected. In case the large equine T wave is erroneously interpreted as QRS, surface electrode positions must be adapted to prevent T wave detection. Shock delivery on a T wave is very likely to result in terminal ventricular fibrillation. Subsequently, shock delivery is started and energy is progressively increased in case cardioversion is not achieved. The author starts at 150 J and increases the energy in steps of 50 J up to 360 J. Failure to restore sinus rhythm might be due to a suboptimal catheter position and might require catheter repositioning. Administration of 5 mg/kg body weight amiodarone intravenously over 30 minutes might lower the threshold for electrical cardioversion when given before shock delivery. One should carefully check the arterial blood pressure during infusion, because amiodarone occasionally leads to hypotension.

After restoration of sinus rhythm, this author prefers to allow 10 minutes of sinus rhythm before the horse goes to recovery to assess the burden of atrial ectopy.

Aftercare

AF induces electrical and contractile remodeling. Reverse remodeling is probably complete within 1 or a few days if the horse presented acute AF (eg, 1-week duration),[13] but will take longer (probably 4–6 weeks) after long-lasting AF (eg. >2 months duration).[14,30] Incomplete recovery could theoretically lead to an increased recurrence risk, but this supposition remains unproven. Follow-up ultrasound examinations are useful to monitor atrial contractile function in the days and weeks after cardioversion.[9,11] Twenty-four-hour ECG recordings allow to assess the presence of APDs or even runs of AT, which are possible triggers for AF recurrence. Preferentially, assessment of contractile function and atrial ectopy should not be done in the first 24 hours after anesthesia. In patients with a high burden of ectopy, oral sotalol treatment (2–3 mg/kg twice a day) is thought to be beneficial to decrease this recurrence risk, but no studies have been performed so far. After the resting period, horses are gradually brought back into normal training and are expected to return to their previous athletic ability. Because recurrence within 1 year is encountered in about 35% of successfully treated cases of lone AF,[9] long-term follow-up of heart rhythm is indicated. ECG recording is ideal. Some owners perform palpation of the apex beat or auscultation to check the regularity of the rhythm. Monitoring heart rate variability parameters, such as the root mean square of the successive differences, recorded at rest and walk, is also useful to identify recurrence of AF.[31,32] Finally, assessing ventricular response rate by a heart rate monitor during a self-defined exercise test is also useful because recurrence of AF will result in markedly increased ventricular rates during a similar type of exercise.

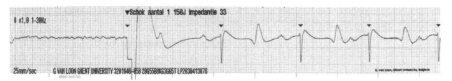

Fig. 12. Transvenous electrical cardioversion of atrial fibrillation. Shock delivery at 150 J synchronized on the R wave terminates atrial fibrillation with immediate restoration of normal sinus rhythm. Correct R wave detection by the defibrillator is indicated by the *small black triangles*.

VENTRICULAR ARRHYTHMIAS

Ventricular arrhythmias originate from the ventricular myocardium. Underlying causes include myocardial damage, systemic disease, hypoxia, acid–base or electrolyte disturbance, drugs, and toxicity. Because the impulse is conducted differently through the ventricles and depends on (slower) cell-to-cell conduction, the resulting QRS complex will have a different morphology and longer duration, depending on the site of origin. Some ectopic impulses probably involve partial conduction over the His bundle and are only slightly different from normal QRS morphology, making them difficult to distinguish from a junctional (nodal) rhythm. Multiple lead ECG recording is recommended because some abnormal ventricular depolarizations are much easier to identify on specific leads (**Fig. 13**).

Ventricular premature depolarizations (VPDs) are isolated beats that occur too early. Most commonly, VPDs are not retrogradely conducted to the atria, do not affect underlying sinoatrial nodal activity, and therefore are followed by a compensatory pause, which means that the RR interval enclosing the VPD equals twice the normal RR interval (**Fig. 14**). Occasionally, a VPD is interpolated, meaning that it occurs in between 2 normal beats, without changing the underlying rhythm. When 3 or more VPDs occur in a row, the rhythm is called VT, which can be paroxysmal (when it terminates spontaneously) or sustained. Monomorphic or uniform VPDs or VT likely originate from 1 focus (**Fig. 15**), whereas polymorphic or multiform rhythms suggest multiple foci or reentry mechanisms and therefore more widespread myocardial disease (**Fig. 16**).

Occasional single VPDs in the absence of structural heart disease are considered to be normal and are commonly found at the end of or during recovery of strenuous (racing) exercise.[2,33,34] Accelerated idioventricular rhythm (also called slow VT) occurs as a slow, monomorphic ectopic rhythm, only slightly faster than sinus rhythm, usually at rates around 50 to 80 bpm (**Fig. 17**). It is generally believed to be benign if no underlying systemic or cardiac disease is present, and when it disappears at increased heart

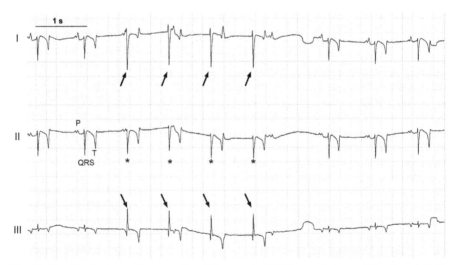

Fig. 13. On this electrocardiogram, the difference in QRS-T morphology of the 4 ventricular ectopic beats is small on lead II (*asterisks*), but much more pronounced on the other leads (*arrows*), indicating that multilead recordings can be helpful in identifying and characterizing arrhythmias.

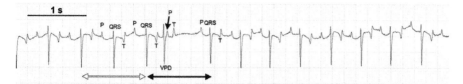

Fig. 14. A ventricular premature depolarization (VPD) with a slightly different QRS morphology is followed by a compensatory pause, which means that the RR interval encompassing the VPD (*black double arrow*) equals twice the normal RR interval (*white double arrow*). Note the normal P wave occurring at a normal PP interval, buried in the ST segment of the VPD, indicating that the VPD was not retrogradely conducted to the atria and did not reset the sinus node.

rates. VPDs represent a potential risk for deterioration into ventricular tachyarrhythmias such as VT, torsade de pointes, or ventricular fibrillation, which may be associated with sudden collapse or even sudden cardiac death. The exact risk is unknown, but recommendations should be biased toward safety for horse and rider. A high number of VPDs, different morphologies, short coupling intervals, and the presence of paroxysmal VT are all considered factors that increase the risk. In particular, the coexistence of myocardial or structural disease (ultrasonographically visible myocardial lesions such as scar tissue, myocardial disease, aortocardiac fistula) or valvular regurgitation (especially aortic regurgitation) with ventricular dilation are considered important risk factors.

Resting ECG, possibly a 24-hour ECG recording, echocardiography, and measurement of the plasma cardiac troponin I or cardiac troponin T concentration should be performed. Except for horses with severe arrhythmia or underlying disease, an exercise test must be performed because exercise may exacerbate or suppress the ectopic rhythm. Horses with occasional VPDs without concomitant underlying disease can be ridden with caution by an adult informed rider.[2] Horses with sustained VT should be rested and treated and may have a good long-term prognosis after successful treatment. If moderate or severe structural heart disease is present, the risk for recurrence of the arrhythmia may be increased.

The treatment of ventricular arrhythmias should target underlying cardiac or systemic causes whenever possible. The treatment of ventricular arrhythmias is mainly based on rest, corticosteroids, and antiarrhythmic drugs. Many antiarrhythmic drugs may have proarrhythmic effects and they are only administered in symptomatic or

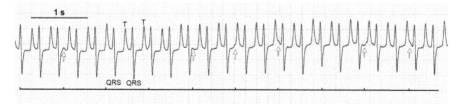

Fig. 15. Sustained monomorphic ventricular tachycardia at a rate of 180 bpm shows wide QRS complexes with an abnormal but similar morphology. A careful analysis of the trace allows to identify partially hidden P waves (*white arrows*) and to determine the underlying regular atrial rate (indicated by the *black dots on the horizontal line* at the bottom), which is 79 bpm. P waves are not associated with the QRS complexes, a phenomenon termed atrioventricular dissociation.

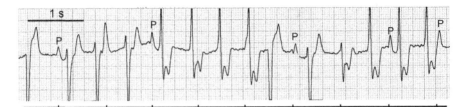

Fig. 16. Polymorphic ventricular tachycardia occurred in this horse after ingestion of *Nerium oleander*. All QRS complexes are abnormal: they are widened, show different morphologies, and have no relation with P waves (P). The underlying regular atrial rhythm is indicated by the *black marks on the horizontal line* at the bottom.

clinical cases or when rapid VT is present.[35] Occasional VPDs may respond to a rest period and a corticosteroid treatment (eg, dexamethasone 0.05–0.2 mg/kg intravenously). In horses with sustained VT, exercise and stress should be avoided and prompt antiarrhythmic treatment is needed.

Lidocaine, a class IB sodium channel blocker, is most commonly used. Treatment is started with a 0.25 to 0.5 mg/kg slow intravenous injection every 5 minutes up to 1.5 mg/kg followed by a constant rate infusion of 0.05 mg/kg/min.[36] The horse's behavior should be carefully watched for adverse effects, such as altered visual function, eye blinking, anxiety, and collapse.[37] These clinical signs might be treated with diazepam, but usually resolve quickly when lidocaine administration is terminated. Phenytoin has similar effects and has been recommended in case of digoxin toxicity. Treatment dose is usually 20 mg/kg orally twice a day for 2 days followed by 10 to 15 mg/kg twice a day. It is recommended to monitor plasma drug concentrations (target 5–10 µg/mL). Magnesium sulfate (2–6 mg/kg/min intravenously, up to a total dose of about 55–100 mg/kg) might be useful, especially to treat or avoid Torsade de pointes. Other drugs to treat ventricular arrhythmias include procainamide, quinidine gluconate, amiodarone, sotalol, propranolol, and propafenone.

After successful treatment of VT, before resuming normal work, at least 4 weeks of normal sinus rhythm should be present followed by a 24-hour ECG recording and an exercise ECG, and another exercise ECG when the horse is back into normal training.[2] In horses treated for complex ventricular arrhythmias with presence of structural heart disease, there is an increased risk for recurrence and ongoing concern about safety. These horses should regularly be followed up and only be used by an informed adult rider.[2]

Accessory Pathway

Accessory pathways resulting in ventricular preexcitation are rare in horses. Under normal circumstances, the AV node is the only electrical connection between the atria and the ventricles. An accessory pathway represents an additional electrical

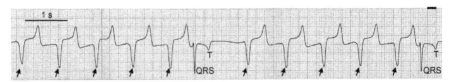

Fig. 17. Accelerated idioventricular rhythm or slow ventricular tachycardia (*black arrows*) at a rate of 68 bpm. Two normal QRS complexes and T waves are present, of which the P wave is buried in the preceding T wave.

conduction pathway. As such, an atrial depolarization will be able to quickly initiate ventricular depolarization, visible on the ECG as a shortened PR interval and a different QRS morphology and duration. Depending on the location of the pathway, a delta wave at the onset of the QRS complex may be present. Little is currently known about the effect on performance or risk for riding. The condition may lead to an electrical circus movement over the pathway and AV node, resulting in supraventricular tachycardia. In the case of AF, conduction toward the ventricles may be increased and may involve a risk.[38]

CONDUCTION DISTURBANCES

First- and second-degree AV block are usually vagal tone mediated and therefore physiologic, as long as they disappear with decreased vagal and increased sympathetic tone (stress or exercise). Advanced second-degree AV block indicates that 3 or more successive P waves are blocked at the AV node, which is considered abnormal. Often, an inappropriate heart rate response during exercise is present, leading to exercise intolerance. The condition may further evolve to third-degree AV block, in which complete AV dissociation is present as P waves are no longer conducted to the ventricles. Ventricular rate now depends on its own lower, intrinsic rhythm. This ventricular escape rhythm may be regular and monomorphic or irregular or polymorphic, with ventricular rates usually between 10 and 35 bpm. The escape QRS morphology and duration depend on the site of origin. Slow ventricular rates cause hypotension, which typically induces a reflex increase in atrial rate (often 45–90 bpm) with many P waves for only a few QRS complexes (**Fig. 18**). These ECG characteristics must be differentiated from (slow) focal AT, for which the QRS complexes have a consistent relation with the preceding P′ wave. Stress or exercise usually has little impact on the ventricular rate in horses with third-degree AV block. Horses are typically exercise intolerant and usually present numerous episodes of collapse when ventricular escape rhythm is insufficient to maintain minimal blood pressure. Horses may present low head carriage, which helps to support a minimal cerebral blood flow. Forcing them to lift the head may induce collapse. Presyncopal signs include increased respiratory effort and flaring the nostrils. Horses that collapse usually fall aside and to the back and may remain recumbent for seconds to minutes.

Third-degree AV block may be caused by primary AV node disease, intoxication, uroperitoneum, or other electrolyte disturbances. Emergency treatment may be attempted by administration of vagolytic drugs such as atropine (0.01–0.02 mg/kg intravenously) or glycopyrolate (0.005–0.01 mg/kg intravenously), although these are rarely effective. In the absence of infection, corticosteroids (dexamethasone 0.05–0.2 mg/kg intravenously) should be administered because it may be effective to

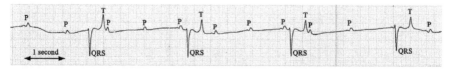

Fig. 18. Third-degree atrioventricular block resulted in atrioventricular dissociation and a slow (junctional) escape rhythm at a rate of 25 bpm. The atrial rate is increased to about 60 bpm, probably as a reflex to systemic hypotension. Note that the term atrioventricular dissociation is a purely descriptive term that simply describes that the P waves are not associated with the QRS complex. This can also be caused by ventricular tachycardia (as shown in **Fig. 15**).

reduce inflammation around the AV node and improve conduction. Very often, however, pacemaker implantation is the only definitive treatment. A standardized approach for implantation via the cephalic vein, using bipolar screw-in electrodes, has been described.[39] The pacemaker type determines the complexity of the implantation procedure. A single chamber ventricular pacemaker only needs 1 ventricular screw-in lead and aims to keep ventricular rate above a minimal value (VVI model). Including a rate adaptive functionality (VVIR model) will enable to increase ventricular rate during physical activity. The optimal system is a dual chamber on-demand pacemaker (DDI model) that delivers a ventricular stimulus through a ventricular lead, for every atrial depolarization detected via an atrial lead. This results in a physiologic change in heart rate as atrial depolarizations are transferred to the ventricles by the pacemaker.

REFERENCES

1. Schwarzwald CC, Kedo M, Birkmann K, et al. Relationship of heart rate and electrocardiographic time intervals to body mass in horses and ponies. J Vet Cardiol 2012;14(2):343–50.
2. Reef VB, Bonagura J, Buhl R, et al. Recommendations for management of equine athletes with cardiovascular abnormalities. J Vet Intern Med 2014;28(3):749–61.
3. Saoudi N, Cosio F, Waldo A, et al. Classification of atrial flutter and regular atrial tachycardia according to electrophysiologic mechanism and anatomic bases: a statement from a joint expert group from the working group of arrhythmias of the European Society of Cardiology and the North American Society of Pacing and Electrophysiology. J Cardiovasc Electrophysiol 2001;12(7):852–66.
4. Broux B, De Clercq D, Decloedt A, et al. Atrial premature depolarization-induced changes in QRS and T wave morphology on resting electrocardiograms in horses. J Vet Intern Med 2016;30(4):1253–9.
5. Slack J, Boston RC, Soma LR, et al. Occurrence of cardiac arrhythmias in Standardbred racehorses. Equine Vet J 2015;47(4):398–404.
6. van Loon G, Boussy T, Vera L, et al. Successful high resolution 3D electroanatomical cardiac mapping in adult horses in sinus rhythm. Paper presented at: ACVIM Forum. Washington, June 8–9, 2017.
7. Christmann U, van Loon G. ECG of the month. J Am Vet Med Assoc 2013;242(2): 165–7.
8. Kraus M, Physick-Sheard PW, Brito LF, et al. Estimates of heritability of atrial fibrillation in the Standardbred racehorse. Equine Vet J 2017;49(6):718–22.
9. Decloedt A, Schwarzwald CC, De Clercq D, et al. Risk factors for recurrence of atrial fibrillation in horses after cardioversion to sinus rhythm. J Vet Intern Med 2015;29(3):946–53.
10. De Clercq D, Decloedt A, Sys SU, et al. Atrial fibrillation cycle length and atrial size in horses with and without recurrence of atrial fibrillation after electrical cardioversion. J Vet Intern Med 2014;28(2):624–9.
11. Decloedt A, Verheyen T, Van der Vekens N, et al. Long-term follow-up of atrial function after cardioversion of atrial fibrillation in horses. Vet J 2013;197(3):583–8.
12. Vandecasteele T, Van den Broeck W, Tay H, et al. 3D reconstruction of the porcine and equine pulmonary veins, supplemented with the identification of telocytes in the horse. Anat Histol Embryol 2018;47(2):145–52.
13. De Clercq D, van Loon G, Tavernier R, et al. Atrial and ventricular electrical and contractile remodeling and reverse remodeling owing to short-term pacing-induced atrial fibrillation in horses. J Vet Intern Med 2008;22(6):1353–9.

14. van Loon G, Tavernier R, Fonteyne W, et al. Pacing induced long-term atrial fibrillation in horses. Europace 2001;2(Suppl):A84.

15. van Loon G, Tavernier R, Duytschaever M, et al. Pacing induced sustained atrial fibrillation in a pony. Can J Vet Res 2000;64(4):254–8.

16. Verheyen T, Decloedt A, Van der Vekens N, et al. Ventricular response during lunging exercise in horses with lone atrial fibrillation. Equine Vet J 2013;45(3): 309–14.

17. Buhl R, Carstensen H, Hesselkilde EZ, et al. Effect of induced chronic atrial fibrillation on exercise performance in Standardbred trotters. J Vet Intern Med 2018; 32(4):1410–9.

18. De Clercq D, Van Loon G, Baert K, et al. Effects of an adapted intravenous amiodarone treatment protocol in horses with atrial fibrillation. Equine Vet J 2007;39(4): 344–9.

19. De Clercq D, van Loon G, Baert K, et al. Intravenous amiodarone treatment in horses with chronic atrial fibrillation. Vet J 2006;172(1):129–34.

20. De Clercq D, Baert K, Croubels S, et al. Evaluation of the pharmacokinetics and bioavailability of intravenously and orally administered amiodarone in horses. Am J Vet Res 2006;67(3):448–54.

21. Carstensen H, Hesselkilde EZ, Fenner M, et al. Time-dependent antiarrhythmic effects of flecainide on induced atrial fibrillation in horses. J Vet Intern Med 2018;32(5):1708–17.

22. Hesselkilde EZ, Carstensen H, Haugaard MM, et al. Effect of flecainide on atrial fibrillatory rate in a large animal model with induced atrial fibrillation. BMC Cardiovasc Disord 2017;17(1):289.

23. Haugaard MM, Pehrson S, Carstensen H, et al. Antiarrhythmic and electrophysiologic effects of flecainide on acutely induced atrial fibrillation in healthy horses. J Vet Intern Med 2015;29(1):339–47.

24. Dembek KA, Hurcombe SD, Schober KE, et al. Sudden death of a horse with supraventricular tachycardia following oral administration of flecainide acetate. J Vet Emerg Crit Care (San Antonio) 2014;24(6):759–63.

25. Robinson SJ, Feary DJ. Sudden death following oral administration of flecainide to horses with naturally occurring atrial fibrillation. Australian Equine Veterinarian 2008;27(3):49–51.

26. van Loon G, Blissitt KJ, Keen JA, et al. Use of intravenous flecainide in horses with naturally-occurring atrial fibrillation. Equine Vet J 2004;36(7):609–14.

27. McGurrin MKJ, Physick-Sheard PW, Kenney DG. Transvenous electrical cardioversion of equine atrial fibrillation: patient factors and clinical results in 72 treatment episodes. J Vet Intern Med 2008;22(3):609–15.

28. De Clercq D, van Loon G, Schauvliege S, et al. Transvenous electrical cardioversion of atrial fibrillation in six horses using custom made cardioversion catheters. Vet J 2008;177(2):198–204.

29. van Loon G, De Clercq D, Tavernier R, et al. Transient complete atrioventricular block following transvenous electrical cardioversion of atrial fibrillation in a horse. Vet J 2005;170(1):124–7.

30. De Clercq D. Pathophysiology and treatment of atrial fibrillation in horses [PhD]. Merelbeke: large animal internal medicine. Belgium (Europe): Ghent University; 2008.

31. Broux B, De Clercq D, Decloedt A, et al. Heart rate variability parameters in horses distinguish atrial fibrillation from sinus rhythm before and after successful electrical cardioversion. Equine Vet J 2017;49(6):723–8.

32. Broux B, De Clercq D, Vera L, et al. Can heart rate variability parameters derived by a heart rate monitor differentiate between atrial fibrillation and sinus rhythm? BMC Vet Res 2018;14(1):320.
33. de Solis CN, Green CM, Sides RH, et al. Arrhythmias in thoroughbreds during and after treadmill and racetrack exercise. J Equine Vet Sci 2016;42:19–24.
34. Ryan N, Marr CM, McGladdery AJ. Survey of cardiac arrhythmias during sub-maximal and maximal exercise in thoroughbred racehorses. Equine Vet J 2005; 37(3):265–8.
35. Sleeper MM. Equine cardiovascular therapeutics. Vet Clin North Am Equine Pract 2017;33(1):163–+.
36. Mitchell KJ. Practical considerations for diagnosis and treatment of ventricular tachycardia in horses. Equine Vet Educ 2017;29(12):670–6.
37. Meyer GA, Lin HC, Hanson RR, et al. Effects of intravenous lidocaine overdose on cardiac electrical activity and blood pressure in the horse. Equine Vet J 2001; 33(5):434–7.
38. Jesty SA, Kraus MS, Johnson AL, et al. An accessory bypass tract masked by the presence of atrial fibrillation in a horse. J Vet Cardiol 2011;13(1):79–83.
39. van Loon G, Fonteyne W, Rottiers H, et al. Dual-chamber pacemaker implantation via the cephalic vein in healthy equids. J Vet Intern Med 2001;15(6):564–71.

Equine Congenital Heart Disease

Brian A. Scansen, DVM, MS

KEYWORDS

- Horse • Cardiac • Ventricular septal defect • Morphologic approach
- Sequential segmental anatomy • Veterinary

KEY POINTS

- Congenital heart disease appears rare in horses, although many forms have been recognized and reported in this species.
- Ventricular septal defect is frequently reported as the most common form of congenital heart disease in the horse and diagnostic findings may guide prognosis.
- The morphologic method and a sequential segmental approach are useful to methodically analyze the congenitally malformed heart.

CARDIAC DEVELOPMENT, FETAL CIRCULATION, AND CONVERSION TO EXTRAUTERINE LIFE

Congenital heart defects represent the eventual outcome of an error or errors during cardiac development. An understanding of congenital heart disease (CHD), therefore, requires an appreciation of normal cardiac development and anatomy, the normal fetal circulation, and the processes by which the fetal circulation matures to the postnatal circulation and extrauterine life.

A detailed description of cardiac development is outlined elsewhere but briefly involves a complex process during which mesodermal cells coalesce to form a primary heart tube that initiates peristaltic activity and forms the first functional organ of the fetus.[1,2] The primary heart tube will then differentiate into primitive cardiac chambers that undergo a looping and septation process to generate a four-chambered, four-valved mammalian heart. Cardiac looping establishes right-left laterality, and errors in this process lead to defects considered within the heterotaxy complexes (situs inversus, atrial isomerism, etc.) whereby a morphologic right atrium may lie on the animal's left side and vice versa.[1] Septation refers to the division of the cardiac chambers. Atrial septation involves fluctuating extension and subsequent fenestration of

Disclosure Statement: No relevant disclosures.
Department of Clinical Sciences, Colorado State University, Campus Delivery 1678, Fort Collins, CO 80523, USA
E-mail address: Brian.Scansen@colostate.edu

Vet Clin Equine 35 (2019) 103–117
https://doi.org/10.1016/j.cveq.2018.11.001
0749-0739/19/© 2018 Elsevier Inc. All rights reserved.
vetequine.theclinics.com

membranes between the right and left atria. The septum primum, or valve of the oval foramen, will remain open in the fetal circulation to permit right to left shunting of oxygen-rich placental blood to the left heart and systemic circulation before closing after birth. Defects in atrial septation lead to the various atrial level shunts including atrial septal defects (ASD) and anomalous pulmonary venous connections. Ventricular septation leads to separation of the subaortic (left) from the subpulmonary (right) ventricles and occurs at 2 levels, the ventricular inflow and the ventricular outflow.[1] The interventricular septum grows up from the ventricular apex to initiate this separation, but definitive closure occurs from the central portion of the developing heart associated with maturation of the endocardial cushions. Deficiencies in the endocardial cushions lead to atrioventricular septal defects (AVSD), whereas errors during ventricular septation lead to ventricular septal defects (VSD). Incomplete or altered looping of the primary heart tube may also affect proper septation of the ventricles. Errors during septation of the outflow tracts have often been termed conotruncal defects in veterinary medicine. However, the term conotruncal has no broadly accepted definition that is scientifically accurate and the term might logically be applied to abnormalities of the semilunar valves that lie between the conus and the arterial trunks.[3] As such, errors during division of the outflow tracts and great vessels are more precisely described as proximal (ventricular outlets), intermediate (arterial roots and valves), and distal (arterial trunks) lesions.[3]

The fetal circulation is not constant but evolves during embryogenesis from the linear peristaltic activity of the primary heart tube to a circulation that relies on 2 important communications (or shunts)—the arterial duct and the oval foramen. Note that there is a trend toward anglicizing many terms in CHD nomenclature from the older latinized form; as such, patent ductus arteriosus (PDA) becomes the patent arterial duct and patent foramen ovale (PFO) becomes the patent oval foramen.[4] Oxygen-rich blood is generated in the placental circulation from the maternal blood supply, returns to the fetal heart via the umbilical vein and venous duct, and then crosses the interatrial septum via the oval foramen. The oval foramen acts as a diverter valve to preferentially send this oxygen-rich blood to the left heart. Systemic venous return from the fetus, containing desaturated hemoglobin, is directed preferentially across the tricuspid valve orifice to the right ventricle (RV) and pulmonary trunk. Because the lungs are not expanded in the fetus and pulmonary vascular resistance is high, the open arterial duct allows deoxygenated blood from the pulmonary trunk to enter the descending aorta where it can return to the placenta via the umbilical artery.

Conversion of fetal circulation to extrauterine life involves closure of the shunts that were necessary to bring oxygenated blood to the left atrium (venous duct and oval foramen) and deoxygenated blood to the descending aorta (arterial duct). Typically, these close in the first 1 to 2 weeks of life, but persistent patency of the arterial duct or oval foramen leads to postnatal complications as discussed later.

THE MORPHOLOGIC METHOD AND A SEQUENTIAL SEGMENTAL APPROACH TO CONGENITAL HEART DISEASE

Acquired heart disease presents in variable form (myocardial, valvar, electrical), but in all cases these are deviations from what was initially a structurally normal heart. However, CHD exists as a much broader spectrum because errors in development can occur in almost innumerable form and complexity. To deal with this complexity, 2 approaches to analyzing and categorizing CHD have developed in the field of pediatric cardiology. The morphologic method assesses the heart as a group of individual segments or building blocks (atria, ventricles, great arteries) that have clearly defined and identifying features.[5–8] The sequential segmental approach to CHD analyzes each segment and connection according to blood flow in a sequential manner (venoatrial connection, atrial morphology, atrioventricular connection, ventricular morphology, ventriculoarterial connection, arterial anomalies). Analyzing each anatomic chamber independently avoids associating adjacent connections as hallmarks of that segment. For example, although the left atrium is expected to receive the pulmonary veins, the chamber is not defined by this arrangement because the pulmonary veins can have an anomalous connection to the right atrium or systemic vasculature. The atria are primarily defined by the extension of pectinate muscles, with the morphologic left atrium characterized by pectinate muscles confined to the appendage, whereas the morphologic right atrium has pectinate muscles that extend around the orifice of the atrioventricular valve.[8] The RV is primarily defined by the coarse trabeculations that line the apex and a prominent moderator band, whereas the morphologic left ventricle has a smooth septal surface and finer, criss-crossing apical trabeculations.[7] The morphologic characteristics of the great vessels are less preserved but the coronary vasculature derives from the aorta, whereas bifurcation after a short main segment is characteristic of the pulmonary trunk. The morphologic method and sequential segmental approaches are complementary to one another and were initially used at autopsy to characterize complex CHD but are now used extensively in pediatric cardiology to classify patients with CHD by imaging (echocardiography, computed tomography, MRI).

Despite reports describing the sequential segmental approach in the veterinary literature,[9–13] widespread adoption of sequential segmental analysis has not occurred. Singular defects (isolated ventricular septal defect, isolated valvar dysplasia, etc) may not require a systematic approach, but this approach is particularly useful for thorough understanding of complex malformations and to assure secondary lesions are not missed. Complex lesions are occasionally encountered in equine cardiology; furthermore, this approach provides a useful framework for CHD classification and understanding. The utility of the morphologic method and a sequential segmental approach to characterizing CHD in the horse was nicely demonstrated in a recent report of complex CHD in a foal.[14]

CAUSE AND PREVALENCE OF CONGENITAL HEART DISEASE IN THE HORSE

The precise cause of CHD in nearly all veterinary species is not known. In roughly 20% of human cases, chromosomal abnormalities, single gene mutations, or teratogens (drug use, toxin exposure, or infectious diseases during pregnancy) are implicated in the genesis of CHD; however, most of the human CHD cases have no identifiable cause.[15] In horses, familial risk for CHD seems to be present with a disproportionate number of Arabians among horses with CHD.[16,17] A familial risk for VSD in the Welsh Mountain pony[18] and Standardbred horse[19] has also been suggested. It is likely that multiple genetic and environmental factors interplay in the development of CHD, with genetic predispositions triggering cardiac maldevelopment when the appropriate epigenetic factors are present. Determining which specific genes and external factors lead to CHD in humans and animals will remain as a focus of research for the foreseeable future.

In humans, CHD is the most common developmental defect occurring in 9 out of every 1000 live births.[20] The prevalence of CHD in the horse is less well-defined, with historical studies compiled by Michaelsson and Ho[16] suggesting a prevalence of 0.03% to 0.2% that compares similarly to studies of dogs reporting prevalence ranges of 0.13% to 0.7%.[21,22] In a series of 6500 equine autopsies, 32 cases of variable forms of CHD were identified for a prevalence of 0.5%.[23] In a series of 3434 horses evaluated in a university hospital, 12 cases of VSD were the only reported incidence of CHD.[24] It is possible that many foals with severe cardiac malformations die during or shortly after birth and before veterinary examination. Others may have clinically silent defects that go undetected. As such, the exact prevalence and relative proportion of equine CHD is unknown.

RECOGNITION OF CONGENITAL HEART DISEASE IN FOALS AND HORSES

Foals with complex or severe CHD may present within the first days to weeks of life due to failure to thrive, dyspnea, cyanosis, or syncope. Signs of CHD can be nonspecific and differentials may include pneumonia, dysmaturity, or sepsis. Growth and maturation of the foal or horse with CHD can also be normal. Recognition of CHD requires that the practitioner considers CHD as a differential for animals displaying nonspecific signs of disease and devotes attention to cardiac auscultation and evaluation of the jugular veins and peripheral arterial pulse to detect abnormalities that may signal CHD is present. Careful auscultation and a thorough physical examination of young horses are therefore important because they may provide the first and earliest clue that CHD is present. Most forms of CHD are associated with a loud heart murmur; care should be taken to listen on both the left and right sides of the thorax because the murmur of a VSD is typically loudest on the right. Rarely, horses with CHD present later in life and often as a result of complications (heart failure, syncope, arrhythmias, cyanosis) from their cardiovascular disorder if it was not detected at an earlier age.

SPECIFIC FORMS OF CONGENITAL HEART DISEASE IN HORSES

Forms of CHD may be subdivided into shunts, valvar dysplasia, vascular malformations, and myocardial or electrical developmental anomalies. Of these, shunting lesions seem to be the most common form of CHD observed in horses.

A shunt is defined as an abnormal communication in the heart or great vessels resulting in mixing of blood between the systemic venous and systemic arterial circulations. The consequences of mixing between the left and right sides of the circulation vary depending on the shunt's magnitude and direction. In a left-to-right shunt (meaning from the systemic arterial circulation to the systemic venous or pulmonary circulation), the signs are principally of volume overload to the receiving chamber—left atrium and ventricle for VSD and PDA or right atrium and ventricle for ASD—because the normal amount of blood flowing to this chamber is augmented by the amount added from the shunt. Conversely, right-to-left shunts (where blood is diverted from the venous system to the systemic arterial system) result in deoxygenated blood entering the systemic arterial circulation, central cyanosis, and erythrocytosis. Chronic, high-volume left-to-right shunts can result in pulmonary vascular remodeling, increased pulmonary vascular resistance, and eventual right-to-left shunt flow if pulmonary vascular resistance exceeds systemic vascular resistance (termed Eisenmenger physiology).

VSD seems to be the defect observed most frequently in horses[23] and, as noted earlier, has increased prevalence in certain breeds.[17-19] Classification schemes for VSDs are variable and ill-defined in animals due to multiple and inconsistent descriptors for the same lesion in the historical literature. A trend in human medicine is to now evaluate these interventricular communications by phenotype, geographic location, and degree of septal malalignment.[25,26] VSDs exist in 1 of 3 phenotypes—perimembranous, doubly committed (these are also commonly termed juxtaarterial), and muscular (**Fig. 1**). The phenotype of a muscular defect is the one completely

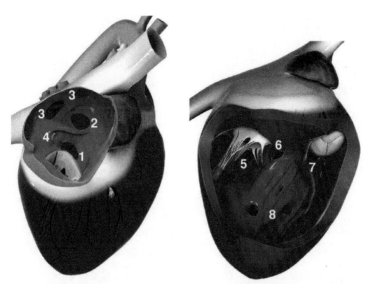

Fig. 1. The anatomic locations of ASDs (*left image*) and VSDs (*right image*). Defects in the ventral interatrial septum above the tricuspid valve are termed primum ASD (1); those in the area of the oval fossa are secundum ASD (2); those high in the dorsal atrial septum near either cranial or caudal vena caval inflow are sinus venosus ASD (3) and may be associated with anomalous pulmonary venous drainage; and an unroofed coronary sinus ASD (4) represents the last location for these defects. Defects in the interventricular septum may geographically lie within the inlet portion of the right ventricle under the septal tricuspid valve leaflet in the setting of an atrioventricular septal defect (5); perimembranous VSDs (6) occur at the cranial aspect of the septal tricuspid valve leaflet, resulting in fibrous continuity of the aortic and tricuspid valves and may extend toward the inlet, outlet, or apex; doubly committed VSDs (7) occur immediately below the pulmonary valve leaving the aortic and pulmonary valves in fibrous continuity; and muscular VSDs (8) can occur anywhere so long as they are completely surrounded by muscle and may be located within the inlet, trabecular/apical, or outlet septum. (*Courtesy of* The Ohio State University, Columbus (OH), USA; with permission.)

surrounded by muscular tissue; that of a perimembranous defect is fibrous continuity between the aortic and tricuspid valve; and the phenotypic feature of a doubly committed defect is fibrous continuity between the aortic and pulmonary valves.[25] Although all VSDs can be classified into 1 of these 3 categories, the phenotype by itself does not fully describe the defect. A VSD is then categorized by geography, meaning where does the interventricular communication open when viewed from the right ventricular perspective—centrally, apically, inlet, or outlet. Last, the degree of septal alignment apparent at the borders of a VSD should be defined to fully categorize the defect. As an example, a VSD with perimembranous phenotype may be observed to extend from the membranous septum to the outlet septum with cranial malalignment (a common VSD in Tetralogy of Fallot [TOF]). **Fig. 2** demonstrates echocardiographic features of a left-to-right shunting perimembranous, central VSD without septal malalignment in a 5-year-old Standardbred. Determining the clinical importance of a VSD can be challenging, with the presence of concurrent defects and the size of the VSD on echocardiography the most useful variables to ascertain. Some investigators have suggested that defects likely to result in hemodynamic derangement in horses are larger than 2.5 cm in a 450 to 500 kg horse or display a ratio of VSD diameter to

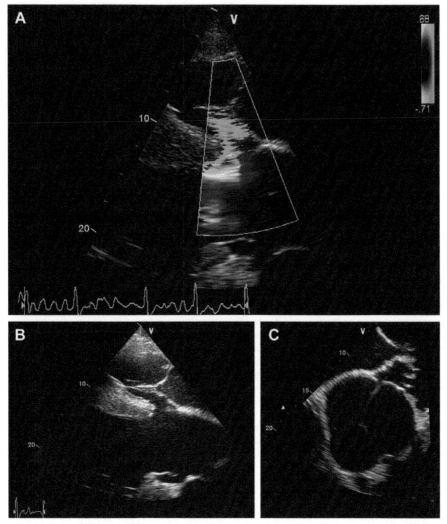

Fig. 2. Right-sided echocardiographic images from a 5-year-old Standardbred racehorse with a left-to-right perimembranous central ventricular septal defect. Color flow Doppler shows the high velocity left-to-right flow from under the aortic valve to the inlet right ventricle on a zoomed long-axis image (*A*), while long-axis (*B*) and close-up short axis (*C*) 2-dimensional images demonstrate echocardiographic drop-out in the area of the membranous septum resulting in aortic to tricuspid valve fibrous continuity.

aortic root diameter greater than 0.4.[19] **Box 1** highlights additional features of VSD that have been associated with a worse prognosis in horses. In foals with large defects, clinical signs of heart failure or pulmonary overcirculation and congestion on thoracic radiographs may be apparent. The grade of heart murmur is not discriminatory as small defects may result in loud murmurs and concurrent CHD may accentuate abnormal auscultatory findings. Small VSDs may be tolerable even in performance horses and, as in children, spontaneous closure is possible.[27]

An ASD is a persistent communication between the left and right atria. It seems to be a relatively rare defect in horses. The left-to-right shunt of an ASD leads to volume

---

Box 1
Diagnostic findings in horses with ventricular septal defect that suggest an unfavorable prognosis

- Physical Examination
  - Resting tachycardia
  - Jugular venous distension
  - Subcutaneous edema
  - Bounding/hyperkinetic arterial pulse
  - Pulmonary crackles
  - Increased respiratory effort

- Echocardiography
  - Left atrial enlargement
  - Left ventricular enlargement
  - Moderate to severe pulmonary artery dilation
  - Right ventricular hypertrophy
  - Prolapse of the aortic root into the defect
  - Malalignment of the aortic root (overriding aorta)
  - Defect measures greater than 2.5 cm in a 450 to 500 kg horse
  - Defect measures greater than 40% of aortic annular diameter
  - Doppler velocity less than 4.5 m/s with good alignment to flow direction
  - Moderate to severe aortic, mitral, or tricuspid regurgitation
  - Concurrent congenital defects

---

overload of the right heart and increases pulmonary blood flow, which can generate a murmur at the left heart base termed "relative pulmonary stenosis." In moderate to large ASDs, right atrial enlargement, right ventricular enlargement, and pulmonary overcirculation develop because the right heart directly receives both the normal systemic venous return as well as the excess volume traversing the shunt. Four forms of ASD are considered, classified by location relative to the interatrial septum (see **Fig. 1**). An example of a small sinus venosus ASD in a 6-year-old Standardbred is shown in **Fig. 3**.

In some animals with concurrent causes for high right atrial pressure, as a consequence of pulmonary stenosis, pulmonary hypertension, or tricuspid valve disease, there may be a shunt at the atrial level without a deficiency in atrial septal tissue. This form of interatrial communication is the PFO, which is reported in several examples of complex CHD in horses. Similarly, most cases of reported ASD in the equine literature note this lesion within a complex of concurrent anomalies,[17,28,29] with mitral/tricuspid stenosis or atresia,[30,31] or as a component of AVSD.[32–35] Isolated ASD is not well described in horses, although it has been reported in the setting of heart failure and atrial fibrillation in a foal.[36]

An AVSD, formerly called endocardial cushion or atrioventricular canal defect, results from maldevelopment of the atrioventricular septum. This tissue comprises portions of the cardiac septae that unify the atrial and ventricular septae and separates the dorsal left ventricle from the ventral right atrium—it is atrial on the right and ventricular on the left. Partial AVSD implies there is only an atrial communication or only a ventricular communication and that both AV valve annuli appear as discrete orifices. A complete AVSD is a defect in which there is a large primum ASD as well as an interventricular communication; furthermore, the AV valve is singular and covers both the right and left sides of the heart with bridging leaflets in between. In all cases—partial, intermediate, and complete—there can also be defects present in the atrioventricular valves, resulting in variable degrees of regurgitation, most notably a cleft in the septal

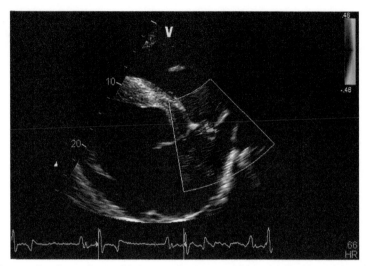

Fig. 3. Long-axis echocardiographic image of a 6-year-old Standardbred racehorse from the right thorax with a sinus venosus atrial septal defect. An aliasing jet of flow from the pulmonary vein can be seen entering the right atrium through a small defect in the dorsal interatrial septum, consistent with a sinus venosus type atrial septal defect. The clinical consequence of this defect is minimal as the shunt volume was estimated to be very low.

leaflet of the left atrioventricular valve that facilitates regurgitation into the left atrium and often the right atrium. Several reports of AVSD exist in the horse.[32–35]

The arterial duct, as discussed earlier, is a normal structure in the fetus that allows for the diversion of blood away from the lungs. Within the first 12 to 24 hrs after birth, the arterial duct begins to constrict in response to increased oxygen tension and is physiologically closed by 3 days postpartum in the horse.[37] If the arterial duct remains open, the normal decrease in pulmonary vascular resistance allows flow from the aorta to the pulmonary artery and excess left-to-right shunt flow through the lungs. Most cases of PDA in horses describe it as a concurrent defect in a heart with other forms of CHD or in very young foals in which patency is expected. Isolated cases of PDA in the horse beyond the neonatal period seem rare.[23] Closure of isolated PDA is advised in other species, either by surgical ligation or by interventional occlusion, and doing so is likely to provide a survival advantage in the horse. The heart murmur of a PDA is a continuous, machinery-type murmur at the left heart base. Diagnosis is confirmed by echocardiography, where continuous turbulent flow can be observed entering the pulmonary trunk (**Fig. 4**).

The prototypical right-to-left shunt is TOF. The 4 components of the tetralogy are right ventricular outflow tract obstruction, right ventricular hypertrophy, VSD, and an overriding aorta (also known as dextroposition). The underlying pathophysiology of this defect is believed to result from incomplete rotation and faulty partitioning of the outflow tracts. Long-standing sequelae of right-to-left shunt flow include erythrocytosis and blood hyperviscosity. Several examples of TOF in horses have been described in the veterinary literature with the Arabian breed often reported.[17,38,39] The extreme form of TOF is atresia of the pulmonary valve, in which pulmonary blood supply depends on patency of the arterial duct or aortopulmonary collateral vessels. Several cases of TOF and TOF with pulmonary atresia exist in the equine literature, most often described in Arabian foals.[16,40] Pulmonary atresia with intact ventricular septum—a less common variant—has also been described.[41]

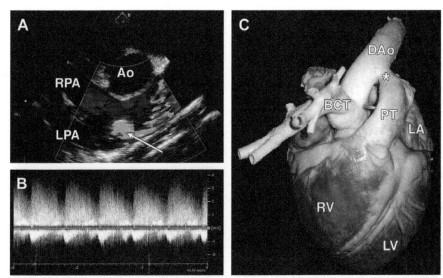

Fig. 4. Echocardiographic images (*A*, *B*) from the right thorax and an autopsy picture (*C*) from a 11-month-old miniature donkey with a patent arterial duct. On transthoracic echocardiography, turbulent flow (*arrow*) is observed entering near the origin of the left pulmonary artery (LPA). Spectral Doppler (*B*) demonstrates continuous, high-velocity flow, suggesting preservation of normal pulmonary arterial pressure. The postmortem specimen (*C*) confirms the vascular connection (*asterisk*) between the descending aorta (DAo) and pulmonary trunk (PT). The cause of death in this animal was unrelated to the heart condition. Ao, aorta; BCT, brachiocephalic trunk; LA, left atrium; LV, left ventricle; RPA, right pulmonary artery; RV, right ventricle.

Sharing many similarities with TOF, double outlet right ventricle (DORV) is a cardiac malformation in which both great vessels arise entirely or predominately from the RV. Clinical signs greatly depend on the magnitude of pulmonary blood flow, with cyanosis related to insufficient pulmonary flow and heart failure associated with excessive left-to-right shunting. A great deal of controversy exists over the precise terminology of this condition. Characteristics of DORV are shared with TOF and transposition of the great arteries (TGA).[42,43] As noted in the Congenital Heart Surgery Nomenclature and Database Project, the degree of aortic positioning over the RV required for the description DORV is variable, with some investigators requiring greater than or equal to 50% of the aorta arising from the RV, whereas others use a standard of greater than or equal to 90%; others confine the term DORV to situations in which aortic-mitral fibrous continuity is lost.[44] There are several forms of DORV, which are predominately related to the position of the interventricular communication relative to the aorta and pulmonary trunk: the defect can be subaortic, subpulmonary, doubly committed, or remote/noncommitted.[8,42] DORV has been sporadically reported in horses[14,45–47], and echocardiographic images of this lesion from a 6-year-old Quarterhorse are shown in **Fig. 5**.

Valvar dysplasia broadly means a malformed valve, which may manifest with features of stenosis, insufficiency, or both. Congenital stenosis is more common in the semilunar valves but may affect the atrioventricular valves as well. For semilunar valve stenosis, obstruction may be subvalvar, valvar, or supravalvar. In order to maintain forward stroke volume, such that the same volume of blood is pumped out of the

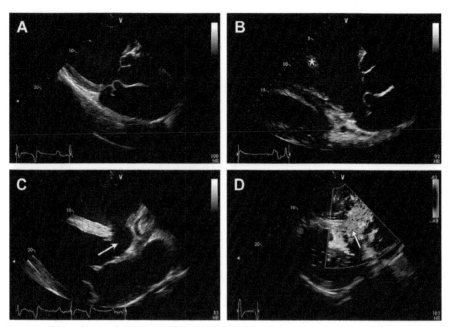

Fig. 5. Echocardiographic images from a 6-year-old Quarterhorse with DORV and valvar aortic and pulmonary stenoses. Both great vessels can be seen arising from the same ventricle when imaged from the right (A) and left thorax (B). The ventricle that derives the great vessels has a large moderator band (*asterisk*) consistent with a morphologic right ventricle. In both the long axis (C) and short axis (D) images from the right thorax, a large interventricular communication (*arrow*) is observed with aliasing left-to-right flow (D).

ventricle with each heartbeat, the blood must accelerate through the narrowing at a higher velocity. This requires that a greater ventricular pressure be generated, which leads to increased ventricular wall stress and the development of concentric hypertrophy. Patients with mild semilunar valve stenosis typically live a normal life, although they may have reduced exercise capacity; those with moderate to severe disease are more likely to experience exercise intolerance, syncope, congestive heart failure, or sudden cardiac death. Atrioventricular valve stenosis presents with a different clinical picture; these lesions lead to progressive atrial enlargement, atrial arrhythmias, and congestive heart failure if untreated. Valvar stenosis seems to be uncommon in horses, although reports exist of pulmonary valve stenosis,[16,38,48–50] subvalvar aortic stenosis,[51] mitral stenosis,[30,52] and tricuspid stenosis.[38] Numerous reports exist of tricuspid atresia in horses,[31,38,53–56] with some investigators suggesting this unique defect is among the most common form of equine CHD.[16,17]

Valvar insufficiency of the pulmonary or aortic valve is relatively common to detect on color Doppler imaging in horses, although it is typically trace or mild and considered physiologic (ie, nonpathologic) in young animals. Insufficiency of the mitral or tricuspid valve can also be observed in normal horses, particularly fit athletes.[57] Less commonly, structural abnormalities in the mitral or tricuspid apparatus are observed resulting in moderate to severe regurgitation (**Fig. 6**). Chronic atrioventricular valve regurgitation leads to atrial and ventricular volume overload and dilation, which may advance to congestive heart failure. Postmortem and echocardiographic findings of dysplastic atrioventricular valves display fused and malformed leaflets with

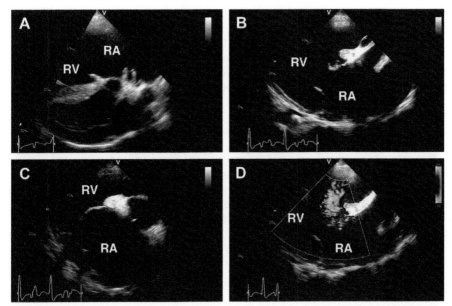

Fig. 6. Echocardiographic images from the right (*A*) and left (*B–D*) lateral thorax of a 2-year-old Standardbred with tricuspid valve dysplasia. In all images, there is moderate to severe enlargement of the right atrium (RA) and RV. The tricuspid valve shows incomplete coaptation (*B*), tethering to a lateral papillary muscle (*C*), and severe regurgitation (*D*).

shortened chordae tendineae. Direct attachment from the papillary muscle to the valve is a common feature. Valve dysplasia characterized by insufficiency is not widely reported in horses, although reports exist for both mitral[58] and tricuspid dysplasia.[17,52]

Several malformations of the major thoracic arteries have been described in horses. Vascular ring anomalies result from variable persistence and regression of the paired pharyngeal arterial arches during development, and a common clinical presentation is a pediatric animal with dysphagia or stridor. The most common form of vascular ring compression in small animals is persistence of the right aortic arch (PRAA) with absence of the left fourth arch. There are also rare reports of PRAA in horses, including surgical correction.[59–61] A vascular ring anomaly associated with dorsal compression of the esophagus from an anomalous vessel has also been reported, although the precise vascular anatomy was not defined.[62]

Other rare arterial malformations include a common arterial trunk, coarctation of the aorta, and TGA. A common arterial trunk is characterized by a single great vessel leaving the heart through a common valve to provide systemic, pulmonary, and coronary circulations. Pulmonary circulation in truncus arteriosus is reduced if there is a restriction or stenosis at the origin of the branch arteries or high-resistance pulmonary vascular disease. Pulmonary blood flow is increased if entry into the branch arteries is unrestricted because the pulmonary circulation originates from a high-pressure vessel. Although there is mixing of blood in common arterial trunk, clinical signs of cyanotic disease could potentially be reduced by relatively higher contributions of oxygenated blood from the left ventricle. Conversely, marked pulmonary overcirculation could lead to pulmonary congestion. Reports in horses with this defect are rare in the veterinary literature.[63–65]

Aortic coarctation is a common affliction of children but rarely seen in veterinary species. The coarctation is a ridge of tissue at the aortic isthmus—the junction of the arch and the descending aorta, where the arterial duct/ligament attaches, distal to the brachiocephalic artery in horses. Rather than a discrete ridge of tissue, tubular hypoplasia refers to segmental narrowing of the aortic arch and is reflected as greater than 50% narrowing compared with the normal aortic diameter. Last, interruption of the aortic arch may be considered the most extreme form of coarctation where the descending aorta is anatomically separated from the arch. In such cases, perfusion of the descending aorta and caudal half of the body is accomplished by ductal flow and the enlargement of collateral vessels. Tubular hypoplasia of the aortic arch has been observed in some horses with complex CHD by the author. Interruption of the aortic arch has been reported in 2 foals.[66]

TGA refers to ventriculoarterial discordance—the aorta arises from the RV and the pulmonary trunk from the left. Using the analogy of an electrical circuit, TGA creates 2 circulations in parallel, rather than in series (the normal arrangement). Without a communication between the systemic and pulmonary circulations, such as a VSD, ASD, or PDA, circulatory collapse occurs shortly after birth. The embryologic basis of TGA remains uncertain, although new research suggests that abnormalities in left-right lateralization and improper spiralization of the heart during development may contribute to it.[67] This defect has been reported in several foals.[68–71]

SUMMARY

CHD represents a small proportion of horses undergoing clinical evaluation; however, the spectrum and complexity of defects that can occur during cardiac development are many. Given this complexity, evaluation of a horse with CHD should optimally be performed in consultation with a specialist trained and experienced in malformations of the heart. A morphologic and sequential segmental approach to CHD assessment is advised, particularly for complex malformations of the equine heart. This review aims to provide a summary of CHD in horses, offering an overview of what lesions should be considered during the evaluation of horses suspected to have CHD. Unfortunately, for many congenital malformations of the heart in horses, therapies are limited because cardiac interventions and cardiac surgery are not routinely pursued in this species.

REFERENCES

1. Gittenberger-de Groot AC, Bartelings MM, Deruiter MC, et al. Basics of cardiac development for the understanding of congenital heart malformations. Pediatr Res 2005;57(2):169–76.
2. Gittenberger-de Groot AC, Bartelings MM, Poelmann RE, et al. Embryology of the heart and its impact on understanding fetal and neonatal heart disease. Semin Fetal Neonatal Med 2013;18(5):237–44.
3. Anderson RH. Unravelling the mysteries surrounding development of the outflow tracts. Cardiol Young 2014;24(4):721–2.
4. Franklin RCG, Beland MJ, Colan SD, et al. Nomenclature for congenital and paediatric cardiac disease: the International Paediatric and Congenital Cardiac Code (IPCCC) and the Eleventh Iteration of the International Classification of Diseases (ICD-11). Cardiol Young 2017;27(10):1872–938.
5. Shinebourne EA, Macartney FJ, Anderson RH. Sequential chamber localization–logical approach to diagnosis in congenital heart disease. Br Heart J 1976;38(4):327–40.
6. Van Praagh R. Terminology of congenital heart disease. Glossary and commentary. Circulation 1977;56(2):139–43.

7. Anderson RH, Shirali G. Sequential segmental analysis. Ann Pediatr Cardiol 2009;2(1):24–35.
8. Ezon DS, Goldberg JF, Kyle WB. Atlas of congenital heart disease. Houston (TX): Ezon Educational Services; 2015.
9. Michaelsson M, Ho SY. Sequential segmental analysis. In: Michaelsson M, Ho SY, editors. Congenital heart malformations in mammals: an illustrated text. London: Imperial College Press; 2000. p. 19–28.
10. Abduch MC, Tonini PL, de Oliveira Domingos Barbusci L, et al. Double-outlet right ventricle associated with discordant atrioventricular connection and dextrocardia in a cat. J Small Anim Pract 2003;44(8):374–7.
11. Schwarzwald CC. Sequential segmental analysis - a systematic approach to the diagnosis of congenital cardiac defects. Equine Vet Educ 2008;20(6):305–9.
12. Scansen BA, Schneider M, Bonagura JD. Sequential segmental classification of feline congenital heart disease. J Vet Cardiol 2015;17(Suppl 1):S10–52.
13. Mitchell KJ, Schwarzwald CC. Echocardiography for the assessment of congenital heart defects in calves. Vet Clin North Am Food Anim Pract 2016;32(1):37–54.
14. Kohnken R, Schober K, Godman J, et al. Double outlet right ventricle with subpulmonary ventricular septal defect (Taussig-Bing anomaly) and other complex congenital cardiac malformations in an American Quarter Horse foal. J Vet Cardiol 2018;20(1):64–72.
15. Blue GM, Kirk EP, Sholler GF, et al. Congenital heart disease: current knowledge about causes and inheritance. Med J Aust 2012;197(3):155–9.
16. Michaelsson M, Ho SY. Horses. In: Congenital heart malformations in mammals. London: Imperial College Press; 2000. p. 43–56.
17. Hall TL, Magdesian KG, Kittleson MD. Congenital cardiac defects in neonatal foals: 18 cases (1992-2007). J Vet Intern Med 2010;24(1):206–12.
18. Marr CM. Cardiac murmurs: congenital heart disease. In: Marr CM, Bowen IM, editors. Cardiology of the horse. 2 editipn. Edinburgh (Scotland): Saunders Elsevier; 2010. p. 193–205.
19. Reef VB. Evaluation of ventricular septal defects in horses using two-dimensional and Doppler echocardiography. Equine Vet J Suppl 1995;(19):86–95.
20. van der Linde D, Konings EE, Slager MA, et al. Birth prevalence of congenital heart disease worldwide: a systematic review and meta-analysis. J Am Coll Cardiol 2011;58(21):2241–7.
21. Patterson DF. Epidemiologic and genetic studies of congenital heart disease in the dog. Circ Res 1968;23(2):171–202.
22. Schrope DP. Prevalence of congenital heart disease in 76,301 mixed-breed dogs and 57,025 mixed-breed cats. J Vet Cardiol 2015;17(3):192–202.
23. Buergelt CD. Equine cardiovascular pathology: an overview. Anim Health Res Rev 2003;4(2):109–29.
24. Leroux AA, Detilleux J, Sandersen CF, et al. Prevalence and risk factors for cardiac diseases in a hospital-based population of 3,434 horses (1994-2011). J Vet Intern Med 2013;27(6):1563–70.
25. Spicer DE, Hsu HH, Co-Vu J, et al. Ventricular septal defect. Orphanet J Rare Dis 2014;9:144.
26. Crucean A, Brawn WJ, Spicer DE, et al. Holes and channels between the ventricles revisited. Cardiol Young 2015;25(6):1099–110.
27. Short DM, Seco OM, Jesty SA, et al. Spontaneous closure of a ventricular septal defect in a horse. J Vet Intern Med 2010;24(6):1515–8.
28. Musselman EE, LoGuidice RJ. Hypoplastic left ventricular syndrome in a foal. J Am Vet Med Assoc 1984;185(5):542–3.

29. Reppas GP, Canfield PJ, Hartley WJ, et al. Multiple congenital cardiac anomalies and idiopathic thoracic aortitis in a horse. Vet Rec 1996;138(1):14–6.
30. Grunberg W, Jaksch W. Lutembacher's syndrome in an aged Lipizzan stallion. Wien Tierarztl Monatsschr 1972;59(6):211–6 [in German].
31. Reef VB, Mann PC, Orsini PG. Echocardiographic detection of tricuspid atresia in two foals. J Am Vet Med Assoc 1987;191(2):225–8.
32. Physick-Sheard PW, Maxie MG, Palmer NC, et al. Atrial septal defect of the persistent ostium primum type with hypoplastic right ventricle in a Welsh pony foal. Can J Comp Med 1985;49(4):429–33.
33. Ecke P, Malik R, Kannegieter NJ. Common atrioventricular canal in a foal. N Z Vet J 1991;39(3):97–8.
34. Kutasi O, Voros K, Biksi I, et al. Common atrioventricular canal in a newborn foal–case report and review of the literature. Acta Vet Hung 2007;55(1):51–65.
35. Kraus MS, Pariaut R, Alcaraz A, et al. Complete atrioventricular canal defect in a foal: Clinical and pathological features. J Vet Cardiol 2005;7(1):59–64.
36. Taylor FG, Wotton PR, Hillyer MH, et al. Atrial septal defect and atrial fibrillation in a foal. Vet Rec 1991;128(4):80–1.
37. Machida N, Yasuda J, Too K, et al. A morphological study on the obliteration processes of the ductus arteriosus in the horse. Equine Vet J 1988;20(4):249–54.
38. Bayly WM, Reed SM, Leathers CW, et al. Multiple congenital heart anomalies in five Arabian foals. J Am Vet Med Assoc 1982;181(7):684–9.
39. Cargile J, Lombard C, Wilson JH, et al. Tetralogy of Fallot and segmental uterine aplasia in a three-year-old Morgan filly. Cornell Vet 1991;81(4):411–8.
40. Vitums A, Bayly WM. Pulmonary atresia with dextroposition of the aorta and ventricular septal defect in three Arabian foals. Vet Pathol 1982;19(2):160–8.
41. Kruger MU, Wunschmann A, Ward C, et al. Pulmonary atresia with intact ventricular septum and hypoplastic right ventricle in an Arabian foal. J Vet Cardiol 2016;18(3):284–9.
42. Mahle WT, Martinez R, Silverman N, et al. Anatomy, echocardiography, and surgical approach to double outlet right ventricle. Cardiol Young 2008;18(Suppl 3):39–51.
43. Anderson RH. How best can we define double outlet right ventricle when describing congenitally malformed hearts? Anat Rec 2013;296(7):993–4.
44. Jacobs ML. Congenital heart surgery nomenclature and database project: tetralogy of fallot. Ann Thorac Surg 2000;69(4 Suppl):S77–82.
45. Vitums A. Origin of the aorta and pulmonary trunk from the right ventricle in a horse. Pathol Vet 1970;7(6):482–91.
46. Chaffin MK, Miller MW, Morris EL. Double outlet right ventricle and other associated congenital cardiac anomalies in an American miniature horse foal. Equine Vet J 1992;24(5):402–6.
47. Fennell L, Church S, Tyrell D, et al. Double-outlet right ventricle in a 10-month-old Friesian filly. Aust Vet J 2009;87(5):204–9.
48. Critchley KL. An interventricular septal defect, pulmonary stenosis and bicuspid pulmonary valve in a Welsh pony foal. Equine Vet J 1976;8(4):176–8.
49. Hinchcliff KW, Adams WM. Critical pulmonary stenosis in a newborn foal. Equine Vet J 1991;23(4):318–20.
50. Gehlen H, Bubeck K, Stadler P. Valvular pulmonic stenosis with normal aortic root and intact ventricular and atrial septa in an Arabian horse. Equine Vet Educ 2001;13(6):286–8.
51. King JM, Flint TJ, Anderson WI. Incomplete subaortic stenotic rings in domestic animals–a newly described congenital anomaly. Cornell Vet 1988;78(3):263–71.

52. McGurrin MK, Physick-Sheard PW, Southorn E. Parachute left atrioventricular valve causing stenosis and regurgitation in a Thoroughbred foal. J Vet Intern Med 2003;17(4):579–82.
53. Rooney JR, Franks WC. Congenital cardiac anomalies in horses. Pathol Vet 1964; 1:454–64.
54. Gumbrell RC. Atresia of the tricuspid valve in a foal. N Z Vet J 1970;18(11):253–6.
55. Button C, Gross DR, Allert JA, et al. Tricuspid atresia in a foal. J Am Vet Med Assoc 1978;172(7):825–30.
56. Meurs KM, Miller MW, Hanson C, et al. Tricuspid valve atresia with main pulmonary artery atresia in an Arabian foal. Equine Vet J 1997;29(2):160–2.
57. Reef VB, Bonagura J, Buhl R, et al. Recommendations for management of equine athletes with cardiovascular abnormalities. J Vet Intern Med 2014;28(3):749–61.
58. Schober KE, Kaufhold J, Kipar A. Mitral valve dysplasia in a foal. Equine Vet J 2000;32(2):170–3.
59. Bartels JE, Vaughan JT. Persistent right aortic arch in the horse. J Am Vet Med Assoc 1969;154(4):406–9.
60. Mackey VS, Large SM, Breznock EM, et al. Surgical correction of a persistent right aortic arch in a foal. Vet Surg 1986;15(4):325–8.
61. Butt TD, MacDonald DG, Crawford WH, et al. Persistent right aortic arch in a yearling horse. Can Vet J 1998;39(11):714–5.
62. Smith TR. Unusual vascular ring anomaly in a foal. Can Vet J 2004;45(12):1016–8.
63. Sojka JE. Persistent truncus arteriosus in a foal. Equine Pract 1987;9(4):19–26.
64. Steyn PF, Holland P, Hoffman J. The angiocardiographic diagnosis of a persistent truncus arteriosus in a foal. J S Afr Vet Assoc 1989;60(2):106–8.
65. Jesty SA, Wilkins PA, Palmer JE, et al. Persistent truncus arteriosus in two Standarbred foals. Equine Vet Educ 2007;19(6):307–11.
66. Scott EA, Chaffee A, Eyster GE, et al. Interruption of aortic arch in two foals. J Am Vet Med Assoc 1978;172(3):347–50.
67. Unolt M, Putotto C, Silvestri LM, et al. Transposition of great arteries: new insights into the pathogenesis. Front Pediatr 2013;1:11.
68. Vitums A, Grant BD, Stone EC, et al. Transposition of the aorta and atresia of the pulmonary trunk in a horse. Cornell Vet 1973;63(1):41–57.
69. McClure JJ, Gaber CE, Watters JW, et al. Complete transposition of the great arteries with ventricular septal defect and pulmonary stenosis in a Thoroughbred foal. Equine Vet J 1983;15(4):377–80.
70. Zamora CS, Vitums A, Nyrop KA, et al. Atresia of the right atrioventricular orifice with complete transposition of the great arteries in a horse. Anat Histol Embryol 1989;18(2):177–82.
71. Sleeper MM, Palmer JE. Echocardiographic diagnosis of transposition of the great arteries in a neonatal foal. Vet Radiol Ultrasound 2005;46(3):259–62.

Equine Acquired Valvular Disease

Celia M. Marr, BVMS, MVM, PhD, FRCVS

KEYWORDS

- Equine • Horse • Degenerative valve disease • Endocarditis • Valvular regurgitation
- Valvular prolapse • Aging

KEY POINTS

- Degenerative myxomatous disease is the commonest form of acquired valvular pathology in the horse, most commonly affecting the aortic and/or mitral valves.
- Valvular regurgitation and likely degenerative valvular pathology are age related. Often this is of minimal clinical relevance and overall life expectancy does not seem to be affected by its presence, although some individuals are more severely affected.
- Valvular prolapse is identified echocardiographically, but a link between this functional abnormality and subsequent structural change has not been established in the horse, although it has been shown in dogs and other species.
- Infective endocarditis is associated with a range of organisms, the presentation includes fever and other systemic signs accompanying valvular regurgitation, and overall the prognosis is poor, warranting aggressive therapy.
- Other forms of acquired inflammatory valvular disease, rupture of one or more chordae tendineae, tearing of valve cusps, and regurgitation relating to primary chamber dilation and dysfunction occur rarely and require investigation with echocardiography to provide a definitive diagnosis.

 Video content accompanies this article at http://www.vetequine.theclinics. com.

INTRODUCTION

Valvular disease is common in horses presented for cardiological investigation.[1] Typically horses with valvular disease have murmurs of valvular regurgitation. The clinician's task is to differentiate horses, in which valvular regurgitation has minimal impact on the horse's performance and its quality of life from other individuals, where valvular regurgitation is associated with moderate or severe valvular pathology. It has been known for many years that horses commonly develop valvular lesions, and

Disclosure Statement: None.
Internal Medicine, Rossdales Equine Hospital and Diagnostic Centre, Cotton End Road, Exning, Newmarket, Suffolk CB8 7NN, UK
E-mail address: celia.marr@rossdales.com

Vet Clin Equine 35 (2019) 119–137
https://doi.org/10.1016/j.cveq.2018.12.001
0749-0739/19/© 2018 Elsevier Inc. All rights reserved.

structurally these are similar to the changes seen in humans and other species with degenerative myxomatous disease. Despite its importance, knowledge of aetiopathogenesis of myxomatous disease in the dog is relatively limited, and understanding of mechanisms involved in the development of this pathology in horses is minimal. Nevertheless, despite many gaps in our knowledge, there is a body of work based on clinical observations of horses with valvular regurgitation, which serves as a useful knowledge base for clinical decision-making. In this article, this work is summarized with the aim of helping clinicians to make evidence-based recommendations for their cases.

DEGENERATIVE VALVULAR DISEASE
Pathology and Pathogenesis

In what remains one of the most important studies ever performed in equine cardiology, a pathologic survey of 1557 equine hearts performed in the early 1970s, it was established that valvular pathology occurs in around one-third of adult horses.[2] The aortic valve was the most common site of valvular pathology and these were usually nodular lesions, which were documented in all 3 cusps with variable cusp involvement in individual cases.[2] In a parallel histologic study, valve lesions were characterized by varying degrees of fibrous thickening with mixed cellular infiltrates,[3] consistent with myxomatous valve disease, a pathology that has been studied far more extensively in dogs and humans[4] than in horses. Myxomatous valvular degeneration involves expansion of the extracellular matrix with glycosaminoglycans and proteoglycans, valvular endothelial and valvular interstitial cell alterations, and loss of the collagen-laden fibrosa layer with altered expression of matrix metalloproteinases and their inhibitors.[4–6] Myxomatous valve disease represents a continuum, in its mildest form consisting of subendothelial accumulation of elastin, laminin, and abnormal collagen, whereas at its more severe form, the pathology can include gross distortion and ballooning of the valve cusps and proximal chordal thickening.[4] Inflammation does not have a major role in myxomatous valve disease.[6]

Myxomatous degeneration is not an inevitable consequence of aging, but aging affects disease progression.[5] In common with other species, equine heart valves are dynamic structures and they contain both contractile and neural elements, which affect their mechanical behavior and function. Aortic valve tone is modified by various endocrine, paracrine, and neuronal mediators such as thromboxane, endothelin-1, serotonin (ie, 5-hydroxytryptamine), and alpha-adrenoreceptor agonists.[7] Equine-specific knowledge is lacking, but in other mammals, aging reduces valvular cell density and leads to collagen remodeling and elastin loss. Serotonin, along with transforming growth factor beta, are key mediators in the pathogenesis of valvular degeneration.[8] Valves become stiffer with age and there is a loss of nerve density in the valves.[9] Valvular endothelial cells, which line the surface of the valve, and valvular interstitial cells are also lost.[10] Myxomatous degeneration is thought to be a response to shear forces created as blood flows across the surface of the valve and repeated impact of the leaflets as they close.[11] There are similarities between age-related valvular change and myxomatous disease, and it is postulated that myxomatous valvular disease in dogs may be an abnormal amplification of the aging process.[5] To what extent that theory applies to horses is unclear. Furthermore, the factors that lead to accelerated aging of the valves have not yet been fully elucidated in other species.

Epidemiology

A large study has demonstrated that physiologic atrioventricular valve regurgitation is common in Thoroughbred racehorses and does not affect racing performance.[12]

But, this epidemiologic information relates to horses in which there is not likely to be valvular pathology, and epidemiologic studies specifically addressing degenerative valvular disease are sparse. The studies that do exist are limited by the fact that they focus on clinical presentation and findings, that is, specific forms of murmurs and/or valvular regurgitation identified echocardiographically, and that valvular pathology cannot be defined.[13–17] Nevertheless, given that degenerative valvular disease is much the most common form of pathology, it is reasonable to assume that it accounts for most of the cases included in existing epidemiologic studies involving general riding horses and middle-aged and geriatric animals. Male sex and increasing age are recognized risk factors for equine aortic regurgitation (AR).[1,15] Small ponies are less likely to have AR compared with other horse types.[15] Similarly, horses older than 15 years were more likely to suffer from MR in a survey of a general horse population in United Kingdom, whereas sex and breed predispositions were not found for MR.[15] The tricuspid and pulmonary valves are not commonly affected by degenerative change and typically tricuspid valve regurgitation (TR) is found in isolation in racehorses[1,12] and other equine athletes. However, both TR[15] and physiologic valvular regurgitation[1] can be associated with left-sided valvular disease.

Geriatric horses have a high prevalence of left-sided cardiac murmurs; usually their owners are unaware of these and often they are of relatively low intensity. In 87 horses older than or equal to 30 years of age in North-West England and North Wales, 36.2% had murmurs of which 28% (7 of 25 horses) were grade 3/6 or higher.[17] Despite this high prevalence, cardiac disease remains a relatively uncommon cause of death. Cardiovascular problems accounted only 6.4% of owner-reported nonsurvival amongst a group of horses with left-sided valvular regurgitation (LSVR) and this prevalence was similar to the prevalence of cardiovascular problems in horses that had not been identified as having LSVR.[16] A longitudinal study of horses with mild MR, primarily Warmbloods used for pleasure and low-level competition, which were reevaluated between 2 and 9 years of initial diagnosis, showed little evidence of clinical progression although there were subtle increases in left ventricular dimensions in the subgroup, which were reevaluated echocardiographically.[13] Another study on riding horses with various forms of valvular regurgitation and reexamined at 2 to 11 years after initial diagnosis concluded that in the horses with mild or moderate heart disease, deterioration was mild.[14] Nevertheless, MR in particular is the most common form of valvular disease associated with congestive heart failure.[1]

Clinical Characterization and Prognosis

Assessment of cases presented for evaluation of potential degenerative valvular disease should include careful clinical examination to characterize all murmurs, assess pulse quality, and document potential signs of congestive heart failure. Echocardiography is the primary tool used to document valvular pathology and assess its severity, but useful additional information can be gleaned from Holter monitoring, exercise testing, and blood pressure measurement.

Aortic regurgitation is typically associated with a decrescendo holodiastolic murmur, which can often be musical in character and is loudest over the aortic valve on the left or right sides and sometimes both sides of the thorax. In the presence of moderate or severe AR, the systolic arterial pressure increases and diastolic pressure decreases, which is reflected by an appreciable change in pulse quality, that is, the pulse becomes hyperkinetic. Clinical characteristics that have been shown to be associated with the onset of exercise intolerance or death within 2 years of identification of AR included abnormal pulse quality, pulse pressure greater than 60 mm Hg measured at the coccygeal artery, and supraventricular premature depolarizations occurring at a rate of greater than 1 per hour. However, as predictors for progression, in general the sensitivity of these criteria was low, indicating that it is difficult for the clinician to identify the horses that will progress. Presence of an AR murmur of grade 4/6 or higher, hyperkinetic pulse quality, and pulse pressure greater than or equal to 60 mm Hg were moderately specific and the presence of ventricular premature depolarizations was highly specific for predicting progression.[15] A more recent study confirmed that noninvasive pulse pressure measurements can be useful in assessing AR severity with a cut off of greater than 67 mm Hg, being highly specific although not very sensitive to differentiate horses with mild-moderate AR from those with severe AR.[18]

In degenerative AR, varying degrees of thickening and nodular changes on the aortic valve cusps may be apparent echocardiographically. The hemodynamic consequences of chronic AR can be inferred from echocardiographic studies, which show left ventricular dilation and changes in global ventricular function reflecting initially increased cardiac output and eventually myocardial failure.[19–21] The echocardiographic assessment of AR severity is based on subjective assessment of the regurgitant jet size, subjective assessment of left ventricular size and shape, and M-mode measurement of the internal diameter of the left ventricle in diastole (**Figs. 1–3**). A grading system has been developed to assign scores to these features (**Table 1**).[20] This is practical and easy to apply, but clinicians should bear in mind that it depends on subjective assessments and allometric scaling[22,23] that has not been validated in every breed, notably Thoroughbreds and Standardbreds, have not yet been investigated. Furthermore, healthy athletic horses may have large ventricles and this should be kept in mind when assessing ventricular size in cases of AR that occur in equine athletes. Additional echocardiographic features that are seen in some, but not all, cases of degenerative AR include high-frequency vibrations on the mitral valve, aortic valve, or septum; early closure of the mitral valve; dilation of the aortic root; and increased fractional shortening (Videos 1–5).[19] A study seeking to identify easily measured objective variables to grade AR severity showed that preejection period (decreasing with severity), stroke volume (increasing with severity), and diastolic decrease in aortic diameter (increasing with severity) were different across severity groups.[20] However, there is a need to validate this work in other centers and patient populations before these variables can be recommended for routine use in severity grading.

Mitral regurgitation is associated with a systolic murmur loudest over the mitral valve on the left side. Radiation, if present, is usually in a caudodorsal direction. Clinical signs associated with severe MR include murmurs of grade 3/6 or greater, loud third heart sound, exercise intolerance, respiratory signs, and congestive heart failure.[24] MR is the most common form of valvular disease associated with atrial fibrillation[1] and ventricular arrhythmias are also common in horses with severe MR.[24] MR is usually classified as mild when there is no left atrial enlargement, and color flow Doppler echocardiography demonstrates 1 or 2 thin regurgitant jets, whose height is subjectively no more than one-third of the height of the left atrium (Videos 6–9).[13] Horses with moderate MR develop increases in pulmonary wedge pressure, particularly at exercise, which may be associated with exercise limitation.[25] Severe MR leads to left atrial, left ventricular, and pulmonary artery dilation, which can lead to pulmonary artery rupture, and affected horses will often show signs of congestive heart failure at rest[24] (**Fig. 4**; see Videos 6–9).

Ambulatory and exercise electrocardiography (ECG) are extremely valuable adjunctive tools in achieving a full assessment of horses with degenerative valvular disease, and both AR and MR can be associated with arrhythmias (see **Fig. 4**, Videos 1–9). In

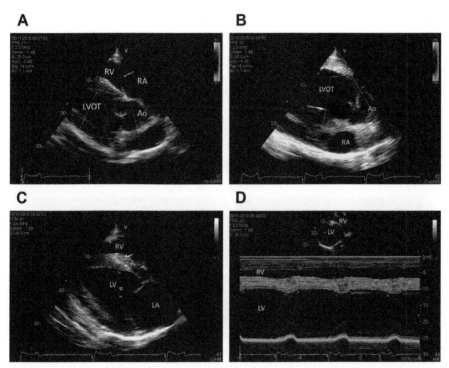

Fig. 1. Right (*A*) and left (*B*) parasternal long-axis images and color Doppler echocardiography of the left ventricular outflow tract (LVOT) and aorta (Ao) from a 7-year-old racing Thoroughbred gelding (495 kg) with no exercise intolerance and a grade 1/6 aortic regurgitation (AR) murmur. There are 2 thin strands of AR seen in the left parasternal image, which are green near the valve cusps and orange at their tips. From the right, only one of these is seen. Together, these occupy a small area and are assigned 1 point (see **Table 1**). (*C*) The right parasternal 4-chamber image shows no signs of enlargement of the left ventricle (LV) with a normal apex shape (1 point). (*D*) An M-mode study of the LV at the chordal level shows that when allometrically scaled to a body weight of 500 kg, the internal diameter of the LV in diastole is 13.1 cm (2 points). Thus, the combined grade is 4, indicating mild AR.[20] LA, left atrium; RA, right atrium; RV, right ventricle. This case is also illustrated in Videos 1–5.

some centers, stress echocardiography is used to attempt to investigate the impact of moderate valvular regurgitation. There is some evidence that tissue Doppler imaging[21] and potentially speckle tracking echocardiography will prove useful in the early detection of left ventricular dysfunction in horses with degenerative valve disease. However, this has not been confirmed in all studies[26] and further work is needed before firm recommendations can be made on how to use these tools for severity grading and prognostication.

VALVULAR PROLAPSE

Valvular prolapse is a functional disorder identified echocardiographically. In dogs and humans, mitral valve prolapse (MVP) is a risk factor for degenerative (ie, myxomatous) mitral valve disease.[27] It is estimated that the prevalence of MVP in humans is around 2.4% and 7% of these patients will develop severe MR, compared with a prevalence of severe MR of 0.5% in patients without MVP.[28] However, MVP does not inevitably lead to myxomatous disease. In horses, MVP is described occasionally both with[24]

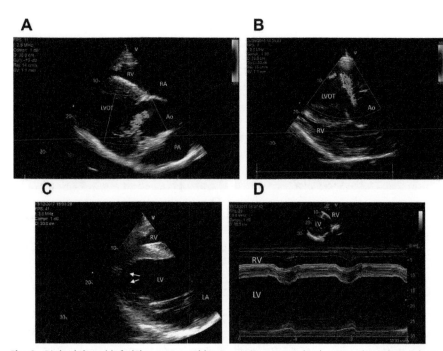

Fig. 2. Right (*A*) and left (*B*) parasternal long-axis images and color Doppler echocardiography of the left ventricular outflow tract (LVOT) and aorta (Ao) from a 17-year-old Thoroughbred stallion (560 kg) with no signs of exercise intolerance and a grade 4/6 aortic regurgitation (AR) murmur detected at the time of annual vaccination. The arterial pulse was slightly hyperkinetic. The regurgitant jet (green) occupies more than one-third of the LVOT (2 points, see **Table 1**). (*C*) The right parasternal 4-chamber image shows subjective enlargement of the left ventricle (LV) with a round apex (*arrows*) (3 points). (*D*) An M-mode study of the LV at the chordal level shows that when allometrically scaled to a body weight of 500 kg, the internal diameter of the LV in diastole is 13.2 cm (2 points). Thus, the combined grade is 7 points, indicating moderate AR.[20] Note, reflecting a hyperdynamic LV, the movement of the septum seen in the M-mode image is slightly more exaggerated in this case compared with the milder case in **Fig. 1**. LA, left atrium; PA, pulmonary artery; RA, right atrium; RV, right ventricle. This case is also illustrated in Videos 1–5.

and without severe MR.[29,30] The echocardiographic identification of MVP in horses is challenging, partly because of the saddle shape of the valve and because apical image planes cannot be achieved in adult horses. Convex bulging of a mitral valve leaflet into the left atrium with a mid-to-late systolic murmur and Doppler echocardiographic evidence of mid-to-late systolic MR suggest MVP (Video 10).[29] In the absence of any other structural changes in the valve, with MVP alone the degree of MR is usually mild. Similarly, horses can have echocardiographic changes suggesting tricuspid valve prolapse[31] but this can be difficult to diagnose confidently due to the restricted imaging planes that are available in the horse.

Physiologic valvular regurgitation is extremely common in equine athletes. In a large echocardiography study including 526 British racehorses, TR was reported in 80% to 90% of mature Thoroughbred racehorses and MR has a prevalence of 40% to 60% in mature Thoroughbred racehorses. Two-year-olds racing on the flat had the lowest prevalence.[12] The relationship between physiologic valvular regurgitation and valvular prolapse is unclear. To some extent, differences in opinion amongst equine clinicians

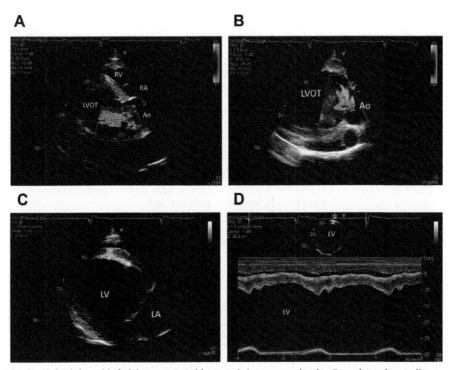

Fig. 3. Right (*A*) and left (*B*) parasternal long-axis images and color Doppler echocardiography of the left ventricular outflow tract (LVOT) and aorta (Ao) from a 20-year-old Thoroughbred stallion (575 kg). Aortic regurgitation (AR) had first been identified 5 years back. The region of interest for color flow Doppler has been positioned near the valve in both of these images and this shows that the regurgitant jet (green) is very wide. The sample volume must be moved in a series of cardiac cycles to fully evaluate the area of LVOT occupied by the jet, which confirmed that this jet was also long, subjectively occupying more than two-thirds of the LVOT (3 points, see **Table 1**). (*C*) The right parasternal 4-chamber image shows the left ventricle (LV) is very large and round (5 points). (*D*) An M-mode study of the LV at the chordal level shows that when allometrically scaled to a body weight of 500 kg, the internal diameter of the LV in diastole is 18.5 cm (3 points). Thus, the combined grade is 11 points, indicating severe AR.[20] Note, the diameter of the LV continues to increase during diastole on the M-mode image, as ventricular filling continues during mid-diastole due to the AR. LA, left atrium; RA, right atrium; RV, right ventricle. This case is also illustrated in Videos 1–5.

may reflect the individuals' interpretation of the term "physiologic regurgitation." Physiologic regurgitation is usually interpreted as meaning that echocardiography demonstrated regurgitation but no evidence of valvular disease, which, depending on the clinicians' preference, may or may not include valvular prolapse. However, it is probably preferable not to conflate the 2 phenomena. In a small study, physiologic regurgitation did not seem to parallel valvular prolapse.[30] Furthermore, physiologic regurgitation in the athlete increases with cardiac adaptation to exercise[32] and it is not known whether mitral and tricuspid valve prolapse is training related.

Aortic valve prolapse (AVP) is also a common echocardiographic finding in horses. Diagnostic criteria of its identification have been developed by consultation amongst equine cardiologists coupled with an optimization study.[33] Aortic valve prolapse can be created artefactually during echocardiography, in particular if there is triangulation of the outflow tract or downward angulation of the septum. Criteria developed to

Table 1
Severity grading system for equine aortic regurgitation

Point	Criteria
	Subjective assessment of the regurgitant jet, based on the size and area of the jet compared with the left ventricular outflow tract in diastole (LVOTd), choosing either left or right parasternal jet-orientated views to maximise the jet size
1	Mild: a small jet that occupies $<^1/_3$ of LVOTd
2	Moderate: a larger jet that occupies $<^2/_3$ of LVOTd
3	SEVERE: very large jet that occupies $>^2/_3$ of LVOTd
	Subjective assessment of left ventricular size in the four-chamber view
1	Normal ventricle, no signs of enlargement, normal apex shape
2	Normally shaped ventricle, mild enlargement, normal apex shape
3	Large ventricle with normal shape, apex slightly rounder than normal
4	Large ventricle, apex with globoid shape
5	Severe enlargement with a very large, rounded ventricle
	M mode measurement of left ventricular internal diameter in diastole, normalised for body weight (BW), that is, measured diameter/$BW^{1/3} \times 500^{1/3}$
1	12–13 cm
2	13–14 cm
3	$\geq$14 cm
Combined grade	
$\leq$4	Mild aortic regurgitation
5–7	Moderate aortic regurgitation
$\geq$8	Severe aortic regurgitation

Data from Ven S, Decloedt A, Van Der Vekens N, et al. Assessing aortic regurgitation severity from 2D, M-mode and pulsed wave Doppler echocardiographic measurements in horses. Vet J 2016;210:34–8.

consistently and repeatedly identify AVP involve visualization of downward displacement of an aortic cusp in 3 consecutive cardiac cycles and in 2 image planes. For the right-sided parasternal long-axis view of the left ventricular outflow tract and aortic valve, the image is obtained from the right fourth intercostal space, with the interventricular septum perpendicular to the ultrasound beam, the walls of the aorta parallel, and 2 aortic valve cusps visible. The optimal short-axis images are also obtained from the right fourth intercostal space, with the aortic valve centered in the middle of the images and all 3 cusps visible, the tricuspid valve in the near field and the pulmonic valve in the far field. Aortic valve prolapse is defined as mild when less than one-third of the cusp prolapsed in the latter half to third of diastole, moderate when the whole cusp prolapses throughout diastole forming a slight curve, and severe when the cusp forms an obvious C shape. Prolapse of any cusp is identified in short-axis images when opposing edges of the cusps meet and then move out of the imaging plane during diastole. These criteria have been found to have good reproducibility and repeatability for identification of AVP (**Fig. 5**).[33] The relationship between AVP and aortic valve disease has not been clarified and, as MVP, it can be seen without other echocardiographic evidence of valvular pathology (see **Fig. 5**; Video 11). Cross-sectional studies in Thoroughbreds suggest increased prevalence is associated with age and training,[34] but currently there is no robust evidence to suggest that AVP is a risk factor for degenerative disease in horses.

INFECTIVE ENDOCARDITIS

Infective endocarditis usually is a bacterial or rarely fungal infection of the valvular or mural endocardium. The most common site of infection is the mitral valve, closely

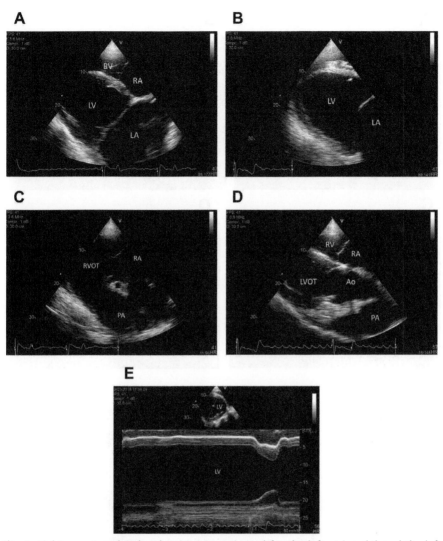

Fig. 4. Right parasternal 4-chamber images optimized for the left atrium (*A*) and the left ventricle (*B*) from a 19-year-old Thoroughbred gelding with severe and long-standing degenerative mitral valve disease. The images show that the mitral valve is diffusely thickened, the left ventricle (LV) is dilated and rounded at the apex, and the left atrium (LA) is dilated. (*C*) Right parasternal long-axis views of the right ventricular outflow tract (RVOT) and (*D*) the left ventricular outflow tract (LVOT) show that the pulmonary artery (PA) is dilated, which is identified by comparing the diameters of the PA and aorta (Ao). (*E*) An M-mode recording confirms LV dilation. Note that the M-mode was obtained during post-examination analysis using an anatomic M-mode tool, which can be very helpful in optimizing placement of the M-mode cursor, particularly when the heart is enlarged as in this case. Also note that the electrocardiographs (ECGs) show atrial fibrillation with a ventricular response rate of 47 to 56 bpm. RA, right atrium; RV, right ventricle. This case is also illustrated in Videos 6–9.

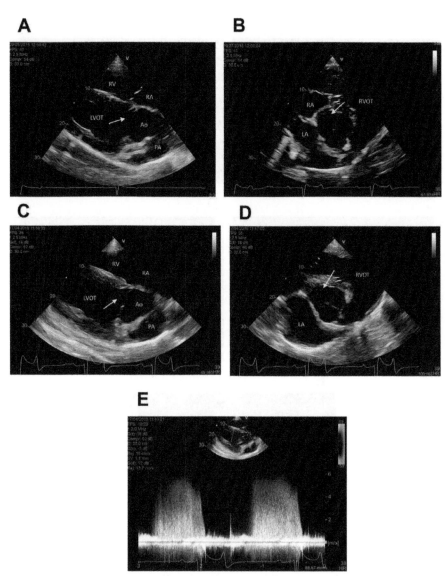

Fig. 5. Aortic valve prolapse (*arrows*) in (*A*) a right parasternal long-axis image of the left ventricular outflow tract (LVOT) and (*B*) a right parasternal short-axis image of the heart base in a 10-year-old horse with no detectable aortic regurgitation. In the long-axis image, the noncoronary cusp is curved throughout diastole, and in the short-axis image, the edge of noncoronary cusp is not opposed with the adjacent right coronary cusp, confirming the prolapse in 2 perpendicular planes, confirming that it is a genuine finding. Similar but more severe changes can be seen in images (*C*) and (*D*) from a 10-year-old Thoroughbred gelding. This horse also has nodular changes on the aortic valve, suggesting degenerative pathology and (*E*) aortic regurgitation, demonstrated here with continuous-wave Doppler echocardiography. Ao, aorta; LA, left atrium; PA, pulmonary artery; RA, right atrium; RV, right ventricle; RVOT, right ventricular outflow tract.

followed by the aortic valve.[35] The tricuspid valve most frequently occurs in horses with septic jugular vein thrombophlebitis.[36,37] Horses of all ages can be affected, but the condition is more common in younger animals and has been reported in males more than females.[35] A combination of endothelial damage and bacteremia are prerequisites for the development of infective endocarditis. However, documented associations between preexisting heart disease and infective endocarditis in horses are limited to one case in a horse with ventricular septal defect.[38] A wide range of organisms have been implicated in equine infective endocarditis, with no single group dominating and *Pasteurella/Actinobacillus spp.*,[36,39] *Pseudomonas spp.*,[40,41] and *Rhodococcus equi*[42,43] being slightly more common in equine reports. In humans, potential routes of infection include dental infection, infection of other body systems, medical procedures, and intravenous drug abuse.[44] Bacteremia is common with equine dental procedures[45] and in horses infective endocarditis has been reported following dental procedures associated with *Fusobacterium necrophorum* in only one case[46] and a mixed growth of *Klebsiella spp,* gram-positive cocci, and gram-positive rods in another.[47]

Clinical signs depend on site and severity of the intracardiac infection, embolization of vegetations to any organ, the presence of bacteremia, and the development of immune-complex disease. Signs can vary in severity from a relatively mild febrile condition to severe systemic signs and heart failure. Presenting signs frequently include fever, shifting leg lameness, and synovial distension.[35] Large vegetative lesions may obstruct the outflow of blood from the chamber, resulting in a murmur of valvular stenosis. More often, vegetations lead to valvular regurgitation. It is important to be aware that with tricuspid valve involvement there may be no murmur.[36,37] Rupture of associated chordae tendineae will exacerbate regurgitation. There may also be concurrent myocarditis with arrhythmias.

Definitive diagnosis of infective endocarditis is established with echocardiography by identifying irregular, hypoechoic to echoic oscillating masses associated with the valve leaflet, chordae tendineae, or mural endocardium (**Fig. 6**, Video 12). Small lesions can be difficult to identify, so echocardiography should not be relied on to definitively rule out the condition. Echocardiography is also used to assess the impact of the lesions by assessing the degree of regurgitation and chamber enlargement. In early cases, there may be minimal chamber enlargement, but repeated echocardiographic examinations may identify its development.[43] Ideally, 3 serial blood cultures at 1-hour intervals should be obtained before treatment with antimicrobials. Assay of cardiac troponin I can be helpful to identify myocardial involvement. Typically, there is neutrophilic leukocytosis with hyperfibrinogenemia, hyperglobulinemia, and anemia of chronic disease. Azotemia may be detected in horses with renal emboli or may be prerenal in horses with low cardiac output.[35]

The prognosis is primarily determined by the valve affected and severity of valvular damage that develops and is also likely to be influenced by the organism involved and the response to antimicrobial treatment. Cases with involvement of the mitral valve have a particularly grave prognosis.[43] Even when bacteriologic cure is achieved, severe valvular regurgitation can ultimately lead to heart failure. Selection of antimicrobials should be broad-spectrum or whenever possible based on culture and sensitivity results. Antibiotics with good tissue penetration should be chosen. This is a life-threatening condition and therefore, despite concerns regarding antimicrobial resistance, treatment with the critically important antimicrobials, fluoroquinolones, macrolides, or cephalosporins is often warranted. Nonsteroidal antiinflammatory drugs are also indicated.

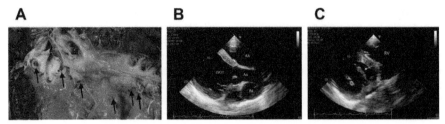

Fig. 6. (*A*) Infective endocarditis most commonly affects the mitral and aortic valve. In this 4-month-old Thoroughbred filly both valves have vegetative lesions (*arrows*). Note the pathologist has removed sections of both valves before this image being captured (*asterisks*). (*B*) A long-axis image of the left ventricular outflow tract shows a shaggy vegetation on the aortic valve from the same filly. Subjective comparison of the diameters of the pulmonary artery (PA) and aorta (Ao) shows the PA is disproportionately large, consistent with pulmonary hypertension. Note there is a reverberation artifact in the right ventricle, likely due to poor skin contact. (*C*) A short-axis image of the mitral valve shows marked thickening of the septal cusp (*arrow*) and vegetations on the nonseptal cusp (*asterisks*). LVOT, left ventricular outflow tract; RA, right atrium. This case is also illustrated in Video 12.

OTHER FORMS OF EQUINE ACQUIRED VALVULAR DISEASES

In comparison with equine degenerative valvular disease, other forms of valvular pathology are fairly rare. Rupture of one or more chordae tendineae can occur spontaneously or be associated with preexisting degenerative disease or infective endocarditis (**Figs. 7** and **8**, Video 13).[24,31,48–50] The mitral valve is the most common site. Tearing of the aortic or pulmonary valve creates similarly catastrophic valvular regurgitation.[51] Because of the rapid change in hemodynamics, horses with ruptured chordae tendineae will often develop signs of acute left-sided heart failure, including coughing, foamy nasal discharge, and moist crackles on auscultation of the lung fields. Sudden death is also possible. Rupture of a chorda tendinea will often create a very honking or musical murmur and flail of the affected valve cusp is visualized echocardiographically.[24] With very acute onset regurgitation associated with ruptured

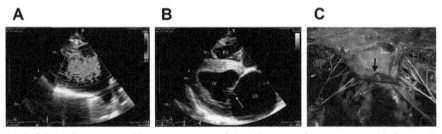

Fig. 7. (*A*) A left parasternal long-axis image of the left atrium from a 5-year-old Thoroughbred gelding with severe mitral regurgitation, displayed in color Doppler mode. The green color depicts turbulent regurgitant flow during systole. (*B*) A flail portion of the septal cusp (*white arrow*) is visible on the septal cusp of the mitral valve, corresponding to (*C*) rupture of a chorda tendinea, confirmed at post mortem (*black arrows*). The upper portion of the rupture chorda has become adherent to the underside of the associated valve leaflet. Note the ECG (*A*) demonstrates rapid atrial fibrillation and both echocardiographic images show marked left atrial (LA) dilation. LA, left atrium; LV, left ventricle; RV, right ventricle. The pathology image was provided by Dr A Foote, Rossdales LLP. This case is also illustrated in Video 13.

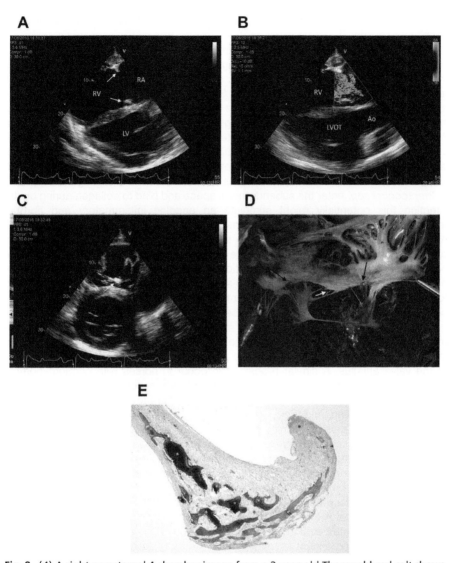

Fig. 8. (*A*) A right parasternal 4-chamber image from a 2-year-old Thoroughbred colt shows severe right ventricular dilation and thickening and distortion of the tricuspid valve (*arrows*) with (*B*) severe tricuspid regurgitation (TR) visible in the right parasternal left ventricular outflow tract (LVOT) image. Green color indicates turbulent systolic regurgitant flow. (*C*) A short-axis image of the level of the atrioventricular valves frozen in systole demonstrates that the tricuspid valve cusps are not opposed and have echogenic modular changes (*arrows*). (*D*) Grossly, the tricuspid valve is markedly thickened and fibrotic with loss of division between the cusps and mineralized nodules near the cusp edges (*black arrows*). There is secondary rupture of a chorda tendinea (*white arrow*), which was not appreciated echocardiographically. (*E*) Histologically, mineralization and ossification are evident (white *asterisks*), but there is only mild evidence of inflammation (black *asterisk*). Ao, aorta; LV, left ventricle; LVOT, left ventricular outflow tract; MV, mitral valve; RA, right atrium; RV, right ventricle; RVOT, right ventricular outflow tract. The pathology images were provided by Dr A Foote, Rossdales LLP. This case is also illustrated in Video 14.

chorda tendinea or semilunar valve cusp tears, chamber dilation may not be evident despite its severity.[31]

Nonseptic valvulitis is also discussed in the equine literature, but relatively little is known of its pathogenesis or epidemiology. In humans, it has long been considered that this is an immune-mediated disease, relating to molecular mimicry and cross-reactivity between antibodies against the Streptococcal M protein and cardiac epitopes.[52] However, more recently, evidence has emerged suggesting that the relevant immunologic target is the Streptococcal group A carbohydrate and that antibodies then cross-react with host contractile proteins. Importantly, these proteins are intracellular and thus are sequestered. Alternative candidate cell surface targets include laminin or other basement membrane proteins. Collagen is also a potential site of inflammation, yet M protein antibody does not cross-react with collagen. However, if *Streptococci spp.* enter the subendothelial space and bind to collagen during acute infection this potentially might stimulate an ongoing inflammatory and fibrotic response within the extracellular space despite healing of the overlying endothelium.[53] Although it is tempting to assume that a similar process might occur in horses, this proposal is entirely speculative. In some horses, extensive valvular pathology can occur accompanied by severe regurgitation and clinical signs, yet it is impossible to determine the pathogenesis. In the end-stage fibrotic valve, it can be very difficult to distinguish an inflammatory cause from congenital dysplasia with echocardiography or indeed pathologic examination (see **Fig 8**; Video 14).

In humans, valvular regurgitation can also arise secondary to ischemic papillary muscle dysfunction[54] and dilation of great vessels[55] or cardiac chambers, whereas in dogs MR is a common consequence of dilated cardiomyopathy and stretching of the valve annulus. A similar process can occur in horses with cardiomyopathy (**Fig 9**) and dilation of the valve annulus can lead to MR secondary to chronic severe AR.[19] Similarly, severe pulmonary hypertension can lead to right heart enlargement, pulmonic regurgitation, and tricuspid annular dilation with secondary TR (see Videos 6–9). Transient or persistent mitral or TR can be observed with papillary muscle ischemia or necrosis, impairing the normal systolic function of the valve apparatus. The aortic root is often dilated in horses with moderate or severe AR.[19,20] However, it is generally assumed that this is a consequence of AR rather than a predisposing pathology and has only been described in horses with echocardiographic evidence of concurrent valvular pathology.[19] In contrast, in humans, aortic root dilation is associated with functional AR in the presence of anatomically normal valve cusps. Aortic root dilation stimulates aortic cusp enlargement, but cusp adaptation and distensibility are limited in prominent asymmetrical aortic root dilation and this leads to progressive AR.[55]

CLINICAL MANAGEMENT OF HORSES WITH ACQUIRED VALVULAR DISEASE

Although horses with severe valvular regurgitation can be managed with drugs including ACE inhibitors,[56,57] pimobendan,[58] and diuretics, the major clinical focus is usually on assessment and prognostication rather than medication. Currently, although there is mounting evidence to support early intervention and treatment of subclinical canine valvular disease in dogs,[59–61] there is no evidence in horses with valvular regurgitation that the early introduction of medication aimed at neuroendocrine targets affects disease progression, preserves performance, or extends life expectancy. Guidelines for the clinical management of athletic horses with cardiovascular abnormalities have been defined in a joint ACVIM/ECEIM consensus statement.[29] Key common elements for all forms of acquired valvular disease are that (1)

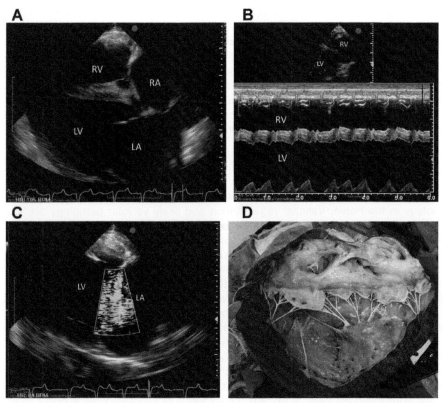

Fig. 9. (*A*) A right parasternal 4-chamber image from a 3-year-old Thoroughbred gelding shows dilation of all chambers and mild thickening of the mitral valve. (*B*) An M-mode echo-cardiogram of the left (LV) and right (RV) ventricle confirms severe biventricular enlarge-ment. Note that the image plane does not truly bisect the RV and, due to cardiomegaly, the LV free wall is not visualized fully on this 30 cm image. Atrial fibrillation is present. (*C*) A left parasternal long-axis image in color Doppler mode demonstrates mitral regurgita-tion secondary to dilation of the mitral valve annulus. (*D*) Post mortem examination confirmed dilation of all 4 chambers and cardiomyopathy of unknown cause. Both the tricuspid and mitral valves showed slight thickening and oedema, which was considered to be secondary changes relating to turbulence. The pathology image was provided by Dr A Foote, Rossdales LLP.

detailed assessment of likely cause and severity is essential to rational clinical decision-making and (2) the impact of cardiac disease both on the horse's perfor-mance and on quality of life and its potential significance with regards rider and driver safety must be given priority. Many horses with MR can perform to their owners' ex-pectations; however, MR can limit performance, be a risk factor for atrial fibrillation (see **Fig 4**) and other arrhythmias, and occasionally lead to heart failure.[1,24] Aortic regurgitation is typically a condition of the older horse, nevertheless in many equestrian sports, middle-aged and older animals remain competitive. In horses with AR that are in work, exercising and ambulatory ECG are important tools with which to identify concurrent, potentially malignant, or fatal ventricular ectopy (see Videos 1–5). Recommendations for both MR and AR include regular monitoring of heart rate and rhythm; annual cardiological reassessment of MR (or if mild, every other year) and biannual reassessment of AR until it is established the condition is stable; and exercising ECG with moderate or severe MR and AR, rapidly progressive regurgitation, and in cases in which atrial fibrillation, ventricular ectopy, or other arrhythmias are suspected. TR is common in athletes,[1,12] whereas valvular pathology is much less frequently seen in this cohort. Recommendations for horses that on initial examination are shown to have structural or motional abnormalities of the tricuspid valve or right-sided chamber dilation is more guarded. Recommendations in the ACVIM/ECEIM consensus statement suggest annual reassessment of moderate and severe TR and urge clinicians to appreciate the high prevalence of training-induced TR in performance horses.[29]

SUMMARY

Degenerative myxomatous disease is the commonest form of acquired valvular pathology in the horse. Valvular regurgitation and likely valvular pathology are age related. Poor prognostic indicators for equine AR specifically include ventricular ectopy, increased pulse pressure (>60 mm Hg), and hyperkinetic pulses. Risk factors for progression of other forms of equine valvular disease remain relatively unexplored. Atrial fibrillation and left atrial dilation can accompany moderate MR, and severe MR can lead to pulmonary hypertension, RV dilation, and congestive heart failure. However, mild degenerative valvular disease often is of minimal clinical relevance and overall life expectancy does not seem to be affected by its presence. Valvular prolapse is an important risk factor for severe valvular regurgitation in other species but a link between this functional abnormality and subsequent structural change has not been established in the horse. Infective endocarditis is associated with a range of organisms, the presentation includes fever and other systemic signs accompanying valvular regurgitation, and overall the prognosis is poor, warranting aggressive therapy. Other forms of valvular disease occur rarely in the horse, and most of these present with relatively severe regurgitation. Management of horses with valvular disease can include palliative medication but is mainly focused on assessment of severity and regular echocardiographic and ECG monitoring.

SUPPLEMENTARY DATA

Supplementary data related to this article can be found online at https://doi.org/10.1016/j.cveq.2018.12.001.

REFERENCES

1. Leroux AA, Detilleux J, Sandersen CF, et al. Prevalence and risk factors for cardiac diseases in a hospital-based population of 3,434 horses (1994-2011). J Vet Intern Med 2013;27(6):1563–70.
2. Else RW, Holmes JR. Cardiac pathology in the horse. 1. gross pathology. Equine Vet J 1972;4(1):1–8.
3. Else RW, Holmes JR. Cardiac pathology in the horse. 2. Microscopic pathology. Equine Vet J 1972;4(2):57–62.
4. Fox PR. Pathology of myxomatous mitral valve disease in the dog. J Vet Cardiol 2012;14(1):103–26.
5. Connell PS, Han RI, Grande-Allen KJ. Differentiating the aging of the mitral valve from human and canine myxomatous degeneration. J Vet Cardiol 2012;14(1):31–45.

6. Aupperle H, Disatian S. Pathology, protein expression and signaling in myxomatous mitral valve degeneration: comparison of dogs and humans. J Vet Cardiol 2012;14(1):59–71.

7. Bowen IM, Marr CM, Chester AH, et al. In-vitro contraction of the equine aortic valve. J Heart Valve Dis 2004;13(4):593–9.

8. Orton EC, Lacerda CM, MacLea HB. Signaling pathways in mitral valve degeneration. J Vet Cardiol 2012;14(1):7–17.

9. Culshaw GJ, French AT, Han RI, et al. Evaluation of innervation of the mitral valves and the effects of myxomatous degeneration in dogs. Am J Vet Res 2010;7(12): 194–202.

10. Corcoran BM, Black A, Anderson H, et al. Identification of surface morphologic changes in the mitral valve leaflets and chordae tendineae of dogs with myxomatous degeneration. Am J Vet Res 2004;65(2):198–206.

11. Richards JM, Farrar EJ, Kornreich BG, et al. The mechanobiology of mitral valve function, degeneration, and repair. J Vet Cardiol 2012;14(1):47–58.

12. Young LE, Rogers K, Wood JL. Heart murmurs and valvular regurgitation in thoroughbred racehorses: epidemiology and associations with athletic performance. J Vet Intern Med 2008;22(2):418–26.

13. Imhasly A, Tschudi PR, Lombard CW, et al. Clinical and echocardiographic features of mild mitral valve regurgitation in 108 horses. Vet J 2010;183(2): 166–71.

14. Gehlen H, et al. A survey of the frequency and development of heart disease in riding-horses - part 2: clinical and echocardiographic follow-up examination. Pferdeheilkunde 2007;4:378–87.

15. Horn JNR. Sympathetic nervous control of cardiac function and its role in equine heart disease. London: 2002.

16. Stevens KB, Marr CM, Horn JN, et al. Effect of left-sided valvular regurgitation on mortality and causes of death among a population of middle-aged and older horses. Vet Rec 2009;164(1):6–10.

17. Ireland JL, McGowan CM, Clegg PD, et al. A survey of health care and disease in geriatric horses aged 30 years or older. Vet J 2012;192(1):57–64.

18. Boegli J, et al. Diagnostic value of noninvasive pulse pressure measurements in horses with aortic regurgitation. J Vet Intern Med 2018;32(2):876.

19. Reef VB, Spencer P. Echocardiographic evaluation of equine aortic insufficiency. Am J Vet Res 1987;48(6):904–9.

20. Ven S, Decloedt A, Van Der Vekens N, et al. Assessing aortic regurgitation severity from 2D, M-mode and pulsed wave Doppler echocardiographic measurements in horses. Vet J 2016;210:34–8.

21. Ven S, Decloedt A, De Clercq D, et al. Detection of subclinical left ventricular dysfunction by tissue Doppler imaging in horses with aortic regurgitation. Equine Vet J 2018;50:587–93.

22. Rovira S, Munoz A, Rodilla V. Allometric scaling of echocardiographic measurements in healthy Spanish foals with different body weight. Res Vet Sci 2009;86: 325–31.

23. Huesler IM, Mitchell KJ, Schwarzwald CC. Echocardiographic assessment of left atrial size and function in warmblood horses: reference intervals, allometric scaling, and agreement of different echocardiographic variables. J Vet Intern Med 2016;30(4):1241–52.

24. Reef VB, Bain FT, Spencer PA. Severe mitral regurgitation in horses: clinical, echocardiographic and pathological findings. Equine Vet J 1998;30(1):18–27.

25. Gehlen H, Bubeck K, Stadler P. Pulmonary artery wedge pressure measurement in healthy warmblood horses and in warmblood horses with mitral valve insufficiencies of various degrees during standardised treadmill exercise. Res Vet Sci 2004;77(3):257–64.

26. Koenig TR, Mitchell KJ, Schwarzwald CC. Echocardiographic assessment of left ventricular function in healthy horses and in horses with heart disease using pulsed-wave tissue doppler imaging. J Vet Intern Med 2017;31(2):556–67.

27. Orton EC. Mitral valve degeneration: still more questions than answers. J Mol Cell Cardiol 2012;14(1):3–5.

28. Freed LA, Levy D, Levine RA, et al. Prevalence and clinical outcome of mitral-valve prolapse. N Engl J Med 1999;341(1):1–7.

29. Reef VB, Bonagura J, Buhl R, et al. Recommendations for management of equine athletes with cardiovascular abnormalities. J Vet Intern Med 2014;28(3):749–61.

30. Marr CM, Reef VB. Physiological valvular regurgitation in clinically normal young racehorses: prevalence and two-dimensional colour flow Doppler echocardiographic characteristics. Equine Vet J Suppl 1995;(19):56–62.

31. Marr CM, Love S, Pirie HM, et al. Confirmation by Doppler echocardiography of valvular regurgitation in a horse with a ruptured chorda tendinea of the mitral valve. Vet Rec 1990;127(15):376–9.

32. Young LE, Wood JL. Effect of age and training on murmurs of atrioventricular valvular regurgitation in young thoroughbreds. Equine Vet J 2000;32(3):195–9.

33. Hallowell GD, Bowen M. Reliability and identification of aortic valve prolapse in the horse. BMC Vet Res 2013;9:9.

34. Hallowell GD. Aortic vavlue prolapse in the horse. Nottingham: 2010.

35. Porter SR, Saegerman C, van Galen G, et al. Vegetative endocarditis in equids (1994–2006). J Vet Intern Med 2008;22(6):1411–6.

36. Maxson AD, Reef VB. Bacterial endocarditis in horses: ten cases (1984-1995). Equine Vet J 1997;29(5):394–9.

37. Ramzan PHL. Vegetative bacterial endocarditis associated with septic tenosynovitis of the digital sheath in a Thoroughbred racehorse. Equine Vet Educ 2000; 12(3):120–3.

38. Froehlich W, et al. Tricuspid valve endocarditis in a horse with ventricular septal defect. Equine Vet Educ 2006;18(4):172–6.

39. Church S, Harrigan KE, Irving AE, et al. Endocarditis caused by Pasteurella caballi in a horse. Aust Vet J 1998;76(8):528–30.

40. Buergelt CD, Cooley AJ, Hines SA, et al. Endocarditis in six horses. Vet Pathol 1985;22(4):333–7.

41. Travers CW, van den Berg JS. Pseudomonas spp. associated vegetative endocarditis in two horses. J S Afr Vet Assoc 1995;66(3):172–6.

42. Collatos C, Clark ES, Reef VB, et al. Septicemia, atrial fibrillation, cardiomegaly, left atrial mass, and Rhodococcus equi septic osteoarthritis in a foal. J Am Vet Med Assoc 1990;197(8):1039–42.

43. Marr CM. Cardiovascular infections. In: Sellon DC, Long MT, editors. Equine infectious diseases. St Louis (MO): Elsevier; 2014. p. 21–41.

44. Stuesse DC, Vlessis AA. Epidemiology of native valve endocarditis. In: Vlessis AA, Bolling SF, editors. Endocarditis: a multidisciplinary approach to modern treatment. Armonk (NY): Futura Publishing; 1999. p. 77–84.

45. Kern I, Bartmann CP, Verspohl J, et al. Bacteraemia before, during and after tooth extraction in horses in the absence of antimicrobial administration. Equine Vet J 2017;49(2):178–82.

46. Bartmann CP, et al. Dentogenous sinusitis caused by gram-negative anaerobes in horses. Tierarztliche Praxis Ausgabe G Grosst Nutzt 2002;30(3):178–83.
47. Verdegaal EJMM, De Heer N, Meerens NM. A right-sided bacterial endocarditis of dental origin in a horse. Equine Vet Educ 2006;18(4):191–5.
48. Brown CM, Bell TG, Paradis MR, et al. Rupture of mitral chordae tendineae in two horses. J Am Vet Med Assoc 1983;182(3):281–3.
49. Holmes JR, Miller PJ. Three cases of ruptured mitral valve chordae in the horse. Equine Vet J 1984;16(2):125–35.
50. Reef VB. Mitral valvular insufficiency associated with ruptured chordae tendineae in three foals. J Am Vet Med Assoc 1987;191(3):329–31.
51. Reimer JM, Reef VB, Sommer M. Echocardiographic detection of pulmonic valve rupture in a horse with right-sided heart failure. J Am Vet Med Assoc 1991;198(5):880–2.
52. Cunningham MW. Rheumatic fever, autoimmunity, and molecular mimicry: the streptococcal connection. Int Rev Immunol 2014;33(4):314–29.
53. Tandon R, Sharma M, Chandrashekhar Y, et al. Revisiting the pathogenesis of rheumatic fever and carditis. Nat Rev Cardiol 2013;10(3):171–7.
54. Pierard LA, Carabello BA. Ischaemic mitral regurgitation: pathophysiology, outcomes and the conundrum of treatment. Eur Heart J 2010;31(24):2996–3005.
55. Kim DH, Handschumacher MD, Levine RA, et al. Aortic valve adaptation to aortic root dilatation: insights into the mechanism of functional aortic regurgitation from 3-dimensional cardiac computed tomography. Circ Cardiovasc Imaging 2014;7(5):828–35.
56. Gehlen H, Vieht JC, Stadler P. Effects of the ACE inhibitor quinapril on echocardiographic variables in horses with mitral valve insufficiency. J Vet Med A Physiol Pathol Clin Med 2003;50(9):460–5.
57. Afonso T, Giguère S, Brown SA, et al. Preliminary investigation of orally administered benazepril in horses with left-sided valvular regurgitation. Equine Vet J 2018;50(4):446–51.
58. Afonso T, Giguère S, Rapoport G, et al. Cardiovascular effects of pimobendan in healthy mature horses. Equine Vet J 2016;48(3):352–6.
59. Summerfield NJ, Boswood A, O'Grady MR, et al. Efficacy of pimobendan in the prevention of congestive heart failure or sudden death in Doberman Pinschers with preclinical dilated cardiomyopathy (the PROTECT Study). J Vet Intern Med 2012;26(6):1337–49.
60. Haggstrom J, Boswood A, O'Grady M, et al. Longitudinal analysis of quality of life, clinical, radiographic, echocardiographic, and laboratory variables in dogs with myxomatous mitral valve disease receiving pimobendan or benazepril: the QUEST study. J Vet Intern Med 2013;27(6):1441–51.
61. Boswood A, Häggström J, Gordon SG, et al. Effect of pimobendan in dogs with preclinical myxomatous mitral valve disease and cardiomegaly: the EPIC study-a randomized clinical trial. J Vet Intern Med 2016;30(6):1765–79.

Pericardial Disease, Myocardial Disease, and Great Vessel Abnormalities in Horses

Annelies Decloedt, DVM, PhD

KEYWORDS

- Pericarditis • Myocarditis • Cardiomyopathy • Aortocardiac fistula
- Aortopulmonary fistula

KEY POINTS

- Pericardial disease, myocardial disease, and great vessel abnormalities are relatively rare in horses compared with other species.
- Pericardial and myocardial disease can be idiopathic or immune-mediated, or the consequence of a wide variety of causes including infectious agents, intoxication, neoplasia, or trauma.
- Aortic rupture is most common in older animals or in the Friesian breed, and can lead to hemopericardium, hemothorax, or formation of an aortocardiac or aortopulmonary fistula.
- As the clinical signs are often nonspecific and vague, the diagnosis is mainly based on echocardiography, electrocardiography, and laboratory analysis.
- The prognosis depends on the etiology and disease stage, ranging from full recovery of athletic function to high case fatality.

 Video content accompanies this article at http://www.vetequine.theclinics.com

INTRODUCTION

Compared with other species, horses rarely develop pericardial, myocardial, or great vessel disease. In human medicine, myocardial ischemia caused by coronary artery disease is globally among the most common causes of death. In small animals, the prevalence of hypertrophic cardiomyopathy is around 15% in cats, and the prevalence of dilated cardiomyopathy is as high as 60% in certain dog breeds.[1,2] The horse is almost free of these diseases, which may be linked to centuries of genetic selection

Disclosure Statement: There are no commercial or financial conflicts of interest.
Department of Large Animal Internal Medicine, Faculty of Veterinary Medicine, Ghent University, Salisburylaan 133, Merelbeke 9820, Belgium
E-mail address: annelies.decloedt@ugent.be

Vet Clin Equine 35 (2019) 139–157
https://doi.org/10.1016/j.cveq.2018.12.005
0749-0739/19/© 2018 Elsevier Inc. All rights reserved.

for performance. Genome-wide sequencing demonstrated that the cardiac system was a key domestication target, with evidence for positive selection for multiple genes for which defects are associated with cardiomyopathy.[3] Pericardial, myocardial, and great vessel diseases have not yet been reported in comprehensive prevalence studies in horses; only isolated case reports or case series are available. However, the equine veterinarian is likely to encounter a horse with pericardial, myocardial, or great vessel disease during his or her career.[4]

The clinical signs are often vague, nonspecific, or related to the underlying etiology. The owner mainly recognizes lethargy, exercise intolerance, or both. Signs on physical examination might include tachycardia, fever, venous distension or jugular pulsation, a weak or bounding arterial pulse, ventral edema, and abnormal cardiac auscultation such as arrhythmia, a murmur, or muffled heart sounds. Sometimes cardiac arrest and sudden death are encountered without preceding warning signs. The prognosis depends on the underlying cause and stage of the disease, and ranges from full recovery and normal athletic function to a poor prognosis with high case fatality rates. However, studies reporting prognosis or mortality in larger groups of affected horses are rare.[5–7] This article focuses on the etiology, diagnosis, prognosis, and treatment of the different types of pericardial, myocardial, and great vessel diseases in horses.

PERICARDIAL DISEASE
Pericarditis

Pericarditis can be effusive, fibrinous, or constrictive, with fibrino-effusive pericarditis as the most common form.[8] Effusive pericarditis is defined as pericardial inflammation resulting in fluid accumulation within the pericardial sac. This leads to cardiac compression (tamponade) when the pressure within the pericardium exceeds the pressure within the heart, resulting in reduced ventricular filling and diastolic dysfunction. Because of the lower right-sided pressures, the main consequence is impaired venous return to the right heart, resulting in clinical signs of right-sided congestive heart failure (CHF). Diastolic filling abruptly ends when the pericardial limits are reached, resulting in decreased cardiac output.[9] Acute pericardial effusion has a greater impact than slowly developing effusion, as the pericardium cannot stretch to accommodate the larger volume. Fibrinous pericarditis is characterized by accumulation of fibrin in the pericardium, with or without free fluid.[8] In constrictive pericarditis, the pericardium is fibrotic and thickened, resulting in cardiac compression.

Pericardial disease is mainly idiopathic, but can also have an immune-mediated, bacterial, or viral origin.[8] Pericardial effusion is also an endpoint in the pathogenesis of multiple diseases such as neoplasia or congestive heart failure, and has been associated with pleuritis or pleuropneumonia (**Table 1**).[8,10,11] Idiopathic pericarditis might in fact have a viral origin in most cases, either through direct cytopathic effects or immune-mediated mechanisms. About one-third of the cases in larger case series is bacterial in origin, with *Actinobacillus* spp. often reported.[12] *Actinobacillus* spp. were also the most commonly identified isolates in the outbreaks of effusive pericarditis in the United States as part of the mare reproductive loss syndrome.[13] The proposed pathogenesis was exposure to eastern tent caterpillars, resulting in alterations of the immune system and secondary opportunistic invasion of commensal pericardiotrophic bacteria.

The clinical signs are related to the underlying condition and impaired ventricular filling, which depends on the amount of effusion and rate of accumulation. In early stages, the signs are often vague and nonspecific, whereas chronic cases might show right-sided CHF. The history includes signs of respiratory or systemic disease, such as fever, depression, lethargy, exercise intolerance, anorexia, weight loss, colic,

Table 1
Potential etiologies of pericardial disease (effusion, pericarditis, mass lesions) in horses

Etiology	Reference
Viral	
Equine herpes Virus-1	8
Bacterial	
Actinobacillus spp. – has been associated with mare reproductive loss syndrome	13,14
Pasteurella spp.	8,13,15
Streptococcus spp.	8
Mycoplasma felis	16
Corynebacterium pseudotuberculosis	17
Clostridium perfringens	18
Rhodococcus equi	19
Other reported results from pericardial culture: *Escherichia coli, Staphylococcus aureus, Pseudomonas* spp., *Acinetobacter, Enterococcus faecalis,* fungi	
Neoplasia	
Lymphoma (most common), mesothelioma, hemangiosarcoma	20
Mass lesion (intra- or extrapericardial) compressing the heart	
Pericardial effusion following systemic neoplastic disease	
Trauma: external, foreign body from gastrointestinal tract or iatrogenic during bone marrow aspiration	21–23
Pericardial effusion associated with myocardial disease (see **Box 1**) or congestive heart failure	
Immune-mediated (or virus-induced) – occasionally associated with vasculitis and hemolytic anemia	8
Idiopathic – often associated with respiratory disease	8,24
Hemopericardium following rib fracture or aortic root rupture	

or ventral edema.[8,24] Physical examination findings include tachycardia, abnormal heart sounds, tachypnea, venous distention or jugular pulsation, ventral edema, weak arterial pulses, pleural effusion, and ascites. Cardiac auscultation reveals mono-, bi-, or classically triphasic pericardial friction rubs in fibrinous pericarditis caused by rubbing of inflamed epicardial and pericardial surfaces, or muffled heart sounds in case of substantial effusion.[8] Electrocardiography (ECG) might show sinus tachycardia or premature complexes, with decreased amplitude of the QRS complexes and occasionally electrical alternans if the heart is swinging in large quantities of pericardial effusion.

Echocardiography is the most useful tool for diagnosis, guidance of pericardiocentesis, and monitoring disease progression or effect of treatment. Pleural fluid is often seen in horses with pericardial disease and should be distinguished from pericardial effusion. In effusive pericarditis, anechoic fluid is present between the pericardium and the epicardium, and the heart may appear to swing from side to side in the fluid (**Fig. 1**, Video 1). The pericardium is visible as an immobile echoic line, with or without fibrin deposition. With pleural effusion, fluid is seen outside the pericardial lining, and the compressed hypoechoic atelectatic lung tip is usually visualized floating in the fluid (**Fig. 2**). Cardiac tamponade caused by pericardial effusion may be detected based on collapse of the right atrium, early diastolic right ventricular (RV) collapse, decreased cardiac chamber dimensions, and impaired diastolic ventricular filling and systolic function. In fibrinous pericarditis, fibrin is visualized in the pericardial sac as shaggy

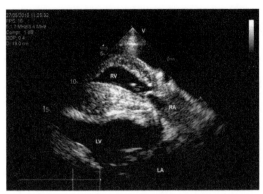

Fig. 1. Right parasternal long-axis 4-chamber view from a 6-year-old Warmblood mare with pericardial effusion following a cardiac glycoside intoxication. The pericardial effusion, indicated by green arrows, is visualized as anechoic fluid separating the pericardium and the epicardium (see Video 1 for corresponding image). LA, left atrium; LV, left ventricle; RA, right atrium; RV, right ventricle.

hypoechoic to hyperechoic strands (**Fig. 3**).[8,22] The diagnosis of constrictive pericarditis can be challenging, as pericardial thickening is more difficult to appreciate. One should be aware that pericardial fat might give the pericardial external surface an irregular and thickened appearance in healthy horses. Echocardiographic signs of pericardial constriction include the abrupt cessation of ventricular filling during early diastole, decreased left ventricular (LV) fractional shortening, and abnormal diastolic motion of the ventricular septum. This might be quantified by tissue Doppler imaging (TDI). Right-sided cardiac catheterization confirms the diagnosis of a constrictive process, with elevated central venous pressure, increased right atrial pressure, increased RV diastolic pressure, and a diastolic dip-and-plateau configuration of RV pressure reflecting the abrupt cessation of diastolic filling.[9,10]

Further diagnostic tests include laboratory analyses. Depending on the etiology, a neutrophilic leukocytosis, hyperfibrinogenemia, hyperproteinemia or anemia

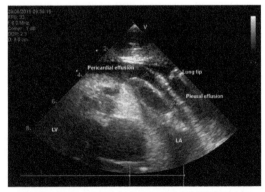

Fig. 2. Left parasternal long-axis view from an 11-year-old Shetland pony with pericardial and pleural effusion. The pericardium, indicated by green arrows, is visible as an immobile echoic line separating pericardial fluid and pleural fluid. The atelectatic lung tip is visible as a hypoechoic structure floating in the pleural fluid. LA, left atrium; LV, left ventricle.

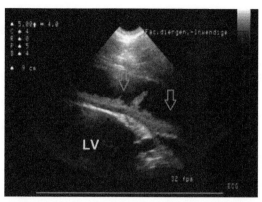

Fig. 3. Left parasternal long-axis view from a Warmblood horse with fibrinous pericarditis. Anechoic pericardial fluid is present, with fibrin visualized on the external surface of the pericardium as shaggy hyperechoic strands (*green arrows*). LV, left ventricle.

might be found. Other hematologic abnormalities are related to CHF and organ hypoperfusion, such as prerenal or renal azotemia, hyponatremia, and hyperkalemia. A sample of pericardial effusion can be acquired through pericardiocentesis or after placing an indwelling tube for pericardial lavage and drainage (**Box 1**).

The treatment of pericardial diseases varies depending on the etiology and clinical signs. The horse should receive stall rest during the course of treatment. Cardiac tamponade is a potentially life-threatening condition, requiring immediate, aggressive treatment by pericardiocentesis or catheter drainage. An indwelling catheter can be left in place to perform drainage, lavage, or local infusion of drugs (see **Box 1**). The use of diuretics is generally contraindicated, because ventricular filling is impaired and cardiac function highly dependent on increased filling pressures. Diuresis would therefore further impair cardiac performance. If cardiac tamponade is absent and the amount of effusion is small, pericardiocentesis or lavage using an indwelling drain might not be necessary or may even be contraindicated because of the risk of cardiac puncture.[4] Pericardiectomy could be attempted in constrictive pericarditis. In 1 case report, constrictive pericarditis and CHF recurred 6 weeks after the intervention.[9] In 2 other cases, attempted thoracoscopic pericardiectomy resulted in fatal hemorrhage and ventricular arrhythmia.[4] However, thoracoscopic transection of the parietal pericardium resulted in full recovery in 2 cases of chronic effusive fibrinous pericarditis.[4]

The prognosis for survival and athletic performance depends on the etiology, severity of the condition, early recognition, and prompt appropriate treatment. Although the prognosis is favorable for idiopathic pericarditis, the prognosis for bacterial pericarditis, especially cardiac or pericardial neoplasia, is guarded to poor. Fibrinous pericarditis might lead to constrictive pericarditis; therefore the prognosis is poor without prompt drainage and lavage. Constrictive pericarditis could also develop as a long-term complication; therefore follow-up by echocardiography is recommended. Thoroughbreds diagnosed with pericarditis at a young age have recently been reported to recover fully and reach their expected athletic potential, if pericarditis was diagnosed early and treated appropriately.[5]

MYOCARDIAL DISEASE

Myocardial disease is rarely diagnosed in horses, although the widespread use of cardiac biomarkers and echocardiography will probably increase the number of detected

---

Box 1
Pericardiocentesis, pericardial lavage, drainage and treatment of pericarditis

- Procedure
  - Always preceded/guided by echocardiography
  - Puncture usually from left fourth to fifth intercostal space dorsal to thoracic vein
  - Needle, Tuohy epidural needle, catheter, teat cannula, or chest tube
  - Continuous ECG monitoring, indwelling intravenous catheter in place to administer anti-arrhythmic drugs if necessary
  - Aseptic preparation, local anesthesia, stab incision of the skin using a scalpel blade
  - Potential complications: arrhythmias, hemorrhage
- Laboratory analysis of pericardial fluid[12]
  - Normal fluid: less than 1500×10^6 nucleated cells/L, protein less than 2.5 g/L
    - Septic pericarditis: ↑ degenerative neutrophils
    - Idiopathic/immune-mediated pericarditis: ↑ protein and nondegenerate neutrophils
    - Neoplasia: tumor cells
  - Bacterial culture/antibiotic sensitivity testing
  - Virus isolation and evaluation of viral titers
  - Plasma cardiac troponin I (cTnI): high concentrations in case of primary myocardial disease
- Lavage/treatment
  - Twice-daily lavage with isotonic fluid at body temperature until:
    - Fluid production reduces (< 1 L over 12 hours or until the volume of fluid drained is less than the volume infused)
    - Clinical signs improve
    - Cytology of the fluid indicates resolution of the inflammatory process
  - Septic pericarditis suspected:
    - Pericardial antimicrobials such as sodium penicillin or gentamicin[8,13]
    - Systemic broad-spectrum antibiotics according to the results of bacterial cultures and antibiotic sensitivity; penicillin and an aminoglycoside or cephalosporins penetrate the pericardium effectively[12]
  - Systemic treatment:
    - Nonsteroidal anti-inflammatory drugs
    - Corticosteroids: use remains controversial, does not appear to reduce the risk of constrictive pericarditis[4]
    - Tissue plasminogen activator (tPA) to promote fibrinolysis[12]
  - Surgical treatment: pericardiectomy

---

cases. Cardiomyopathy could be the consequence of a wide variety of causes (**Table 2**). Myocarditis is defined as focal or diffuse myocardial inflammation with degenerative or necrotic cardiomyocytes and infiltration of inflammatory cells, as a consequence of local or systemic disease. This can be caused by infection with viruses, bacteria, and fungi (see **Table 2**). Myocardial fibrosis is defined as a marked increase of collagen deposition in myocardial tissue, suspected by echocardiography and confirmed at postmortem examination (**Fig. 4**).[25] Fibrosis probably results from a local ischemic event or is the end stage of myocarditis. Although it might be an incidental finding, horses with myocardial fibrosis in conjunction with ventricular arrhythmia should be excluded from rigorous athletic work.[26]

Although myocardial disease is generally rare, some conditions are more frequently described in horses. Horses are susceptible to myocardial damage caused by ionophores, which are used as coccidiostats in poultry and growth promotors in ruminants.[6,7,41,42] Toxicity results from disruption of the transmembrane ion concentration gradients and electrical potentials, eventually leading to cell death. The clinical effects depend on the amount ingested, with LD_{50} of monensin estimated between 2 to 3 mg/kg bwt, and the LD_{50} of lasalocid estimated at 21.5 mg/kg bwt.[7] Ingestion

Table 2
Potential etiology of myocardial disease in horses

Etiology	Reference
Viral	27
Equine Herpesvirus-1	
Equine infectious anemia	
Equine viral arteritis	
Equine influenza	
Morbillivirus	
Eastern equine encephalomyelitis	
African horse sickness (cardiac form)	
Bacterial – has also been associated with pericarditis, pericardial abscess, endocarditis, sepsis	28
Endotoxemia (eg, associated with colic/diarrhea)	29
Streptococcus spp.	30
Staphylococcus spp.	
Clostridium chauvoei	
Borrelia burgdorferi	31
Piroplasmosis	32
Leptospirosis	33
Neorickettsia risticii	
Fungal	34
Parasites	
Strongylus vulgaris – statistically associated with focal ischaemic lesions in the myocardium	35
Onchocerca	
Nutritional	
Vitamin E and selenium deficiency: white muscle disease, predominantly in foals in selenium deficient areas, occasionally in adult horses	36–38
Copper deficiency/molybdenum toxicosis	39
Toxins and drugs	
Snake venom: rattlesnake, viper	40
Ionophores: Monensin, lasalocid, salinomycin	6,7,41–43
Plants containing cardiac glycosides: Digitalis spp. (foxglove), Taxus spp. (yew), Pimelea species, Nerium oleander, Adonis aestivalis (summer pheasant's eye), Lily of valley, Rhododendron, Eonymus	44–46
Other plant associated intoxications: Malva parviflora (marshmallow), atypical myopathy/seasonal pasture myopathy caused by ingestion of hypoglycin-A from seeds of maple trees (Acer spp.)	47,48
Cantharidin (blister beetle)	49
Sodium fluoroactetate rodenticides	
Heavy metals	
Neoplasia	
Lipoma	50
Pulmonary carcinoma	51
Hemangioma/hemangiosarcoma	52
Lymphoma/lymphosarcoma	53–55
Melanoma	56
Mesothelioma	
Chronic systemic hypertension	57,58
Laminitis, chronic pain	
Equine metabolic syndrome	
Chronic renal failure, renal neoplasia	
Pheochromocytoma/catecholamines	59

(continued on next page)

Table 2 *(continued)*	
Etiology	**Reference**
Genetic	
Glycogen branching enzyme deficiency	60
Idiopathic (potentially genetic)	
Dilated cardiomyopathy (phenotype also seen in end-stage myocarditis, toxic cardiomyopathy, or cardiomyopathy after longstanding tachyarrhythmia)	
Hypertrophic cardiomyopathy (phenotype also seen with other myocardial diseases leading LV hypertrophy such as acute myocarditis, chronic hypertension, chronic digitalis intoxication, neoplasia, amyloidosis)	61
Tachycardia-induced cardiomyopathy	62
Arrhythmogenic RV cardiomyopathy (ARVC)	63,64
Other possible causes of myocardial insult	
Trauma leading to myocardial degeneration/necrosis	
Immune-mediated	
Hypoxia	
Ischemic (embolic) myocardial fibrosis	25
Amyloidosis	65
Hyperthermia/heat shock	
Acute hemorrhage	66

of large amounts results in acute or subacute death, whereas smaller amounts lead to signs of muscular, cardiac, and neurologic damage.

Cardiac glycosides might also cause feed-associated cardiomyopathy. Over 40 different plant species contain cardiac glycosides, and accidental intake of green or dried plant material is potentially toxic. Cardiac glycosides are gastrointestinal irritants and cause accumulation of sodium in excitable cells.[45] Death usually occurs within 12 to 36 hours after ingestion, but horses that survive the first hours might present signs

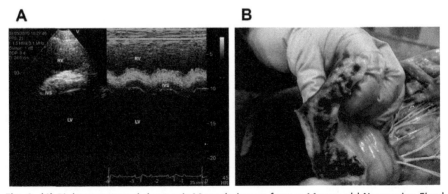

Fig. 4. (*A*) Right parasternal short-axis M-mode image from a 14-year-old Norwegian Fjord with myocardial fibrosis following lasalocid intoxication. Hyperechoic myocardial fibrosis is visualized in the interventricular septum. (*B*) Postmortem cross-section of the interventricular septum, demonstrating multifocal pale areas in the myocardium. Histologic analysis confirmed myocardial fibrosis. LV, left ventricle; IVS, interventricular septum; RV, right ventricle.

of cardiomyopathy. Chronic exposure might result in LV hypertrophy associated with ventricular arrhythmias.

Myocardial damage also occurs in horses with atypical myopathy, an acute and often fatal rhabdomyolysis that results from ingestion of hypoglycin-A from seeds of maple trees (*Acer* spp.) on pasture and that mainly affects the skeletal musculature.[48] Cardiomyopathy caused by intoxication should be considered even if only 1 horse in a group is clinically affected, because individual susceptibility to toxins and the amount of ingested toxins may vary largely. Examination of barn or pasture mates is advised to early identify subclinically affected horses.

Dilated cardiomyopathy is characterized by increased inner dimensions and decreased LV contractile function that cannot be attributed to valvular, vascular, congenital, or coronary disease. Dilated cardiomyopathy is either idiopathic (possibly with a genetic background, although this has not been documented in horses) or develops as a chronic stage of myocarditis, after toxic myocardial injury, or as a consequence of sustained ventricular tachycardia. Tachycardia-induced cardiomyopathy is usually reversible with antiarrhythmic treatment.[62] Primary hypertrophic cardiomyopathy has only been supposed in one recent case report in a Clydesdale gelding.[61] Concentric LV hypertrophy, characterized by increased relative wall thickness, can also be found in horses with systemic hypertension caused by chronic laminitis, renal disease, equine metabolic syndrome or chronic pain and with acute myocarditis, amyloid infiltration, neoplasia, or chronic digitalis exposure.[57,58,65,67]

The clinical signs of myocardial disease are variable, as they result from the underlying cause and the impact on myocardial function. In many horses, myocardial disease is subclinical. Sometimes, myocardial dysfunction leads to poor performance, exercise intolerance, weakness, ataxia, syncope, respiratory distress, congestive heart failure, or sudden death.[7,40] Signs primarily related to the underlying systemic disease or intoxication include fever, inappetence, colic, diarrhea, sweating, weakness, lethargy, signs of respiratory disease, or shock. In some horses, the clinical signs become apparent only after the horse seems to have recovered from a systemic disease and is brought back into training. The physical examination is either normal or reveals tachycardia, tachypnea, a weak pulse, venous distention, ventral edema, cardiac murmur, or arrhythmia.

The final diagnosis is based on ECG, echocardiography, and laboratory analysis. ECG might show ventricular premature depolarizations or ventricular tachycardia, but sinus tachycardia, atrial premature depolarizations, atrial fibrillation, and conduction disturbances such as advanced second degree atrioventricular block or atrial standstill could also be present.[7,29,32,48,66] However, it is important to realize that most horses with arrhythmias do not have evidence of myocarditis or cardiomyopathy as an underlying cause.

Echocardiography usually demonstrates abnormal myocardial function. Cardiac glycoside intoxication might enhance inotropy (**Fig. 5**, Video 2), whereas most other causative agents will result in contractile dysfunction, characterized by ventricular dilation and abnormal wall motion.[38] This can be quantified by decreased fractional shortening or ejection fraction and prolonged pre-ejection period (**Fig. 6**, Video 3). Subtle LV systolic dysfunction or impaired diastolic relaxation and reduced ventricular filling might be detected using advanced echocardiographic techniques such as TDI or 2-dimensional speckle tracking (2DST) (see **Fig. 6**; **Fig. 7**).[38,41,48] Echocardiography can also reveal altered cardiac dimensions and morphology. The relative wall thickness is increased in acute myocarditis (myocardial edema and cell infiltration), cardiac glycoside intoxication and hypertensive, hypertrophic or infiltrative

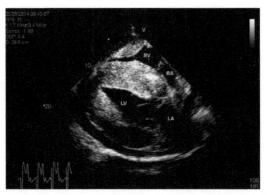

Fig. 5. Right parasternal long-axis 4-chamber view from a 7-year-old Akhal Teke stallion with cardiac glycoside intoxication. Relative wall thickness was increased, and the left ventricle seemed hypercontractile. Pericardial effusion is visible (see Video 2 for corresponding right parasternal long-axis 4-chamber view). RA, right atrium; RV, right ventricle; LA, left atrium; LV, left ventricle.

cardiomyopathy; athletic heart and pseudohypertrophy from severe volume depletion must be excluded. Relative wall thickness is decreased, associated with LV dilation, in the chronic stages of myocarditis, dilated cardiomyopathy, or tachycardia-induced cardiomyopathy.[7,43,62] Focal or diffuse lesions are visualized as hypo- or hyperechoic regions in the myocardium, although these might only become apparent in the subacute or chronic stages (see **Fig. 4**). Color flow mapping might reveal valvular regurgitation secondary to cardiac dilation or papillary muscle dysfunction.

A definite diagnosis of myocardial histologic abnormalities can be made using transvenous endomyocardial biopsies. A safe and minimally invasive ultrasound-guided approach for serial right atrial and ventricular biopsies through the jugular vein has been described. However, this technique has so far mainly been used for research purposes.[68]

Laboratory analysis should include specific biomarkers for myocardial damage such as plasma cTnI or cardiac troponin T (cTnT) concentrations, although elevations of nonspecific markers of myocardial cell injury can also be found. The increase in cTnI can be modest or very high (up to 816 ng/mL in a fatal case of lasalocid intoxication, reference <0.10 ng/mL).[7] Serum, urine, gastrointestinal, and feed samples should be collected for diagnostic testing (eg, digoxin or ionophore concentrations, serology and polymerase chain reaction [PCR] to search for infectious agents, toxicology screening). The environment should be checked for toxic plants.

Postmortem findings in horses with myocardial disease include focal or diffuse myocardial abnormalities such as thinning or thickening, pale color, or fibrosis. Histology confirms myocardial inflammation, necrosis, fibrosis, or calcification.[7]

The therapy aims at tackling the underlying cause, inhibiting life-threatening arrhythmias, and treating heart failure. Myocardial disease should always be treated with stall rest for at least 1 month, and cardiac function and rhythm should be re-examined before rigorous training is resumed. All further contact with toxins should be avoided, and activated charcoal or mineral oil could be administered to reduce absorption in cases of recent uptake of toxins. Depending on the etiology, antibiotics, vitamin E and selenium supplementation, or corticosteroids might be administered, as well as supportive therapy provided. Heart failure could be treated by diuretics, positive

A

B

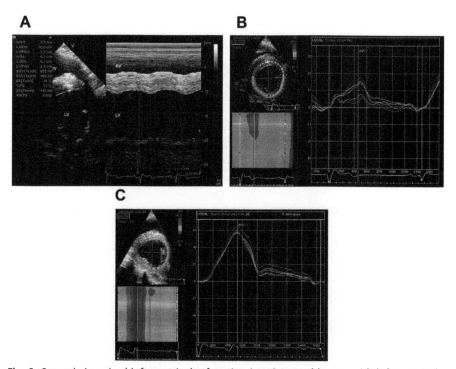

C

Fig. 6. Severely impaired left ventricular function in a 9-year-old pony with left ventricular dysfunction following ionophore intoxication. (*A*) Right parasternal short-axis M-mode image demonstrating left ventricular dilation and decreased fractional shortening (see Video 3 for corresponding right parasternal long-axis 4-chamber view). LV, left ventricle; RV, right ventricle. (*B*) Traces of the 2-dimensional speckle tracking curves showing severely decreased left ventricular peak radial strain values, compared with an age-matched normal horse (*C*). Radial strain is a measure of deformation of the myocardial wall, expressed as a percentage relative to the initial wall thickness. Top left: 2-dimensional grayscale image showing the tracked region of interest. Bottom left: parametric color-coded M-mode. Right: segmental radial strain traces, with colors of the traces corresponding to the colors of the segmented region of interest. An ECG is plotted, with the start and end of the cycle marked by yellow dots. The time of aortic valve closure (AVC) is calculated automatically by the software and indicated by a green vertical line.

inotropic agents and angiotensin converting enzyme (ACE) inhibitors. Positive inotropic agents should be used with caution, however, as they could aggravate ventricular arrhythmias and are contraindicated in horses with an ionophore or cardiac glycoside intoxication. Antiarrhythmic drugs are necessary in case of life-threatening arrhythmias.

Echocardiographic evaluation of myocardial function might have prognostic value. The prognosis is fair to good in the case of myocardial disease causing arrhythmias with normal or mildly depressed myocardial function. In 1 report on ionophore intoxication, horses exhibiting low fractional shortening and ventricular dyskinesis were less likely to survive or return to their previous performance level. However, some horses fully recovered.[6,7] Follow-up using echocardiography, ambulatory ECG and stress ECG are necessary to confirm the absence of permanent myocardial scarring and exercise-induced arrhythmias, as these might compromise rider safety.

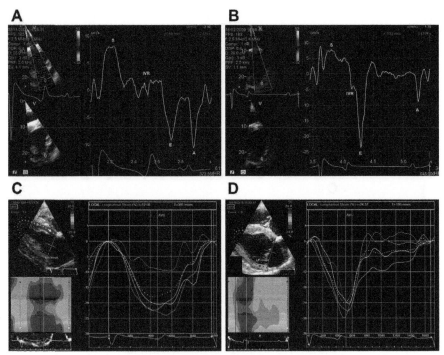

Fig. 7. Altered LV function in an 8-year old Warmblood horse with atypical myopathy. (*A*) Tissue Doppler velocity curve of the LV free wall from a short-axis image at papillary muscle level demonstrating the systolic (S), early diastolic (E), and late diastolic (A) peak velocity. Diastolic wall motion abnormality is characterized by a prolonged isovolumic relaxation period (IVR) and decreased E/A ratio with E/A inversion. (*B*) Tissue Doppler velocity curve in an age- and body weight-matched healthy horse with a normal IVR and E/A ratio. (*C*) Longitudinal strain curves obtained with 2-dimensional speckle tracking from a modified 4-chamber view. The strain curves show a prolonged contraction and biphasic wall motion, with increased mechanical dispersion of contraction. Longitudinal strain is a measure of deformation of the myocardial wall, expressed as a percentage relative to the initial wall thickness. (*D*) Longitudinal strain curves in an age- and body weight-matched healthy horse, showing simultaneous contraction of the different myocardial segments. For further explanations see legend of **Fig. 6.**

GREAT VESSEL ABNORMALITIES

Great vessel disease is an uncommon diagnosis in horses, although pulmonary or aortic rupture has been reported as a relatively frequent cause of sudden death.[69] However, aortic rupture was the cause of sudden death in only 1% of racehorses in a multicenter study.[70] Several terms are used to describe arterial vascular disease. A true aortic aneurysm is defined as a focal increased cross-sectional diameter of the aorta caused by dilation of the entire vessel wall, which can occur at different locations along the tract of the aorta. In contrast, a pseudoaneurysm or aortic dissection is an accumulation of blood between the outer layers of the arterial wall after aortic rupture. Aortic root rupture is defined as rupture of the aorta in the region of the sinus of Valsalva. This might occur following an aneurysm or spontaneously, and results in hemopericardium with acute sudden death or an aortocardiac fistula. In Friesian horses, aortic rupture typically occurs near the ligamentum arteriosum in the absence of an aneurysm.

Aortic Aneurysm

Aneurysm of the right sinus of Valsalva has been reported in horses as an acquired condition, a congenital anomaly, or associated with chronic aortic regurgitation.[71,72] In most cases, aneurysms were detected postmortem after aortic rupture. Antemortem diagnosis is possible using echocardiography, which reveals aortic root dilation (**Fig. 8**, Video 4). These horses are considered unsafe to ride because of the risk of sudden rupture.

Aortic Root Rupture and Aortocardiac Fistula

Aortic root rupture with or without aneurysmal dilation is commonly reported in older horses of all breeds, predominantly stallions.[73] Rupture typically occurs in the right sinus of Valsalva and occasionally in the noncoronary sinus. It has been associated with degenerative lesions in the media of the aorta combined with hypertension during breeding.[72,73] In some cases, aortic root rupture has been associated with chronic aortic regurgitation, but the 2 conditions might be unrelated.[74] Aortic root rupture could result in hemopericardium or formation of a pseudoaneurysm. The aortic sinus could also rupture into a dissecting tract through the ventricular septum or into the right heart chambers, creating an aortocardiac fistula.[74]

Presenting signs in horses with aortocardiac fistulas are acute-onset poor performance, exercise intolerance, sustained tachycardia, and pain or distress that often resembles colic. In the case of dissection of the interventricular septum, horses usually show rapid monomorphic ventricular tachycardia.[74] If the aorta ruptures to the right atrium or ventricle, right-sided CHF usually develops. Physical examination reveals a right-sided continuous low-pitched machinery murmur in case of a typical aortocardiac fistula. The arterial pulses are bounding with rapid diastolic run-off.

Echocardiography is the method of choice for diagnosis, using 2-dimensional imaging and Doppler interrogation to detect turbulent flow caused by left-to-right shunting (**Fig. 9**, Videos 5 and 6).

The management consists of box rest, antiarrhythmic treatment in case of life-threatening arrhythmias, and supportive treatment in case of CHF. Successful occlusion of the fistula using an Amplatzer device has been described in literature and

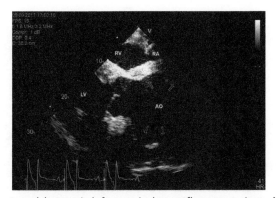

Fig. 8. Right parasternal long-axis left ventricular outflow tract view, showing an aortic aneurysm in a 9-year-old Warmblood mare at 4 months of gestation (see Video 4 for corresponding image). The focal dilation of the aorta is indicated by green arrows. The mare foaled at term without complications. AO, aorta; LV, left ventricle; RA, right atrium; RV, right ventricle.

performed at the author's clinic.[75] However, this was unsuccessful in the longer term. The prognosis of aortocardiac fistulas is guarded, as these horses are not considered safe to ride.[26] Horses that survive the acute event and the concurrent arrhythmias might live for weeks to months before CHF develops, with 1 horse reported alive after 4 years.[74]

Aortic Rupture and Aortopulmonary Fistula

Friesian horses are predisposed to develop aortic rupture, with or without formation of a pseudoaneurysm and/or aortopulmonary fistula.[76] The prevalence of aortic rupture has been estimated at 2%, and this might even be an underestimate. The underlying pathogenesis is probably a hereditary connective tissue disorder, resulting in a higher rate of collagen degradation in the aortic media.[77] Thoracic aortic rupture leads to immediate massive hemorrhage and is fatal. Aortopulmonary fistulas are associated with aortic rupture proximal to the ligamentum arteriosum.[76] Presenting signs are recurrent colic, increased rectal temperature, tachycardia, and respiratory signs. If the horse survives the acute phase, right-sided CHF develops. Physical examination reveals a grade 1 to 3/6 systolic and/or diastolic murmur dorsal to the aortic valve region. The arterial pulses are bounding with a carotid water-hammer pulse.[76]

Diagnosis of an aortopulmonary fistula by echocardiography is challenging, as visualizing the shunt requires nonstandard tilted imaging planes from the left third intercostal space (**Fig. 10**, Video 7).[78] If echocardiography is inconclusive, cardiac catheterization could be performed to confirm pulmonary hypertension and shunting of oxygenated blood.

The management for horses with an aortopulmonary fistula consists of box rest, antiarrhythmic treatment in case of life-threatening arrhythmias, and supportive treatment in case of CHF. The prognosis for horses is guarded. These horses are not considered safe to ride or drive.[26]

Pulmonary Artery Rupture

Pulmonary artery rupture usually occurs after long-standing pulmonary hypertension caused by left-sided heart failure or left-to-right shunting with pulmonary artery

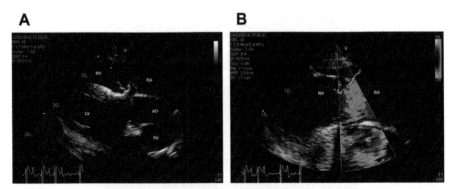

Fig. 9. Aortocardiac fistula with dissection into the right atrium in a 5-year-old Warmblood mare with atrial fibrillation. An unusual fibrous portion of the fistula at the right atrial side, probably consisting of disrupted endocardium, was seen. Right parasternal long-axis left ventricular outflow tract view, 2-dimensional image (A) and color flow Doppler showing turbulent flow caused by the left-to-right shunt (B) (see Videos 5 and 6 for corresponding images). AO, aorta; LV, left ventricle; RA, right atrium; RV, right ventricle; PA, pulmonary artery.

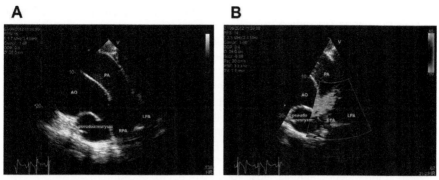

Fig. 10. Aorto-pulmonary fistula in a 4-year-old Friesian gelding. Left parasternal oblique view showing the left and right branch of the pulmonary artery (*A*), with turbulent flow entering the pulmonary artery visualized by color flow Doppler imaging (*B*) (see Video 7 for corresponding image). AO, aorta; LPA, left branch of the pulmonary artery; PA, pulmonary artery; RPA, right branch of the pulmonary artery.

dilation.[79,80] As this is a catastrophic event, horses at risk are considered unsafe for riding or driving.[26] Therefore, echocardiographic monitoring of pulmonary artery diameters should be performed in horses with severe mitral regurgitation and left-to-right shunts.

SUPPLEMENTARY DATA

Supplementary data related to this article can be found online at https://doi.org/10.1016/j.cveq.2018.12.005.

REFERENCES

1. Luis Fuentes V, Wilkie LJ. Asymptomatic hypertrophic cardiomyopathy: diagnosis and therapy. Vet Clin North Am Small Anim Pract 2017;47(5):1041–54.
2. Wess G, Domenech O, Dukes-McEwan J, et al. European Society of Veterinary Cardiology screening guidelines for dilated cardiomyopathy in Doberman Pinschers. J Vet Cardiol 2017;19(5):405–15.
3. Schubert M, Jonsson H, Chang D, et al. Prehistoric genomes reveal the genetic foundation and cost of horse domestication. Proc Natl Acad Sci U S A 2014; 111(52):E5661–9.
4. Reimer J. Management of equine pericarditis. Equine Vet Educ 2013;25(7): 334–8.
5. Sprayberry KA, Slovis NM. Sales performance and athletic outcome in young Thoroughbreds with pericarditis. Equine Vet J 2017;49(6):729–33.
6. Hughes KJ, Hoffmann KL, Hodgson DR. Long-term assessment of horses and ponies post exposure to monensin sodium in commercial feed. Equine Vet J 2009;41(1):47–52.
7. Decloedt A, Verheyen T, De Clercq D, et al. Acute and long-term cardiomyopathy and delayed neurotoxicity after accidental lasalocid poisoning in horses. J Vet Intern Med 2012;26(4):1005–11.
8. Worth LT, Reef VB. Pericarditis in horses: 18 cases (1986-1995). J Am Vet Med Assoc 1998;212(2):248–53.
9. Hardy J, Robertson JT, Reed SM. Constrictive pericarditis in a mare - attempted treatment by partial pericardiectomy. Equine Vet J 1992;24(2):151–4.

10. Wagner PC, Miller RA, Merritt F, et al. Constrictive pericarditis in horse. J Equine Med Surg 1977;1(7–8):242–7.

11. Bernard W, Reef VB, Clark ES, et al. Pericarditis in horses - 6 cases (1982-1986). J Am Vet Med Assoc 1990;196(3):468–71.

12. Marr CM. Cardiovascular infections. In: Sellon DC, Long M, editors. Equine infectious diseases. 2nd edition. Philadelphia: Saunders Elsevier; 2013. p. 21–41.

13. Bolin DC, Donahue JM, Vickers ML, et al. Microbiologic and pathologic findings in an epidemic of equine pericarditis. J Vet Diagn Invest 2005;17(1):38–44.

14. Alcott CJ, Howard J, Wong D, et al. Fibrinous pericarditis and cardiac tamponade in a 3-week-old pony foal. Equine Vet Educ 2013;25(7):328–33.

15. Armstrong SK, Raidal SL, Hughes KJ. Fibrinous pericarditis and pericardial effusion in three neonatal foals. Aust Vet J 2014;92(10):392–9.

16. Morley PS, ChirinoTrejo M, Petrie L, et al. Pericarditis and pleuritis caused by *Mycoplasma felis* in a horse. Equine Vet J 1996;28(3):237–40.

17. Perkins SL, Magdesian G, Thomas WP, et al. Pericarditis and pleuritis caused by *Corynebacterium pseudotuberculosis* in a horse. J Am Vet Med Assoc 2004; 224(7):1133–+.

18. May KA, Cheramie HS, Howard RD, et al. Purulent pericarditis as a sequela to clostridial myositis in a horse. Equine Vet J 2002;34(6):636–40.

19. Reuss SM, Chaffin MK, Cohen ND. Extrapulmonary disorders associated with *Rhodococcus equi* infection in foals: 150 cases (1987-2007). J Am Vet Med Assoc 2009;235(7):855–63.

20. Davis EG, Rush BR. Diagnostic challenges: equine thoracic neoplasia. Equine Vet Educ 2013;25(2):96–107.

21. Bertone JJ, Dill SG. Traumatic gastropericarditis in a horse. J Am Vet Med Assoc 1985;187(7):742–3.

22. Voros K, Felkai C, Szilagyi Z, et al. Two-dimensional echocardiographically guided pericardiocentesis in a horse with traumatic pericarditis. J Am Vet Med Assoc 1991;198(11):1953–6.

23. Durando MM, Zarucco L, Schaer TP, et al. Pneumopericardium in a horse secondary to sternal bone marrow aspiration. Equine Vet Educ 2006;18(2):75–9.

24. Freestone JF, Thomas WP, Carlson GP, et al. Idiopathic effusive pericarditis with tamponade in the horse. Equine Vet J 1987;19(1):38–42.

25. Coudry V, Jean D, Desbois C, et al. Myocardial fibrosis in a horse with polymorphic ventricular tachycardia observed during general anesthesia. Can Vet J 2007;48(6):623–6.

26. Reef VB, Bonagura J, Buhl R, et al. Recommendations for management of equine athletes with cardiovascular abnormalities. J Vet Intern Med 2014;28(3):749–61.

27. Jesty SA, Reef VB. Septicemia and cardiovascular infections in horses. Vet Clin North Am Equine Pract 2006;22(2):481–+.

28. Slack JA, McGuirk SM, Erb HN, et al. Biochemical markers of cardiac injury in normal, surviving septic, or nonsurviving septic neonatal foals. J Vet Intern Med 2005;19(4):577–80.

29. Nostell K, Brojer J, Hoglund K, et al. Cardiac troponin I and the occurrence of cardiac arrhythmias in horses with experimentally induced endotoxaemia. Vet J 2012;192(2):171–5.

30. Dolente BA, Seco OM, Lewis ML. Streptococcal toxic shock in a horse. J Am Vet Med Assoc 2000;217(1):64–7.

31. Chang YF, Novosol V, McDonough SP, et al. Experimental infection of ponies with *Borrelia burgdorferi* by exposure to *Ixodid* ticks. Vet Pathol 2000;37(1):68–76.

32. Diana A, Guglielmini C, Candini D, et al. Cardiac arrhythmias associated with piroplasmosis in the horse: a case report. Vet J 2007;174(1):193–5.
33. Verma A, Stevenson B, Adler B. Leptospirosis in horses. Vet Microbiol 2013; 167(1–2):61–6.
34. Peet RL, Mcdermott J, Williams JM, et al. Fungal myocarditis and nephritis in a horse. Aust Vet J 1981;57(9):439–40.
35. Cranley JJ, McCullagh KG. Ischaemic myocardial fibrosis and aortic strongylosis in the horse. Equine Vet J 1981;13(1):35–42.
36. Barigye R, Dyer NW, Newell TK. Fatal myocardial degeneration in an adult Quarter Horse with vitamin E deficiency. J Equine Vet Sci 2007;27(9):405–8.
37. Dill SG, Rebhun WC. White muscle disease in foals. Compend Contin Educ Pract Vet 7(suppl) 1985;7(11):S627–36.
38. Schefer KD, Hagen R, Ringer SK, et al. Laboratory, electrocardiographic, and echocardiographic detection of myocardial damage and dysfunction in an Arabian mare with nutritional masseter myodegeneration. J Vet Intern Med 2011;25(5):1171–80.
39. Ladefoged O, Sturup S. Copper deficiency in cattle, sheep and horses caused by excess molybdenum from fly-ash - a case-report. Vet Hum Toxicol 1995; 37(1):63–5.
40. Tirosh-Levy S, Solomovich R, Comte J, et al. Daboia (Vipera) palaestinae envenomation in horses: clinical and hematological signs, risk factors for mortality and construction of a novel severity scoring system. Toxicon 2017;137:58–64.
41. Decloedt A, Verheyen T, Sys S, et al. Tissue Doppler imaging and 2-dimensional speckle tracking of left ventricular function in horses exposed to lasalocid. J Vet Intern Med 2012;26(5):1209–16.
42. Aleman M, Magdesian KG, Peterson TS, et al. Salinomycin toxicosis in horses. J Am Vet Med Assoc 2007;230(12):1822–6.
43. Peek SF, Marques FD, Morgan J, et al. Atypical acute monensin toxicosis and delayed cardiomyopathy in Belgian draft horses. J Vet Intern Med 2004;18(5): 761–4.
44. Tiwary AK, Puschner B, Kinde H, et al. Diagnosis of taxus (yew) poisoning in a horse. J Vet Diagn Invest 2005;17(3):252–5.
45. Hughes KJ, Dart AJ, Hodgson DR. Suspected Nerium oleander (oleander) poisoning in a horse. Aust Vet J 2002;80(7):412–5.
46. Renier AC, Kass PH, Magdesian KG, et al. Oleander toxicosis in equids: 30 cases (1995-2010). J Am Vet Med Assoc 2013;242(4):540–9.
47. Bauquier J, Stent A, Gibney J, et al. Evidence for marsh mallow (Malva parviflora) toxicosis causing myocardial disease and myopathy in four horses. Equine Vet J 2017;49(3):307–13.
48. Verheyen T, Decloedt A, De Clercq D, et al. Cardiac changes in horses with atypical myopathy. J Vet Intern Med 2012;26(4):1019–26.
49. Helman RG, Edwards WC. Clinical features of blister beetle poisoning in equids: 70 cases (1983-1996). J Am Vet Med Assoc 1997;211(8):1018–&.
50. Baker D, Kreeger J. Infiltrative lipoma in the heart of a horse. Cornell Vet 1987; 77(3):258–62.
51. Dill SG, Moise NS, Meschter CL. Cardiac-failure in a stallion secondary to metastasis of an anaplastic pulmonary-carcinoma. Equine Vet J 1986;18(5):414–7.
52. Delesalle C, van Loon G, Nollet H, et al. Tumor-induced ventricular arrhythmia in a horse. J Vet Intern Med 2002;16(5):612–7.
53. Sweeney RW, Hamir AN, Fisher RR. Lymphosarcoma with urinary-bladder infiltration in a horse. J Am Vet Med Assoc 1991;199(9):1177–8.

54. Reef VB, Dyson SS, Beech J. Lymphosarcoma and associated immune-mediated hemolytic-anemia and thrombocytopenia in horses. J Am Vet Med Assoc 1984; 184(3):313–7.
55. Southwood LL, Schott HC, Henry CJ, et al. Disseminated hemangiosarcoma in the horse: 35 cases. J Vet Intern Med 2000;14(1):105–9.
56. Kovac M, Ueberschar S, Nowak M, et al. Aortic valve insufficiency and myocardial melanoma in a horse. Pferdeheilkunde 2005;21(5):408–12.
57. de Solis CN, Slack J, Boston RC, et al. Hypertensive cardiomyopathy in horses: 5 cases (1995-2011). J Am Vet Med Assoc 2013;243(1):126–30.
58. Rugh KS, Garner HE, Sprouse RF, et al. Left-ventricular hypertrophy in chronically hypertensive ponies. Lab Anim Sci 1987;37(3):335–8.
59. Dufourni A, De Clercq D, Vera L, et al. Pheochromocytoma in a horse with polymorphic ventricular tachycardia. Vlaams Diergen Tijds 2017;86(4):241–9.
60. Valberg SJ, Ward TL, Rush B, et al. Glycogen branching enzyme deficiency in Quarter Horse foals. J Vet Intern Med 2001;15(6):572–80.
61. Cullimore AM, Lester GD, Secombe CJ, et al. Hypertrophic cardiomyopathy in a Clydesdale gelding. Aust Vet J 2018;96(6):212–5.
62. Stern JA, Doreste YR, Barnett S, et al. Resolution of sustained narrow complex ventricular tachycardia and tachycardia-induced cardiomyopathy in a Quarter Horse following quinidine therapy. J Vet Cardiol 2012;14(3):445–51.
63. Raftery AG, Garcia NC, Thompson H, et al. Arrhythmogenic right ventricular cardiomyopathy secondary to adipose infiltration as a cause of episodic collapse in a horse. Irish Vet J 2015;68:24.
64. Freel KM, Morrison LR, Thompson H, et al. Arrhythmogenic right ventricular cardiomyopathy as a cause of unexpected cardiac death in two horses. Vet Rec 2010;166(23):718–22.
65. Nout YS, Hinchcliff KW, Bonagura JD, et al. Cardiac amyloidosis in a horse. J Vet Intern Med 2003;17(4):588–92.
66. Navas de Solis C, Dallap Schaer BL, Boston R, et al. Myocardial insult and arrhythmias after acute hemorrhage in horses. J Vet Emerg Crit Care 2015;25(2):248–55.
67. Heliczer N, Gerber V, Bruckmaier R, et al. Cardiovascular findings in ponies with equine metabolic syndrome. J Am Vet Med Assoc 2017;250(9):1027–35.
68. Decloedt A, De Clercq D, Ven S, et al. Right atrial and right ventricular ultrasound-guided biopsy technique in standing horses. Equine Vet J 2015;48(3):346–51.
69. de Solis CN, Althaus F, Basieux N, et al. Sudden death in sport and riding horses during and immediately after exercise: a case series. Equine Vet J 2018;50(5):644–8.
70. Lyle CH, Uzal FA, McGorum BC, et al. Sudden death in racing Thoroughbred horses: an international multicentre study of post mortem findings. Equine Vet J 2011;43(3):324–31.
71. Sleeper MM, Durando MM, Miller M, et al. Aortic root disease in four horses. J Am Vet Med Assoc 2001;219(4):491–6, 459.
72. Lester GD, Lombard CW, Ackerman N. Echocardiographic detection of a dissecting aortic root aneurysm in a Thoroughbred stallion. Vet Radiol Ultrasound 1992;33(4):202–5.
73. Rooney JR, Prickett ME, Crowe MW. Aortic ring rupture in stallions. Pathol Vet 1967;4(3):268–&.
74. Marr CM, Reef VB, Brazil TJ, et al. Aorto-cardiac fistulas in seven horses. Vet Radiol Ultrasound 1998;39(1):22–31.

75. Javsicas LH, Giguere S, Maisenbacher HW, et al. Percutaneous transcatheter closure of an aorto-cardiac fistula in a Thoroughbred stallion using an Amplatzer occluder device. J Vet Intern Med 2010;24(4):994–8.

76. Ploeg M, Saey V, de Bruijn CM, et al. Aortic rupture and aorto-pulmonary fistulation in the Friesian horse: characterisation of the clinical and gross post mortem findings in 24 cases. Equine Vet J 2013;45(1):101–6.

77. Saey V, Tang J, Ducatelle R, et al. Elevated urinary excretion of free pyridinoline in Friesian horses suggests a breed-specific increase in collagen degradation. BMC Vet Res 2018;14:139.

78. Vandecasteele T, Cornillie P, Van Steenkiste G, et al. Echocardiographic identification of atrial-related structures and vessels in horses validated by computed tomography of casted hearts. Equine Vet J 2018;51(1):90–6.

79. Buergelt CD, Carmichael JA, Tashjian RJ, et al. Spontaneous rupture of left pulmonary artery in a horse with patent ductus arteriosus. J Am Vet Med Assoc 1970;157(3):313–20.

80. Reef VB, Bain FT, Spencer PA. Severe mitral regurgitation in horses: clinical, echocardiographic and pathological findings. Equine Vet J 1998;30(1):18–27.

Cardiovascular Response to Exercise and Training, Exercise Testing in Horses

Cristobal Navas de Solis, LV, PhD

KEYWORDS

- Exercise testing • Exercise physiology • Training • Cardiovascular adaptations
- Poor performance

KEY POINTS

- Exercise testing is a useful clinical tool that can help veterinarians assess poor performance, fitness, and performance potential and prevent injuries.
- Different exercise tests should be used to evaluate horses performing in different disciplines and levels.
- Exercise tests that simultaneously assess several body systems can be beneficial when assessing poor performance, because this is often a multifactorial problem with signs not detectable at rest.
- Historical questionnaires, lameness examinations, respiratory sampling, dynamic upper airway endoscopy, exercising electrocardiograms, echocardiograms, and measurement of laboratory values are useful components of exercise tests.
- Common diseases detected during exercise tests are lameness, inflammatory airway disease/equine asthma, upper airway obstruction, myopathies, and exercising arrhythmias. Myocardial dysfunction, electrolyte abnormalities, and neurologic disease are less commonly detected.

INTRODUCTION

The physiology of exercise and training is fascinating, and hundreds of interesting studies have given insight into its mechanisms. Exercise testing is a useful clinical tool that can help veterinarians assess poor performance, fitness, and performance potential and prevent injuries. The most clinically applicable aspects of the cardiovascular response to exercise are highlighted here, as a comprehensive review is beyond the scope of this article.

Department of Large Animal Clinical Sciences, Texas A&M University, 4475 TAMU, College Station, TX 77843-4475, USA
E-mail address: crisnavasdes@gmail.com

Vet Clin Equine 35 (2019) 159–173
https://doi.org/10.1016/j.cveq.2018.11.003
0749-0739/19/© 2018 Elsevier Inc. All rights reserved.

CARDIOVASCULAR ADAPTATIONS WITH TRAINING AND CHANGES DURING EXERCISE

The most popular cardiovascular adaptation with training is the cardiac hypertrophy as part of "athlete's heart." There have been stories of racehorses with extremely large hearts; Secretariat's heart was estimated to weigh 10 kg, whereas the heart of an untrained horse may be approximately half this size (0.9% of body weight).[1] The relevance of hypertrophy is the relationship of cardiac size with stroke volume (SV), and therefore, with maximal oxygen consumption (VO_{2max}), the main parameter that allows estimation of aerobic athletic capacity. Maximal oxygen consumption (VO_{2max}) is the amount of oxygen that the horse can transport through the respiratory system into the arterial blood and by the cardiovascular system to the muscles for energy production. Considering the variables that affect VO_{2max} helps explain that cardiovascular changes play an important role in the 10% to 20% increase in VO_{2max} that occurs with training.[2,3]

There is no correlation between VO_{2max} and maximal heart rate during exercise (HR_{max}), but there is a correlation between percentage of VO_{2max} and percentage of HR_{max} and between VO_{2max} and velocity at HR_{max}. The HR_{max} does not change with training and is individual specific, making the increase in SV the main reason for the increase of cardiac output (CO) that occurs with training. HR during submaximal exercise, the speed at a given HR or at HR_{max}, or recovery of heart rate after exercise (HR_{rec})[4] can change with training. Measurements of VO_{2max} and blood gases during exercise are currently difficult to obtain for most clinicians and will not be discussed in this review. It is possible that soon technological advances will make these measurements more widely available.[5]

It is not possible to understand equine cardiovascular changes without considering the splenic reservoir. The spleen of a thoroughbred may store more than 12 L of blood with a PCV of 80% that can be mobilized by a sympathetic stimulus to raise the PCV up to 60% to 70%.[6] The spleen contracts more during higher speeds and when the anaerobic threshold is crossed,[7] mimicking autotransfusions or blood doping. The high PCV increases the oxygen-carrying capacity during exercise despite the decrease in partial pressure of oxygen in the arterial blood caused by diffusion limitations, hypoventilation, and ventilation/perfusion mismatch.

Two other relevant cardiovascular changes with exercise are changes in pulmonary and systemic arterial pressures. Mean pulmonary arterial pressure may increase from resting values of 20 to 40 mm Hg to 90 to 140 mm Hg during exercise. The increase of pulmonary arterial pressure may be one of the main factors contributing to exercise induced pulmonary hemorrhage (EIPH) in racehorses. Systemic systolic pressure may increase from 130 to 230 mm Hg and, interestingly for the clinician, this can be dampened by administration of common drugs used to treat cardiac disease, like ACE inhibitors.[8]

The autonomic nervous system balances sympathetic and parasympathetic tone and plays an important role in cardiovascular function. Resting heart rate (HR) decreases with training in some horses and not in others, but heart rate variability (HRV)-based markers of parasympathetic tone do not, suggesting full activation of the parasympathetic nervous activity even without training.[9] The use of HRV to assess progression of training or overtraining is an attractive concept. A higher sympathetic tone has been shown in competition when compared with sports horses used for pleasure riding.[10] Training programs based on HRV increased running velocity and performance in human endurance athletes.[11,12] These techniques may have potential if easy-to-follow, validated, and standardized protocols, devices, and reference values are designed and described. The rapid progression of wearable technologies is likely to solve this problem in the near future.

EXERCISE TESTS
Introduction, Goals, and Description

In high-level human athletes, exercise testing programs are routinely used to monitor health, maximize performance, and minimize injuries. Exercise tests in horses have been used to study physiology, predict or assess performance and fitness, monitor response to training and readiness for competition, or assess underperformance or disease. Exercise tests on treadmills allow for controlled conditions and intensive monitoring, but treadmills are not accessible to most clinicians and do not replicate conditions that horses will face during their usual activities.[13] Field exercise tests are becoming more common because of newer technology allowing acquisition of much of the information than can be obtained on treadmills. There are currently many different types of exercise tests used in different disciplines but no gold-standard protocols. Validation and standardization are not easy because of the costs involved in these projects, influence of different circumstances (temperature humidity, footing, riders), limitations in access to horses in active training, variability in talent, training levels, and routines of horses. **Table 1** shows a nonexhaustive description of exercise tests used for horses of different disciplines. Other reviews with different and more complete lists have been published.[14–16]

Tests can be performed at submaximal speeds or until fatigue (maximal speeds). Single-step exercise tests have been used particularly in racehorses because of the difficulty to control and sample these horses in a safe way that does not interfere with their training routines. Incremental exercise tests may not give complete information in disciplines in which technically demanding exercise or jumps are a key component.

Performing comprehensive exercise tests that simultaneously assess several body systems can be beneficial when assessing poor performance because this is often a multifactorial problem, in which signs may not be detected at rest. Different protocols that include historical questionnaires, lameness examinations, exercising electrocardiograms (ECG), echocardiograms, respiratory sampling, dynamic upper airway endoscopy, and measurement of laboratory values (lactate, SAA, CK, electrolytes, cardiac troponins [cTn], and so forth) have been described. Common diseases that can be detected using exercise tests are lameness, inflammatory airway disease (IAD)/equine asthma, upper airway obstruction, myopathies, and exercising arrhythmias. Myocardial dysfunction, electrolyte abnormalities, and neurologic disease are less commonly detected, and poor ability and unsuitable rider are more difficult to judge and discuss.[18,22,25] In studies assessing endurance[18] and sports horses performing poorly,[19] higher HR and lactate concentrations during exercise tests and/or slower HR_{rec} were detected. The differences in HR and lactate concentrations were considered to be due to the multiple subclinical diseases, because the training level between groups was comparable.

Upper and lower respiratory tract obstruction is a common cause of poor performance. The use of dynamic endoscopy and the development of overground endoscopes have facilitated the diagnosis of problems that were previously less recognized. Different upper respiratory tract disorders have been traditionally thought to occur independently, but it now appears that multiple or complex forms of collapse are present in many horses.[26] IAD/equine asthma is a common lower airway disease causing poor performance in horses. It has been speculated that there could be a relationship between the presence of respiratory disease and the presence of exercising

Table 1
Exercise test for horses of different disciplines

Discipline	Protocol	Reference
Eventing (field)	Walk (4 min, 400 m), trot (4 min, 600 m), 1000 m at 400 m/min, 1000 m at 500 m/min, 1000 m at 600 m/min, 1000 m at 700 m/min, or individual maximal speed. Walk 5 min between steps	Munsters et al,[60] 2013
Eventing (field)	Walk (5 min, 500 m), trot (20 min, 5000 m), 1000 m at 400 m/min, 1000 m at 500 m/min, 1000 m at 600 m/min. Walk 5 min between steps	Muñoz et al,[17] 1998
Endurance (field)	Walk (10 min), trot (10 min), 27 km at 22 km/h, 1500 m at 27 km/h, 1500 m at 32 km/h, 10 min walk. Slow-trot (700 m) between steps	Fraipont et al,[18] 2011
Endurance (treadmill)	Walk (5 min), trot (5 min), 3 min at 27 km/h, 3 min at 30 km/h, 3 min at 32 km/h, 10 min walk. 2 min trot at 12.6 km/h between steps. 4% incline	Fraipont et al,[18] 2011
Dressage/show jumping (field)	Trot (2 min), working trot (2 min), canter (2 min), extended canter (2 min). No warm up or rest periods	Van Erck Westegren et al,[19] 2014
Show jumping (field)	850 m at 240 m/min, 850 m at 320 m/min, 850 m at 400 m/min, 850 m at 480 m/min, 850 m at 560 m/min	Munk et al,[20] 2014
Show jumping (field)	Elliptical arena with 16 jumps spaced 3 m (5 long sides, 3 short sides). 4.8 laps in 90 s with jumps at 40 cm, stop for blood draw, repeat with jumps in long side raised to 60 cm, repeat with jumps long side raised to 85 cm	Munk et al,[20] 2014
Show jumping (field)	Jump a course with 11 (2 doubles) jumps adjusted to individual's level	Munk et al,[20] 2014
Eventing/show jumping/ dressage (treadmill)	Walk, trot, and brief canter warm up (30 min), trot (210 m/min 1-2 min and 240 min/min 1.5 min), 360 m/min (1 min), 420 m/min (1 min), 480 m/min (1 min), 540 m/min (1 min). Incline 6% and tests stopped if lactate exceeded 4 mmol/L. Stop 5 min then walk	Bitschnau et al,[21] 2010
Reining (field)	Walk (5 min), trot (5 min), lope (5 min to the left), gallop (1 min to the left), lope (5 min to the right), gallop (1 min to the right), walk (1 min), 4 sets of 4 spins (walk 1 min between sets), walk (1 min), 2 sets of 2 stops 80 m gallop between stops (walk for 1 min between sets). Walk 10 min	Navas de Solis et al,[22] 2018
Standardbred racehorse (field)	3 min at 440–500 m/min (age dependent), 3 min after increasing speed by 40–80 m/min, 3 min increasing speed by 40–80 m/min	Couroucé et al,[23] 1999
Thoroughbred racehorse (field)	Trot (1000 m at 250 m/min), 600–800 m 400 m/min, 6–800 min 460 m/min, 6–800 m 550 m/min, 6–800 m 660 m/min 1 min rest between steps	Kobayashi et al,[24] 1999

(continued on next page)

Table 1 (continued)		
Discipline	Protocol	Reference
Standardbred (treadmill)	1600 m at 7 m/s, stop to place scope, 400 m at 9 m/s, 400 m at 10 m/s, 1600 m at 11–14 m/s, 10 m/s for 400, stop. 0° incline	Martin et al,[25] 2000
Thoroughbred (treadmill)	1600 m at 7 m/s, stop to place scope and elevate 3°, 400 m at 9 m/s, 400 m at 11 m/s, 400 m at 12 m/s, 1600 m at 2–14.5 m/s, 10 m/s for 400 at 0° incline	Martin et al,[25] 2000

arrhythmias, perhaps associated with worsening hypoxemia and resulting myocardial hypoxia or with pulmonary arterial/right ventricular hypertension.[25,27] This plausible relationship and its mechanisms have not been proven or the risk quantified.

Exercising Electrocardiogram

Exercise ECGs are important components of cardiovascular assessment.[28] Aortic regurgitation, arrhythmias, syncope, hypertensive response to exercise, acute coronary syndrome, chest pain, and myocardial disease are some cardiovascular indications for exercise testing in humans.[29] Arrhythmias during or immediately after exercise are common in equine athletes, and their importance varies from irrelevant to life threatening. The relationship of exercising arrhythmias with sudden death is particularly relevant to equine clinicians. Sudden death is more commonly reported in higher-level eventing horses and thoroughbred racehorses.[30–32] The incidence of sudden death is 28.7/100,000 starts in thoroughbred racehorses and 14/100,000 starts in eventers. This amount contrasts with a reported incidence of 0.5 to 4/100,000 human athletes per year. Preparticipation screening has been useful in decreasing the number of sudden deaths associated with sports[33] in humans, and the development of preparticipation screening programs in equine medicine would be attractive. Currently, horses receive physical examinations and lameness examinations before certain types of equestrian events (mainly eventing and endurance), but cardiovascular screening rarely extends beyond auscultation. Because of the frequency of exercising arrhythmias in horses, exercise tests are candidates to be part of these programs.

It has been recommended that work intensity during an exercise test should be at or slightly exceeding the horse's customary activities and that some method of inducing unexpected sympathetic stimulation should be included to identify an inappropriate HR, aberrant impulse conduction, or ectopic beats associated with adrenergic stimulation.[28] Occurrence of arrhythmias is influenced by the intensity of the exercise,[32,34] and perhaps, circumstances like the type of test (treadmill vs field)[34] or the presence of sudden HR accelerations or decelerations[35] should be considered. It has been questioned if a single bout of exercise is enough to rule out the presence of arrhythmias, but how many tests are needed is an unanswered question.

Atrial fibrillation (AF) is the most common clinically relevant arrhythmia of the horse, and the effect of exercise in horses with AF deserves special mention. A traditional rule of thumb is that HRs of horses in AF during exercise are approximately 50 beats/min higher than when exercising in sinus rhythm. In a group of standardbred trotters,[36] a 1.56 m/s decrease in maximal velocity and increase in HR_{max} from 226 ± 11/min to 311 ± 27/min was observed on exercise tests on the treadmill after AF induction. Rapid ventricular response with wide complex tachycardia was observed in this study and in a previous study in which only mild exercise was performed on a lunge line.[37]

In humans and dogs,[38,39] frequent and/or complex ventricular arrhythmias occur in trained athletes, and detraining can reverse this process. Fibrosis is a common mechanism mentioned in the discussion surrounding the athlete's heart, and arrhythmia development and proposed mechanisms for the deconditioning effect are reversal of changes related to autonomic nervous system. An effect of training and detraining on exercising arrhythmias or pathologic effects of athlete's heart in horses have not been demonstrated to the best of the author's knowledge.

Echocardiograms

Heart size and valvular regurgitation increase with training.[40,41] In a study in which 348 horses were studied for poor performance, all 102 cardiac murmurs detected were considered to be physiologic or associated with clinically unimportant regurgitations.[25] The absence of clinical relevance is likely due to the type of cases collected in this study and helps one understand that although cardiac murmurs can be associated with relevant acquired or congenital heart disease, the presence of murmurs without significant underlying cardiac disease is common in equine athletes.

The increase in size of the left ventricle in equine athletes is due to an increase in both wall thickness and internal diameter (eccentric hypertrophy). Most horses are used in sports disciplines with a larger endurance component. The relative change in size is therefore in keeping with the traditional Morganroth hypothesis[42] that proposes that endurance-trained athletes exhibit eccentric hypertrophy, whereas hypertrophy in resistance-trained athletes is concentric. Athlete's heart in horses can be differentiated from pathologic myocardial hypertrophy (eg, with hypertensive and infiltrative disease or pseudohypertrophy related to dehydration or endotoxemia) by the presence of a normal relative wall thickness in athletes. A larger heart size is correlated with larger maximal oxygen uptake and better performance in thoroughbred racehorses and elite or advanced endurance and eventing horses have larger hearts than less successful horses.[40,41,43–45]

Stress echocardiograms are performed in the immediate postexercise period to assess exercise-induced myocardial dysfunction as a cause of poor performance. The goal is to obtain selected right parasternal views[46–48] within 2 minutes of exercise and with HRs that exceed 100/min. Obtaining the echocardiographic views rapidly requires optimal conditions and is more commonly performed after treadmill tests. Hypokinesis or segmental areas of myocardial hypokinesis, dyskinesis, or akinesis are the described abnormalities.[25] These abnormalities are thought to be consequences of exercise-induced myocardial ischemia or hypoxia, preexisting myocardial disease, or myocarditis.[25] More sophisticated analysis using quantitative and 2-dimensional speckle tracking has been described.[48] The idea of pharmacologic stress testing has been studied but does not reproduce the effects of exercise and causes larger increases in plasma cTn concentrations than exercise.[47,49] Cardiac dimensions and function have been shown to change differently than in routine exercise tests if tests are performed in hot humid conditions[50] or after prolonged endurance exercise.[51]

Cardiac Troponins

The most common cardiac biomarkers measured in association with exercise tests in horses are cTn. The elimination half-life of intravenously[52] administered cTnI in horses is very short (0.47 hours) and longer (6.4 hours) when postexercise kinetics are calculated.[53] Horses experience a postexercise increase in cTnI[53] and cTnT[54] with peaks occurring 2 to 6 hours postexercise and values returning to normal at 24 hours. Ranges are specific of the assay, and clinicians need to consider this when interpreting results. In a recent study, cTnT preexercise was (median and interquartile range) 4.0 (2.9–6.5) ng/L, and postexercise, the 99th percentile upper reference limit was

23.2 ng/L[54] when using a high sensitivity assay (Roche Cobas-e601 Analyzer). CTnI preexercise was 1.33 ± 0.6 ng/L, and it peaked at 11.96 ± 9.41 ng/L when using a high sensitivity assay (Abbott ARCHITECT STAT). In the same study, cTnI concentrations were below the limit of detection of the assay, and peak was between 39 and 51 ng/L using a Siemens Dimension Vista assay. Systemic concentrations of cTnI increased in endurance horses competing in both 80- and 160-km endurance races (74 ± 10 ng/L and 79 ± 20 ng/L, respectively) compared with resting concentrations (23 ± 8 ng/L) using a Stratus CS assay. The degree of increase was not greater in nonfinishing horses.[55] It is plausible that mild increases in the groups of normal horses described above represent physiologic changes, and larger increases of cTn in horses with cardiovascular disease (arrhythmias or collapse) or poor performance require different interpretation.

Lactate and Heart Rate

Blood lactate is the result of anaerobic metabolism, and an increase during exercise signals that muscle energy demands are not being met by oxygen supply and that fatigue will soon follow. Fatigue can be interpreted as a mechanism to protect health, and therefore, detection of excessive lactatemia during exercise could be a tool for injury prevention.[21] Accuracy and precision of several portable analyzers (Lactate Plus, Nova Biomedical, Waltham(MA), USA, Lactate Pro, KDK, Japan(ceased product), Lactate Scout, EKF Diagnostics Cardiff, England, for example) have been[56] reported, and despite all of them showing inaccuracy at high lactate concentrations and/or with high packed cell volumes (PCVs), they seem acceptable for clinical use if the limitations are recognized. Electrocardiographic equipment or HR monitors that are coupled with GPS technology make it easier to associate velocity with HR. The relationship between velocity and lactate can be approximated by an exponential curve and the relationship between velocity and HR (between HRs of approximately 120–210/min) by linear regression. At least 4 results at incremental speeds are recommended for calculations of parameters that describe these relationships. Plotting results on spreadsheets give the clinician an easy-to-use visual estimation of these parameters, and calculations can be used to obtain values that are more accurate. Lactate concentration after a single bout of strenuous, submaximal exercise has not been shown to be as informative as performance predictors, although lactate concentration after exercise at 10 m/s was negatively correlated with maximal velocity in trotters ($r = -0.66$, $P<.001$) and Timeform rating in thoroughbreds ($r = -0.68$, <0.01).[57]

The most commonly used parameters that associate velocity, lactate, and HR are V_{La4} (speed at which the blood lactate concentration reaches 4 mmol/L) and V_{200} (speed at which HR reaches 200/min). In horses exercising at lower intensities, analogous values of velocity at lactate of 2 mmol/L (V_{La2}) or HR of 150/min (V_{150}), 160/min (V_{160}), and so forth, have been used. V_{La4} is often considered to represent the change from aerobic to anaerobic work or the onset of lactate accumulation. V_{La2} is accepted by many as the work intensity using aerobic metabolism for energy production, and a steady-state lactate concentration of 2 mmol/L is considered normal during aerobic work. The interpretation of V_{La2} and V_{La4} is a simplification to assist clinicians, and calculation of individualized and refined values to determine the anaerobic threshold or maximum lactate steady-state concentrations has been suggested.[58]

It has been proposed that "the only single informative biochemical blood variable of benefit for positive performance diagnosis of sport horses in practice is lactate."[59] However, a single measure that could assess or guide training response or progression does not exist[60] and "no measurement or combination of measurements will ever be perfectly correlated with the ability to perform."[2] The use of plasma lactate

Table 2
Lactate, heart rate, and recovery of heart rate = heart rate at a time point × min after exercise

Discipline	Level	Lactate	HR	HR$_{rec}$	Reference
Eventing (cross country competition)	CCI***	19.1 ± 4.2 mmol/L (after competition)	171 ± 19/min (HR$_{mean}$)		White et al,[67] 1995
Eventing (cross country competition)	CCI****	22.4 ± 11 mmol/L (after competition)	188 ± 11/min (HR$_{mean}$)		Marlin et al,[68] 1995
Eventing (cross country competition)	CCI*	9 mmol/L (after competition)	163.2/min (HR$_{mean}$)		Muñoz et al,[69] 1999
Eventing (cross country competition)	CCI***/CCI****	10.2 ± 4.2 mmol/L (after competition)	195 ± 8/min (HR$_{mean}$)		Serrano et al,[70] 2002
Eventing (field test)	CCI***/****	10.3 ± 0.4 m/s (V$_{LA4}$)	11.4 ± 0.8 m/s (V$_{200}$)	107 ± 19/min (HR$_{rec5}$) 88 ± 11/min (HR$_{rec10}$)	Munsters et al,[60] 2013
Eventing (field test)	CCI***	8.3 ± 0.5 m/s (V$_{LA4}$)	11.1 ± 1.5 m/s (V$_{200}$)		Serrano et al,[71] 2001
Eventing (field test)	Untrained	8.3 ± 0.5 m/s (V$_{LA4}$)	11.4 ± 0.8 m/s (V$_{200}$)		
Eventing (field test)	CCI*/CCI***	9.7 ± 0.73 m/s (V$_{LA4}$)	10.8 ± 0.80 m/s (V$_{200}$)	81 ± 7.7/min (HR$_{rec10}$)	Lorello et al,[10] 2017
Endurance (field test)		6.6 ± 1.79 m/s (V$_{LA2}$)	11 ± 1.8 m/s (V$_{200}$)	74 ± 12/min (HR$_{rec10}$)	Lorello et al,[10] 2017
Endurance (field test)	All levels good performance	9.4 ± 2 m/s (V$_{LA4}$)	13 ± 2.0 m/s (V$_{200}$)	80/min (HR$_{rec5}$) 71/min (HR$_{rec10}$)	Fraipont et al,[18] 2011
	All levels underperforming	8.4 ± 2.1 m/s (V$_{LA4}$)	10.6 ± 1.8 m/s (V$_{200}$)	89/min (HR$_{rec5}$) 80/min (HR$_{rec10}$)	
	All levels eliminated	6.6 ± 1.9 m/s (V$_{LA4}$)	10.0 ± 1.2 m/s (V$_{200}$)	92/min (HR$_{rec5}$) 85/min (HR$_{rec10}$)	
Endurance (field test)	60–90 km	5.2 ± 1.3 m/s (V$_{LA2}$) 7.5 ± 1.7 m/s (V$_{LA4}$)	6.75 ± 1 m/s (V$_{160}$) 9.6 ± 1.3 m/s (V$_{200}$)	142 ± 15.9/min (HR$_{rec2}$) 172 ± 13.7/min (HR$_{rec4}$)	Frapoint et al,[72] 2012
	≥120 km	6.2 ± 1 m/s (V$_{LA2}$) 9.7 ± 0.7 m/s (V$_{LA4}$)	8.4 ± 1 m/s (V$_{160}$) 11.9 ± 0.9 m/s (V$_{200}$)	138 ± 6.25/min (HR$_{rec2}$) 176 ± 15.6/min (HR$_{rec4}$)	

Warmbloods (field test)	Miscellaneous good performers	1.5 mmol/L (after step 1)	97/min (after step 1)		Van Erck Westegren et al,[19] 2014
	Miscellaneous lameness	2 mmol/L (after step 4) 2 mmol/L (after step 1) 2.5 mmol/L (after step 4)	127/min (after step 4) 105/min (after step 1) 142/min (after step 4)		
	Miscellaneous cardiovascular/lower airway disease	2.5/2.3 mmol/L (after step 1) 4.7/3.5 mmol/L (after step 4)	106/min (after step 1) 154/min (after step 4)		
Reining (field test)	Low level	2.7 ± 1.5 mmol/L (after test)	176 ± 14 (end of test = after sliding stops)	47/min (HRrec10)	Navas de Solis et al,[22] 2018
French trotters (field test)	2 y old 3 y old ≥6 y old	9.2 ± 0.5 m/s (VLA4) 9.8 ± 0.7 m/s (VLA4) 10.4 ± 0.5 m/s (VLA4)	9 ± 0.6 m/s (V200) 9.8 ± 0.6 m/s (V200) 10.7 ± 0.6 m/s (V200)		Courouce et al,[73] 2002
Jumping	National Junior Championship	9.04 ± 0.9 mmol/L (after competition)	191.4 ± 3.8/min (HRmax)	101.5 ± 7/min (HRrec2)	Art et al,[74] 1990
Dressage	Elementary		102 ± 13/min (HRmean) 132 ± 20/min (HRmax)		Williams et al,[75] 2009
	Medium		107 ± 8/min (HRmean) 132 ± 10/min (HRmax)		
Thoroughbred racehorse (treadmill 6° incline)	2 y old 3–4 y old	7 ± 1.1 m/s (VLA4) 7.9 ± 0.5 m/s (VLA4)	7.8 ± 0.5 m/s (V200) 8.8 ± 0.1 m/s (V200)		Rose et al,[76] 1990

The specific parameter for each study is reported in parentheses.

Abbreviations: HR160, velocity when HR reaches 160; HRmean, average HR during a given exercise session; V200, velocity when HR reaches 200; VLA2, velocity when lactate reaches 2 mmol/L; VLA4, velocity when lactate reaches 4 mmol/L.

* Denote the CCI level.

concentrations to guide conditioning is attractive and has recently been reviewed.[58] These parameters derived from lactate and HR measurements and speed or intensity of exercise are more useful if measured serially and in a standardized fashion.[13] Higher than expected HR or lactate or unexpected changes may signal subclinical problems but rarely point out the cause. Higher lactate concentrations and HR are found during exercise tests of less fit horses and with clinical problems such as lameness (or pain), muscular disease, upper airway disease, lower airway disease, or cardiac disease. V_{La4} and V_{200} are frequently similar in healthy, trained horses with a good cardiac response to exercise.[15] HR is more labile than lactate because of effects of excitement or physical discomfort. It has been suggested that if V_{200} is significantly lower than V_{La4}, musculoskeletal injury or cardiovascular disease may be suspected and that a decrease in V_{La4} in fit individuals is common with respiratory disease.[13,15]

In a recent study, eventers with higher V_{LA4} and V_{200} were less likely to become injured than those with lower V_{LA4} and V_{200}.[16] Horses that became injured showed higher peak HRs during condition training (200 ± 10/min) than horses that stayed sound (186 ± 12/min). The investigators concluded that increased HR could be an early sign of lameness and that V_{LA4} and V_{200} can be used to prevent injuries. The heterogeneity of exercise tests makes it impossible to currently report universal cutoff values. Eventers with V_{LA4} lower than the average speed required for their level of exercise have been considered unfit to compete. **Table 2** can serve as a guide to clinicians, but specific values for level, type of exercise test, weather, footing, and so forth are needed to give recommendations in specific populations. More detailed and different tables have been published.[13,14,60,61]

Approximate HR ranges during exercise are 60 to 80/min at the walk, 80 to 120/min at the trot, 110 to 150/min at the canter, 150 to 180/min at a hand gallop, and greater than 180/min at the gallop with peak HRs that can reach 210 to 240/min[62] HR increases up to 120/min are mediated by parasympathetic withdrawal, whereas further increases are associated with sympathetic activity.[63] HR_{rec} is easy to obtain and useful for the clinician and rider. Recovery is usually very rapid in the first minute after exercise, followed by a slower decline. Conflicting evidence can be found in the literature about the relevance of HR_{rec}. HR_{rec} has been correlated with time form ratings,[57] performance in human cyclists,[64] and used in endurance rides as part of the criteria to determine if a horse is fit to continue in competition. The cardiac recovery index (CRI) is a popular tool in endurance rides. Horses are not presented to a vet gate until the HR is lower than 60 to 64/min. HR is obtained at presentation to the vet gate. Then the horse is trotted 30 m out and back, and 1 minute after the horse started the trot, HR is taken again. The difference between the 2 HRs is the CRI. Elimination rate was significantly higher in horses with presenting HRs ≥60/min or CRI ≥4.[65] A horse has a 70% chance of being eliminated at the subsequent vet gate of an endurance race if its cardiac recovery time is longer than 11 min at vet gate 1 or 2, or longer than 13 min at vet gates 3 or 4.[66]

SUMMARY

Exercise testing is a useful clinical tool that can help veterinarians assess poor performance, fitness, and performance potential and prevent injuries. Different types of exercise tests should be used to evaluate horses performing in different disciplines and levels. Lack of standardization and gaps in knowledge about interpretation in some parameters commonly obtained during exercise tests can be limitations of exercise tests. Exercise tests that simultaneously assess several body systems can be beneficial when assessing poor performance because this is a multifactorial problem with signs not detectable at rest. Historical questionnaires, lameness examinations, respiratory sampling, dynamic upper airway endoscopy, exercising ECGs, echocardiograms, and measurement of laboratory values are useful components of exercise tests. Common diseases detected during exercise tests are lameness, IAD/equine asthma, upper airway obstruction, myopathies, and exercising arrhythmias. Myocardial dysfunction, electrolyte abnormalities, and neurologic disease are less commonly detected.

REFERENCES

1. Poole D, Erickson H. Heart and vessels: function during exercise and training adaptations. In: Kenneth W, Hinchcliff KW, Kaneps AJ, Geor RJ, editors. Equine sports medicine and surgery. St Louis (MO): Elsevier Saunders; 2014. p. 667–94.
2. Evans DL. Training and fitness in athletic horses. RIRDC report 2000. Available at: https://rirdc.infoservices.com.au/downloads/00-00.
3. Evans DL. Physiology of equine performance and associated tests of function. Equine Vet J 2007;39:373–83.
4. Hada T, Ohmura H, Mukai K, et al. Utilisation of the time constant calculated from heart rate recovery after exercise for evaluation of autonomic activity in horses. Equine Vet J Suppl 2006;(36):141–5.
5. Sides RH, Kirkpatrick R, Renner E, et al. Validation of masks for determination of VO2 max in horses exercising at high intensity. Equine Vet J 2018;50:91–7.
6. Persson SGB. On blood volume and working capacity in horses. Acta Vet Scand 1967;Suppl:1–189.
7. Piccione G, Giannetto C, Fazio F, et al. Haematological response to different workload in jumper horses. Bulg J Vet Med 2007;10:21–8.
8. Muñoz A, Esgueva M, Gómez-Díez M, et al. Modulation of acute transient exercise-induced hypertension after oral administration of four angiotensin-converting enzyme inhibitors in normotensive horses. Vet J 2016;208:33–7.
9. Kuwahara M, Hiraga A, Kai M, et al. Influence of training on autonomic nervous function in horses: evaluation by power spectral analysis of heart rate variability. Equine Vet J Suppl 1999;(30):178–80.
10. Lorello O, Ramseyer A, Burger D, et al. Repeated measurements of markers of autonomic tone over a training season in eventing horses. J Equine Vet Sci 2017;53:38–44.
11. Kiviniemi AM, Hautala AJ, Kinnunen H, et al. Endurance training guided individually by daily heart rate variability measurements. Eur J Appl Physiol 2007;101: 743.
12. Plews DJ, Laursen PB, Stanley J, et al. Training adaptation and heart rate variability in elite endurance athletes: opening the door to effective monitoring. Sports Med 2013;43:773.
13. Couroucé-Malblanc A, Hodgson DR. Clinical exercise testing. In: Hodgson DR, McKeever KH, McGowan CM, editors. The athletic horse, principles and practice of equine sports medicine. St Louis (MO): Elsevier Saunders; 2014. p. 366–78.
14. Couroucé-Malblanc A, van Erck-Westergren E. Exercise testing in the field. In: Hinchcliff KW, Kaneps AJ, Geor RJ, editors. Equine sports medicine and surgery. Edinburgh (United Kingdom): Elsevier Saunders; 2014. p. 25–42.
15. De Maré L, Boshuizen B, Plancke L, et al. Standardized exercise tests in horses: current situation and future perspectives. Vlaams Diergeneeskd Tijdschr 2017; 86:63–72.

16. Munsters CC, van Iwaarden A, van Weeren R, et al. Exercise testing in Warmblood sport horses under field conditions. Vet J 2014;202:11–9.

17. Muñoz A, Riber C, Santisteban R, et al. Investigation of standardized exercise tests according to fitness level for three-day event horses. J Equine Vet Sci 1998;9:1–7.

18. Fraipont A, Van Erck E, Ramery E, et al. Subclinical diseases underlying poor performance in endurance horses: diagnostic methods and predictive tests. Vet Rec 2011;169:154.

19. Van Erck Westegren E. Value of field trials to investigate poor performance in sport horses. Equine Vet J 2014;46(Suppl 46):14.

20. Munk R, Hedegaard L, Möller S, et al. Training of horses used for show jumping and its effect on VLa4. Equine Vet J 2014;46:8.

21. Bitschnau C, Wiestner T, Trachsel DS, et al. Performance parameters and post exercise heart rate recovery in Warmblood sports horses of different performance levels. Equine Vet J Suppl 2010;3:17–22.

22. Navas de Solis C, Sampson SN, McKay T, et al. Standardised exercise testing in 17 reining horses: musculoskeletal, respiratory, cardiac and clinicopathological findings. Equine Vet Educ 2018;30:262–7.

23. Couroucé A, Geffroy O, Barrey E, et al. Comparison of exercise tests in French trotters under training track, racetrack and treadmill conditions. Equine Vet J Suppl 1999;(30):528–32.

24. Kobayashi M, Kuribara K, Amada A. Application of V200 values for evaluation of training effects in the young thoroughbred under field conditions. Equine Vet J Suppl 1999;(30):159–62.

25. Martin BB Jr, Reef VB, Parente EJ, et al. Causes of poor performance of horses during training, racing, or showing: 348 cases (1992-1996). J Am Vet Med Assoc 2000;216:554–8.

26. Lane JG, Bladon B, Little DRM, et al. Dynamic obstructions of the equine upper respiratory tract. Part 1: observations during high-speed treadmill endoscopy of 600 Thoroughbred racehorses. Equine Vet J 2006;38:393–9.

27. Decloedt A, Borowicz H, Slowikowska M, et al. Right ventricular function during acute exacerbation of severe equine asthma. Equine Vet J 2017;49:603–8.

28. Reef VB, Bonagura J, Buhl R, et al. Recommendations for management of equine athletes with cardiovascular abnormalities. J Vet Intern Med 2014;28:749–61.

29. Fletcher GF, Mills WC, Taylor WC. Update on exercise stress testing. Am Fam Physician 2006;15:1749–54.

30. de Solis CN, Althaus F, Basieux N, et al. Sudden death in sport and riding horses during and immediately after exercise: a case series. Equine Vet J 2018;50(5):644–8.

31. Comyn I, Bathe AP, Foote A, et al. Analysis of sudden death and fatal musculoskeletal injury during FEI three-day eventing. Equine Vet J 2017;49:9.

32. Ryan N, Marr CM, McGladdery AJ. Survey of cardiac arrhythmias during submaximal and maximal exercise in Thoroughbred racehorses. Equine Vet J 2005;37:265–8.

33. Pelliccia A, Maron BJ. Preparticipation cardiovascularevaluation of the competitive athlete: perspectives from the 30-year Italian experience. Am J Cardiol 1995;75:827–9.

34. Navas de Solis C, Green CM, Sides RH, et al. Arrhythmias in thoroughbreds during and after treadmill and racetrack exercise. J Equine Vet Sci 2016;42:19–24.

35. Physick-Sheard PW, McGurrin MK. Ventricular arrhythmias during race recovery in Standardbred Racehorses and associations with autonomic activity. J Vet Intern Med 2010;24:1158–66.
36. Buhl R, Carstensen H, Hesselkilde EZ, et al. Effect of induced chronic atrial fibrillation on exercise performance in Standardbred trotters. J Vet Intern Med 2018; 32(4):1410–9.
37. Verheyen T, Decloedt A, van der Vekens N, et al. Ventricular response during lungeing exercise in horses with lone atrial fibrillation. Equine Vet J 2013;45:309–14.
38. Biffi A, Maron BJ, Verdile L, et al. Impact of physical deconditioning on ventricular tachyarrhythmias in trained athletes. J Am Coll Cardiol 2004;44:1053–8.
39. Jesty SA, Johns B, Potter E, et al. Mechanisms for sudden cardiac death in endurance athletes: support for exerciseinduced arrhythmogenesis. J Vet Intern Med 2015;28:1351–2.
40. Young LE. Cardiac response to training in 2-year-old thoroughbreds: an echocardiographic study. Equine Vet J Suppl 1999;30:195–8.
41. Buhl R, Ersboll AK. Echocardiographic evaluation of changes in left ventricular size and valvular regurgitation associated with physical training during and after maturity in Standardbred trotters. J Am Vet Med Assoc 2012;240:205–12.
42. Morganroth J, Maron BJ, Henry WL, et al. Comparative left ventricular dimensions in trained athletes. Ann Intern Med 1975;82(4):521–4.
43. Young LE, Marlin DJ, Deaton C, et al. Heart size estimated by echocardiography correlates with maximal oxygen uptake. Equine Vet J Suppl 2002;34:467–71.
44. Sleeper MM, Durando MM, Holbrook TC, et al. Comparison of echocardiographic measurements in elite and nonelite Arabian endurance horses. Am J Vet Res 2014;75:893–8.
45. Wijnberg I, Maarsse J, Kampen Wand Veraa S. Cardiac morphology and heart murmurs in elite eventing and dressage horses. Equine Vet J 2014;46:26.
46. Reef VB. Stress echocardiography and its role in performance assessment. Vet Clin North Am Equine Pract 2001;17:179–89.
47. Decloedt A, De Clercq D, Ven S, et al. Right ventricular function during pharmacological and exercise stress testing in horses. Vet J 2017;227:8–14.
48. Schefer KD, Bitschnau C, Weishaupt MA, et al. Quantitative analysis of stress echocardiograms in healthy horses with 2-dimensional (2D) echocardiography, anatomical M-mode, tissue Doppler imaging, and 2D speckle tracking. J Vet Intern Med 2010;24:918–31.
49. Durando MM, Slack J, Reef VB, et al. Right ventricular pressure dynamics and stress echocardiography in pharmacological and exercise stress testing. Equine Vet J Suppl 2006;36:183–92.
50. Marr CM, Bright JM, Marlin DJ, et al. Pre- and post exercise echocardiography in horses performing treadmill exercise in cool and hot/humid conditions. Equine Vet J Suppl 1999;30:131–6.
51. Flethøj M, Schwarzwald CC, Haugaard MM, et al. Left ventricular function after prolonged exercise in equine endurance athletes. J Vet Intern Med 2016;30: 1260–9.
52. Kraus MS, Kaufer BB, Damiani A, et al. Elimination half-life of intravenously administered equine cardiac troponin I in healthy ponies. Equine Vet J 2013; 45:56–9.
53. Rossi TM, Kavsak PA, Maxie MG, et al. Post-exercise cardiac troponin I release and clearance in normal Standardbred racehorses. Equine Vet J 2019;51: 97–101.

54. Shields E, Seiden-Long I, Massie S, et al. 24-hour kinetics of cardiac troponin-t using a "high-sensitivity" assay in thoroughbred Chuckwagon racing geldings after race and associated clinical sampling guidelines. J Vet Intern Med 2018;32: 433–40.
55. Holbrook TC, Birks EK, Sleeper MM, et al. Endurance exercise is associated with increased plasma cardiac troponin I in horses. Equine Vet J Suppl 2006;(36): 27–31.
56. Hauss AA, Stablein CK, Fisher AL, et al. Validation of the lactate plus lactate meter in the horse and its use in a conditioning program. J Equine Vet Sci 2014;34: 1064–8.
57. Evans DL, Harris RC, Snow DH. Correlation of racing performance with blood lactate and heart rate after exercise in thoroughbred horses. Equine Vet J 1993;25:441–5.
58. Campbell EH. Lactate-driven equine conditioning programmes. Vet J 2011;190: 199–207.
59. Lindner A. Use of blood biochemistry for positive performance diagnosis of sport horses in practice. Revue Méd Vét 2000;151:611–8.
60. Munsters CCBM, van den Broek J, Welling E, et al. A prospective study on a cohort of horses and ponies selected for participation in the European Eventing Championship: reasons for withdrawal and predictive value of fitness tests. BMC Vet Res 2013;9:182.
61. Allen KJ, Erck-Westergren E, Franklin SH. Exercise testing in the equine athlete. Equine Vet Educ 2016;28:89–98.
62. Allen KJ, Young LE, Franklin SH. Evaluation of heart rate and rhythm during exercise. Equine Vet Educ 2016;28:99–112.
63. Hamlin RL, Klepinger WL, Gilpin KW, et al. Autonomic control of hem rate in the horse. Am J Physiol 1972;222:976–8.
64. Lamberts RP, Swart J, Capostagno B, et al. Heart rate recovery as a guide to monitor fatigue and predict changes in performance parameters. Scand J Med Sci Sports 2010;20:449–57.
65. Robert C, Benamou-Smith A, Leclerc JL. Use of the recovery check in long-distance endurance rides. Equine Vet J Suppl 2002;34:106–11.
66. Younes M, Robert C, Cottin F, et al. Speed and cardiac recovery variables predict the probability of elimination in equine endurance events. PLoS One 2015;10(8): e0137013.
67. White SL, Williamson LH, Maykuth P, et al. Heart rate and lactate concentration during two different cross country events. Equine Vet J 1995;27:463–7.
68. Marlin DJ, Harris PA, Schroter RC, et al. Physiological, metabolic and biochemical responses of horses competing in the speed and endurance phase of a CCI*****3-day-event. Equine Vet J Suppl 1995;20:37–46.
69. Muñoz A, Riber C, Santisteban R, et al. Cardiovascular and metabolic adaptations in horses competing in cross-country events. J Vet Med Sci 1999;61:13–20.
70. Serrano MG, Evans DL, Hodgson JL. Heart rate and blood lactate responses during exercise in preparation for eventing competition. Equine Vet J 2002;34:135–9.
71. Serrano MG, Evans DL, Hodgson JL. Heart rate and blood Lactateconcentrations in a field fitness test for event horses. Aus Equine Vet J 2001;19:154–60.
72. Fraipont A, Van Erck E, Ramery E, et al. Assessing fitness in endurance horses. Can Vet J 2012;53:311–4.
73. Courouce A, Chretien M, Valette JP. Physiological variables measured under field conditions according to age and state of training in French Trotters. Equine Vet J 2002;34:91–7.

74. Art T, Amory H, Desmecht D, et al. Effect of show jumping on heart rate, blood lactate and other plasma biochemical values. Equine Vet J Suppl 1990;(9):78–82.
75. Williams J, Chandler RE, Marlin D. Heart rates of horses during competitive dressage. Comp Exerc Physiol 2009;6:7–15.
76. Rose RJ, Hendrickson DK, Knight PK. Clinical exercise testing in the normal thoroughbred racehorse. Aust Vet J 1990;67:345–8.

Cardiovascular Causes of Poor Performance and Exercise Intolerance and Assessment of Safety in the Equine Athlete

Mary M. Durando, DVM, PhD

KEYWORDS

• Equine • Exercise intolerance • Cardiac • Arrhythmias • Poor performance

KEY POINTS

- Cardiovascular diseases are an important cause of poor performance or exercise intolerance in the equine athlete, and arrhythmias are the most common cardiac abnormality likely to affect performance and safety.
- Because athletic horses have a high prevalence of valvular regurgitation and resting arrhythmias, the clinical importance of some abnormalities encountered on resting examination is not always clear.
- Conversely, the horse may have a normal resting examination, and exercise induce arrhythmias that may affect performance and safety.
- Often a dynamic examination is required to determine if the cardiovascular system is contributing to the reduced athletic potential or if observed abnormalities at rest are important.
- Because many causes of poor performance are multifactorial, examination of all body systems likely to contribute should be evaluated.

INTRODUCTION

Equine veterinarians are frequently asked to examine horses for reduced performance. Most horses are used for athletic purposes, therefore they must be able to perform at a certain level safely for their owner. There is an inherent risk associated with equine activities. If the horse has the potential for weakness or collapse, the risk is magnified. Therefore any decrease in performance ability, or any problem presenting a safety concern warrants veterinary examination.

Disclosure Statement: No disclosures or conflicts of interest.
Equine Sports Medicine Consultants, LLC, 40 East Main Street, Suite 232, Newark, DE 19711, USA
E-mail address: Mdurando2004@yahoo.com

Determining the cause of poor performance can be challenging for several reasons:

- The musculoskeletal and respiratory systems are more commonly affected, with a lower index of suspicion for cardiovascular causes.
- Horses have a high prevalence of cardiac murmurs and arrhythmias, many of which are not clinically important.
- Because of tremendous cardiopulmonary reserve, horses may be normal at rest or during low intensity work, and clinical signs only become apparent when their cardiovascular system is maximally stressed.
- Evaluation under dynamic conditions can be challenging, or unavailable.

CAUSES OF REDUCED PERFORMANCE/EXERCISE INTOLERANCE

Any abnormality of cardiac function or structure has the potential to cause poor performance. The effect on performance will depend on the severity of the cardiac disease, and the discipline the horse performs. Those horses that perform work requiring predominantly muscular ability and coordination, with less aerobic demand (ie, dressage, show hunter), will be able to tolerate more dysfunction than a horse that is required to perform sports using their entire cardiac reserve (ie, racing, eventing). Regardless of the discipline, if they are severely affected, performance will be impacted.

Most abnormalities reduce cardiac output by decreasing stroke volume or affecting heart rate. If cardiac output is reduced sufficiently, performance will be decreased. Some cardiac abnormalities can also result in increased pulmonary vascular pressures (causing exercise-induced pulmonary hemorrhage or pulmonary edema), which also affects performance. The effect on performance in more severe diseases is clearcut; however, the impact of a particular abnormality that is more subtle can be surprisingly difficult to discern. In addition, many cases of decreased performance ability are multifactorial in origin.[1,2] Therefore, the clinical relevance of cardiac abnormalities found in consort with abnormalities of other body systems can be difficult to determine.

This article will focus on some of the more common causes of exercise intolerance that are encountered, including arrhythmias and valvular regurgitation. However it is important to remember that severe abnormalities resulting from any cardiac disease can cause exercise intolerance.

Arrhythmias

Resting arrhythmias are frequently encountered in equine veterinary medicine. Vagally mediated bradyarrhythmias such as second-degree atrioventricular block and sinus block occur commonly in fit, athletic horses at rest. They are almost always a normal finding if overridden by exercise or sympathetic stimulation. Horses with no evidence of primary cardiac disease may also have occasional arrhythmias such as atrial premature complexes. In most cases, occasional isolated premature complexes at rest do not affect performance if they disappear with exercise.

Arrhythmias can also occur when there are fluctuations in autonomic control over heart rate and rhythm. This may be at the beginning of exercise, during transitions in exercise intensity, or during the early recovery period.[3,4] Arrhythmias seen during these periods of heart rate transitions may be clinically unimportant, particularly if isolated and infrequent. The more complex arrhythmias that can be seen occasionally in the immediate post-exercise period are more concerning, although an exact impact on performance or risk they present is not clear.

Uncertainty exists over the importance of isolated premature complexes occurring at maximal heart rate and exercise intensity. Arrhythmias occurring during peak exercise are more concerning than those seen at rest or during rapid changes in heart rate, as they are more likely to affect performance. Ventricular arrhythmias will decrease intracardiac pressures (**Fig. 1**), and cardiac output. Therefore horses performing work requiring maximal cardiac output will be affected by these arrhythmias. Although atrial fibrillation (AF) or ventricular tachycardia affect performance, the effect of isolated premature complexes are more controversial. Martin and colleagues[2] suggested that greater than 2 isolated premature depolarizations during maximal exercise, or greater than 5 pairs or paroxysms of premature depolarizations occurring in the immediate post-exercise period are clinically relevant. A study evaluating cardiac

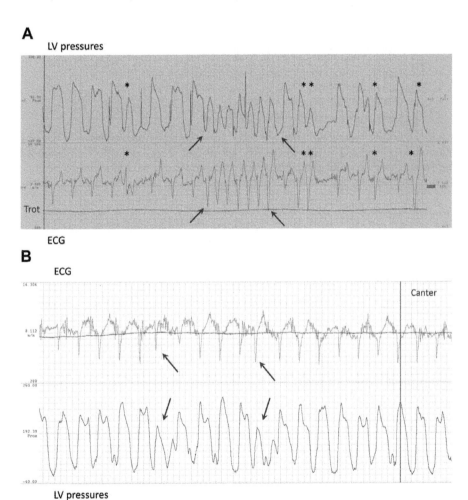

Fig. 1. The effect of ventricular arrhythmias on intracardiac pressures. Simultaneous ECGs and left ventricular (LV) pressure tracings show the effect of ventricular premature complexes (VPCs) on LV pressures. (*A*) The horse is trotting at 3.7 m/s on a treadmill. The top panel shows the LV pressures and the bottom panel shows the ECG. (*B*) Similar depiction as (*A*). The horse is cantering at 8.1 m/s. The ECG is on the top panel and the LV pressures are on the bottom panel. Arrows and asterisks mark arrhythmias.

arrhythmias during treadmill exercise in poorly performing Thoroughbred racehorses showed that 22/88 (25%) had arrhythmias that would be considered clinically relevant by the criteria of Martin and colleagues.[5] Whether these arrhythmias were secondary to other problems, and the exact relationship to affect performance was not evaluated. Arrhythmias may be found in consort with other body system abnormalities, making the determination of specific effect on performance difficult.

A few studies have evaluated cardiac rhythm in normally performing horses in various settings during[3,4,6–8] and after exercise.[9,10] These studies have shown arrhythmias to be fairly prevalent in healthy athletes. The studies evaluating horses during training sessions showed the majority of these arrhythmias occurred at slow speeds, during heart rate transitions, or in the immediate post-exercise recovery period, and not during peak exercise.

The following factors interfere with classifying type (supraventricular vs ventricular) and number of arrhythmias on an exercising electrocardiogram (ECG), which makes clinical interpretation of exercising ECGs difficult:

- Motion artifact (from respiration, footfall, ECG, and rider movement) (**Fig. 2**)
- Definition of prematurity (% RR-interval variability cutoff)[11]
- Lack of multi-lead ECG systems (**Fig. 3**)
- High heart rates at maximal exercise (**Fig. 4**)

A recent study evaluating intra- and inter-observer agreement between observers interpreting exercising ECGs found the agreement to be poor.[12] For the above mentioned reasons, published cutoffs for the number of premature complexes and types of arrhythmias that are clinically important become difficult to apply in practice.

Atrial fibrillation

Atrial fibrillation is the most common pathologic arrhythmia affecting performance in horses.[13–15] It can be self-terminating (paroxysmal), lasting minutes to days,[15,16] or sustained, requiring cardioversion to abolish. A detailed discussion of AF can be found in Gunther van Loon's article, "Cardiac Arrhythmias in Horses," in this issue.

Exercise intolerance or abrupt decreases in performance are common findings in horses with AF.[13,14,17–19] When it occurs during peak exercise, this can be seen as sudden slowing during a race, or pulling up during any exertion. Often these horses pull up in distress, and may vocalize or have epistaxis or hemoptysis. They will have a very rapid, irregular heart rate and rhythm, and a prolonged heart rate recovery. AF can also cause dyspnea, weakness, ataxia, or syncope, although collapse is uncommonly reported.[15,20] Collapse is thought most likely to occur if a rapid ventricular response with wide complex tachycardia is present during exercise or extreme sympathetic stimulation. This has been reported in horses with AF, potentially placing them at an increased risk for sudden death (SD).[21] A recent study reported a decrease in velocity and an increase in maximum heart rate in horses after induced AF compared with control runs before induction of AF, when exercising on a treadmill.[22] In addition, a high percentage of these horses had abnormal QRS complexes.

Paroxysmal AF has also been detected in horses after racing or at the termination of exercise, without an obvious effect on performance. In these situations, it is likely to have been triggered in the immediate post-exercise period.[9,15] Conversely, paroxysmal AF may be missed as a cause of exercise intolerance in some horses, as they could be in sinus rhythm by the time of examination, if there has been a delay before auscultation.

AF has also been associated with heavy exercise-induced pulmonary hemorrhage and epistaxis secondary to rapid increases in pulmonary vascular pressures caused

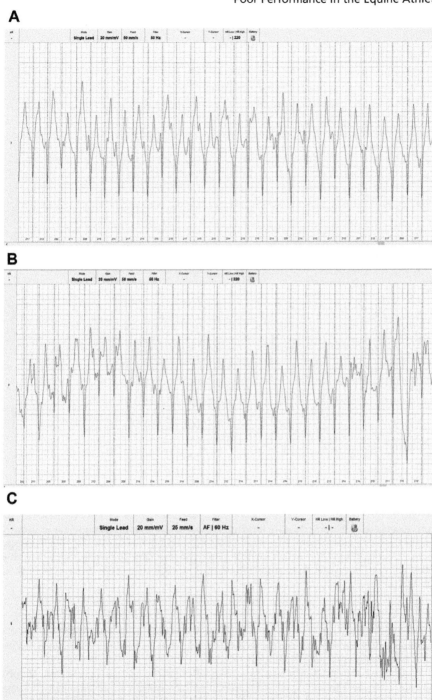

Fig. 2. Base apex ECG recordings during exercise. (*A*) and (*B*) ECG recorded from a galloping horse. Although this trace is of sufficient quality to easily detect QRS-T complexes and is relatively artifact free, there is still motion artifact caused by footfall and respiration that is unavoidable. (*B*) Motion associated with jumps. (*C*) ECG recorded from a galloping horse. This recording shows massive motion artifact and is unreadable.

A

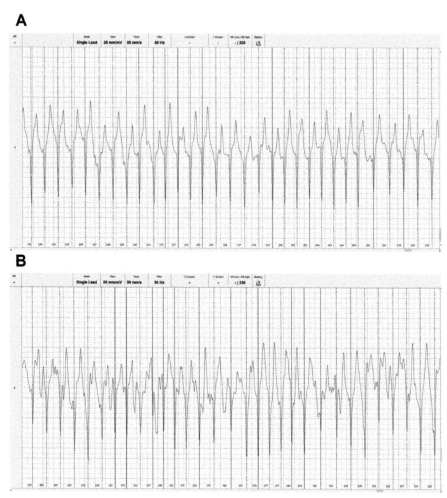

B

Fig. 3. Examples of rhythms that are difficult to classify whether supraventricular or ventricular from a single lead system. Base apex ECGs recorded on 2 horses during high-intensity exercise (A, B). Note the irregular rhythm; although the QRS complexes are not visibly different from the surrounding sinus complexes, it is difficult to definitively classify their origin.

by the arrhythmia.[13,15,23,24] Any performance horse with a history of acute exercise intolerance and epistaxis or hempoptysis should have a cardiac evaluation, emphasizing exercise-associated rhythm disorders.

AF can also be an incidental finding, particularly in those horses that perform at submaximal exercise intensities, where maximal cardiac output is not required.[13,14] The atrial contribution to ventricular filling is considered to be ~10% to 30%; therefore, in less-demanding sports, the required cardiac output may be unaffected. In these situations, an increase in heart rate will compensate for the decrease in stroke volume, allowing submaximal exercise to be unaffected. However, if the horse is required to have maximal cardiac output to perform adequately, it will be unable to increase heart rate enough to meet demands.

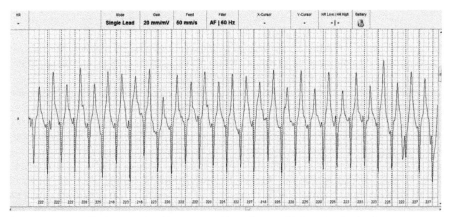

Fig. 4. Base apex ECG at maximal heart rate. Note that at this heart rate the P waves cannot be distinguished.

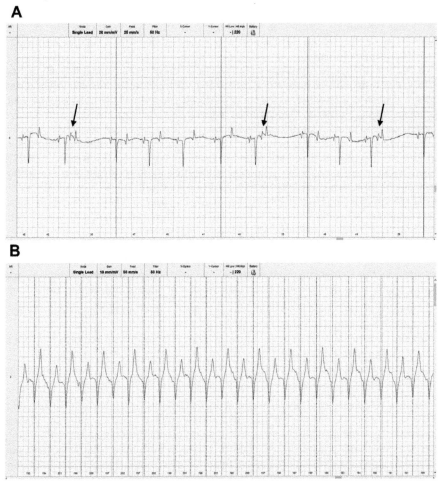

Fig. 5. Base apex ECG recorded from a horse with supraventricular premature complexes (SVPCs). (*A*) Recording at rest. Note the premature P waves (*arrows*) buried in the preceding QRS-T that are non-conducted. (*B*) The same horse during exercise. Note the regular R-R interval with no premature complexes.

Other supraventricular arrhythmias

Supraventricular premature complexes (SVPC) are ectopic beats that originate above the ventricles. See Gunther van Loon's article, "Cardiac Arrhythmias in Horses," for a detailed discussion of supraventricular arrhythmias.

A horse with SVPCs documented at rest should have an exercise test to determine persistence during exercise. Often, the increased sinus rate occurring during exercise will override the ectopic focus (**Fig. 5**). If overridden with exercise, performance will not be affected. However in some horses the frequency of SVPCs will increase with exercise, and may reduce exercise tolerance.[25,26] The impact of isolated SVPCs occurring during maximal exercise is debatable.[6] An occasional isolated SVPC is unlikely to affect cardiac output and performance; however larger numbers, or short bursts of supraventricular tachycardia (SVT), may do so. Frequent SVPCs may also be a risk factor for AF development.[27] SVPCs are also seen during heart rate transitions and fluctuations in autonomic tone, and are unlikely to affect performance.[4,7,8]

Ventricular arrhythmias

Ventricular premature complexes (VPCs) originate from the ventricles (**Fig. 6**). See Gunther van Loon's article, "Cardiac Arrhythmias in Horses," for a detailed discussion of ventricular arrhythmias.

Ventricular premature complexes are thought to be of more clinical relevance than SVPCs, and potentially to have more impact on performance. Occasional VPCs at rest that are abolished with exercise are not considered important, if no obvious underlying pathology exists. However, if they persist or increase in number during exercise, have a short coupling interval, or differing morphologies, they are cause for concern from a safety and performance standpoint. Multiple VPCs likely decrease cardiac output during exercise (see **Fig. 1**). This can cause a sudden drop in exercise tolerance, which, if it were to occur at the wrong time, such as at the start of a jump, could be devastating. Ventricular premature complexes also have the potential to trigger ventricular tachycardia, which could be life threatening, especially if triggered during exercise. Arrhythmias occurring only post-exercise are not likely to affect performance; however, their role in SD occurring immediately after exercise is unknown.

Several studies have reported a higher number of VPCs than previously thought to be acceptable in horses exercising in field conditions.[3,4] However, most of these occurred in the immediate post-exercise period or at submaximal exercise, and were thought to be due to sympathetic stimulation or fluctuations in autonomic tone.

- Show jumpers—less than 3 VPCs/horse seen in 5/34 horses during exercise; 2 horses had single VPCs during recovery[7]
- Dressage horses—2 isolated VPCs in 1/26 horses during exercise; no VPCs observed during recovery[8]
- Racing Standardbreds—1 VPC in 1/26 horses during racing; 6/26 horses had VPCs during recovery[6]

Very few VPCs occurred during maximal work in these field studies, suggesting that, in normal horses, once they have reached a steady state at maximal exercise, minimal numbers of premature beats persist. If increased numbers are seen during maximal exercise, the horse should be considered unsafe to perform at that level, because of the risk of precipitating a more malignant arrhythmia (ventricular tachycardia or ventricular fibrillation).[27]

The large variation of arrhythmias seen during warm-up and recovery portions of exercise in normally performing horses is likely dependent on the type of exercise performed during the test and the discipline of the horse. These data suggest less

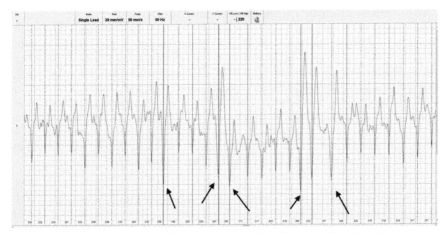

Fig. 6. Base apex ECG recorded from a horse with VPCs (*arrows*) during high-intensity exercise.

importance should be attached to isolated arrhythmias seen during these volatile portions of exercise. However, multiple or malignant VPCs or numerous SVPCs or SVT occurring at peak exercise would be considered abnormal, and likely affect performance and safety. During peak exercise, most studies had similar findings (regardless of discipline) of less than 4 isolated SVPCs or VPCs, except for the findings in racing Standardbreds regarding SVPCs.[6] The reason for the large number of SVPCs seen in horses during racing in that study is not known. However the number of VPCs seen in that study was similar to other studies, suggesting that VPCs are not seen in high numbers during peak exercise. Unfortunately, an exact cutoff number that is abnormal or will definitively reduce performance is not known.

Bradyarrhythmias

Bradyarrhythmias (sinus bradycardia, sinus block, and second-degree atrioventricular block), are common in fit athletic horses, and are a normal finding, as long as sympathetic stimulation restores sinus rhythm at an appropriate heart rate. They are common because of the high resting vagal tone of most athletic horses and do not affect performance. Uncommonly, advanced second- or third-degree atrioventricular block occurs. This is always pathologic, and causes exercise intolerance or even collapse.

Valvular Regurgitation

Cardiac murmurs are frequently detected in athletic horses[28–32] and may be encountered during examination for poor performance. These murmurs can be normal physiologic murmurs or may be associated with valvular regurgitation or other structural abnormalities.

Although the effect of severe valvular regurgitation on performance is obvious, the importance of mild-moderate valvular regurgitation is often unclear. Athletic horses that are performing well have a high prevalence of mild valvular regurgitation. The presence and amount of regurgitation has been shown to increase with training in normally performing athletes, because of normal physiologic remodeling.[31,33–35] This adaptation to training can result in valvular regurgitation.[29,31,33] The frequency of occurrence of murmurs of valvular regurgitation ranges from 1% to 48%, depending on the population of horses studied, whereas the incidence of valvular regurgitation based on color flow Doppler imaging ranges from 31% to 86%.[8,28,30,31,33,36,37] Most of these were trivial to mild in severity. Because of the frequent detection of murmurs associated with regurgitation, as well as the high prevalence of mild valvular regurgitation, it can be challenging to determine their role in association with poor performance. Studies have shown no significant association between the presence of murmurs and performance in racehorses,[31,33] and Young and colleagues did not find a correlation of murmur score or regurgitant grade with performance.[33] However, in this study most of the horses had only trivial-mild regurgitation. In addition, the number of elite horses was low, and few of those had clinically relevant regurgitation.[33] In horses with loud murmurs and signs consistent with heart failure or signs of respiratory compromise, the cardiac disease will clearly affect performance.

Mitral regurgitation

Mitral regurgitation (MR) is common in horses of all ages; the majority are mild and do not affect performance, providing the valve morphology and function remain normal. Young and Wood reported that 58% of National Hunt horses had MR.[36] If mitral valve disease worsens, it is more likely to affect performance than disease at other valves. However, depending on the sport the horse is used for, if the MR is only mild to moderate it may not be important to the horse's potential.[33,38] If regurgitation is more severe, the left atrium (LA) will undergo pressure- and volume-related dilation. This can lead to pulmonary hypertension and edema, which will also compromise athletic ability. MR can also affect performance by the association with arrhythmias caused by the enlarging LA. Atrial arrhythmias (especially AF) can occur secondary to an enlarged LA and may be the cause of reduced performance. Therefore, any horses with murmurs consistent with MR and accompanying respiratory signs, elevated heart rate, or irregular cardiac rhythm are of concern.

Aortic regurgitation

Aortic regurgitation is common in older horses and is usually the result of slowly progressive degenerative valve disease. If the amount of regurgitation is mild when first observed in an older horse, with no left ventricular (LV) enlargement, it is unlikely to affect performance. However, it is usually a progressive disease, so the horse should be monitored for increasing volume overload. Larger insufficiencies are likely to result in LV enlargement, which can be associated with ventricular arrhythmias. As the LV becomes enlarged, it can stretch the mitral valve annulus, causing secondary MR. As both progress, congestive heart failure can result. Independent of development of congestive heart failure, ventricular arrhythmias associated with the enlarging LV can cause exercise intolerance, weakness, or collapse, and can also cause SD by triggering fatal ventricular fibrillation.

The intensity of a diastolic murmur does not correlate with the severity of the regurgitation, and can vary at different auscultation times. Therefore, this is not a good indicator of the amount of regurgitation and the likely effect on performance. The presence of bounding peripheral pulses or a new left-sided systolic murmur consistent with MR are much more important. If these findings are present, performance and safety are more likely to be affected than if only a loud murmur is present, and the horse must be critically evaluated. As LV enlargement progresses, rider and horse safety during exercise become the biggest concern. For these horses, an exercise ECG is required to determine safety of horse and rider for exercise.[27]

Tricuspid regurgitation

Tricuspid regurgitation (TR) is common in athletes, particularly National Hunt horses in the United Kingdom and Standardbreds.[31,36] Horses can usually tolerate mild or moderate TR without a negative effect on performance. If it results in right atrial enlargement, there is a risk for AF.

Velocity of the regurgitant jet can be used to assess relative chamber pressures in the right ventricle. If the velocity of the TR jet is >3.5 m/s, this indicates that the right ventricle likely has increased systolic pressures. In the absence of pulmonic stenosis (which is rare), this implies that the pulmonary artery pressures are also elevated. Although this is not a sensitive indicator of pulmonary hypertension, clinically relevant pulmonary disease or significant left-sided cardiac disease causing pulmonary hypertension should be ruled out. If either of those is found along with TR, there will be a larger effect on performance.

Miscellaneous Causes

Any cardiac abnormality has the potential to affect performance. Less common diseases, such as congenital cardiac disease (particularly VSDs), myocarditis, and aortic root disease/aortocardiac fistulas can result in reduced athletic ability and exercise intolerance, and, if severe, can result in SD. These are covered in detail in Brian A. Scansen's article, "Equine Congenital Heart Disease," in this issue and Annelies Decloedt's article, "Pericardial Disease, Myocardial Disease, and Great Vessel Abnormalities in Horses," in this issue.

COLLAPSE AND SUDDEN DEATH

Collapse is a sudden loss of postural tone, with or without loss of consciousness, resulting in recumbency or near recumbency.[20] Both cardiac and non-cardiac causes can cause collapse, which can occur at rest or during exercise. A retrospective study evaluating causes of collapse found that 20% (5/25 cases) were because of cardiac causes.[20] Most of these were arrhythmogenic (4/5). A presumptive diagnosis was made in 8/25 cases and no diagnosis could be found in 6/25 cases, emphasizing that causes of collapse are often undetermined in the horse.

Sudden death is defined as acute death in a closely observed and apparently healthy horse, in the absence of obvious catastrophic injury or trauma likely to have contributed to death.[39] Collapse and SD can result from similar causes, and collapse may progress rapidly to SD. Sudden cardiac death (SCD) is sudden death from loss of cardiac function.[40,41] A recent paper reviewed SCD in horses.[42]

Post mortem findings after SD have been investigated in horses.[40,43–48] However, the cause is not always clear. In 1 large multicenter study, which collated data from several countries performing necropsies on SD cases during racing, a definitive cause was found in only 53% of cases (143/268).[40] Of the definitively diagnosed cases, 56% (80/143) were determined to be from cardiopulmonary failure; however, only 20% (16/80) of those were attributed to cardiac lesions alone (6% of all cases). Only 2 cases were due to aortic rupture (1% of all cases). A presumptive cause was recorded in 25% of cases, with 54% of those suggested to be from cardiopulmonary failure. However, differences in interpretation by the pathologist and in necropsy protocols may result in different conclusions. In addition, histopathologic lesions do not necessarily equate with cause of death. Twenty-two percent of cases were unexplained. However, even in cases without gross or histologic lesions, fatal arrhythmia or other acute myocardial disease may still be suspected. Indications of cell death may not occur for 12 hours after total ischemia, and arrhythmias may be functional in nature (ie, accessory pathways or ion channelopathies). Therefore, the role of cardiac dysfunction, and, in particular, fatal arrhythmias, is often undetermined. Kiryu and colleagues,[46] investigating arrhythmias as a cause of SD in horses, described 5 horses with SCD. All horses had cardiac histologic abnormalities and 1 horse had documented arrhythmias leading to ventricular fibrillation and cardiac arrest. Vascular sclerosis leading to fibrotic and fibroplastic changes at or near the conduction system were presumed to lead to fatal arrhythmias.

Many other physiologic factors occur rapidly during intense exercise, including tremendously increased pulmonary artery pressure that may promote right ventricular remodeling, changes in vagal and sympathetic tone, and changes in electrolyte, blood volume, and acid-base status, all of which may contribute to arrhythmogenesis. However, the role of these factors in SCD and the assessment of an individual's particular risk for SCD are currently not available.

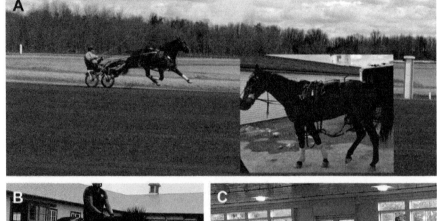
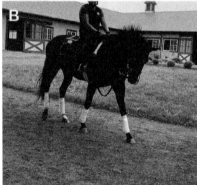
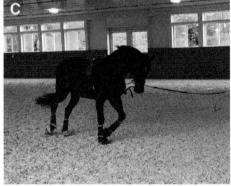

Fig. 7. Examples of field tests in equine athletes. (*A*) A Standardbred with poor performance instrumented with ECG and dynamic endoscopy. (*B*) A Thoroughbred with exercise intolerance instrumented with ECG and dynamic endoscopy. (*C*) Cardiac rhythm evaluation of a stallion with supraventricular premature complexes and mild left-sided cardiac enlargement.

ASSESSMENT OF SAFETY

Determination of the cause of poor performance as well as assessment of safety often requires some type of exercise testing.[27]

The nature of the diagnostic tests and the type of exercise performed depend on the suspected causes, the discipline of the horse, and the exercise intensity at which it has a problem. Because the causes of exercise intolerance can be multifactorial and other body systems may influence risk of collapse or SD, it is usually best to fully evaluate all likely body systems during work.

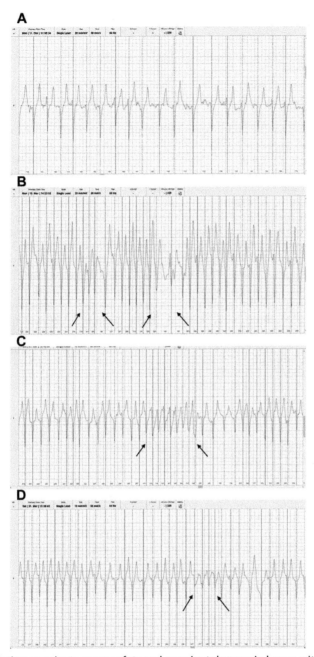

Fig. 8. ECG during exercise to assess safety and exercise tolerance in horses with atrial fibrillation (AF). (*A*) A horse with adequate exercise tolerance for its job requirements. (*B*) A horse in atrial fibrillation, without clinical exercise intolerance. Note the rapid instantaneous heart rates and the abnormal QRS complexes (*arrows*). (*C*) A racehorse horse with atrial fibrillation that was to be "re-purposed" to a riding horse. Note the rapid instantaneous heart rates and the abnormal QRS complexes (*arrows*). (*D*) The rhythm and rate response (*arrows*) to sympathetic stimulation (walking by a group of young foals galloping in a field) in the same horse as (*C*). Note that horses in AF are not considered safe to use and should be cardioverted or retired if the exercising heart rate during sustained maximal exercise exceeds 220 beats/min or if concurrent ventricular arrhythmias are detected during exercise or with sympathetic stimulation.

A thorough history and physical examination should be performed first to rule out overt abnormalities. They also prioritize the next diagnostic steps. Resting upper airway endoscopy, thoracic ultrasound, echocardiogram, and ECG may be indicated. If the results of these tests are normal or equivocal, an exercise test is needed to further elucidate a cause of poor performance or safety to perform.

Exercise testing can be performed on a high-speed treadmill, during lunging, or during ridden or driven exercise (**Fig. 7**). For those situations whereby collapse is a possibility, any type of ridden or driven exercise should be avoided. Lunging or treadmill tests avoid rider safety issues, although risks to the horse should be fully discussed with the owner. The goal of exercise testing is to reproduce the situations that induce the problem or, in the case of poor exercise performance, mimic the type of exercise the horse has had difficulty performing.[27,49] If collapse is not a concern, the choice of exercise test (field vs treadmill) depends on the available facilities. There are pros and cons to both types. Treadmill testing allows a larger variety of instrumentation (ie, arterial blood gas and pressure measurements); however, this may not mimic the intended use of the horse. Upper airway function and heart rhythm can be readily evaluated in the field during the type of exercise associated with problems (see **Fig. 7**). Although there is controversy surrounding the importance of some ECG findings during exercise, exercising ECGs allow screening for those arrhythmias that are clearly more concerning and present a known risk to horse and rider (such as ventricular tachycardia or ventricular ectopy in horses in AF) (**Fig. 8**).

REFERENCES

1. Morris EA, Seeherman HJ. Clinical evaluation of poor performance in the racehorse: the results of 275 evaluations. Equine Vet J 1991;23(3):169–74.
2. Martin BB Jr, Reef VB, Parente EJ, et al. Causes of poor performance of horses during training, racing, or showing: 348 cases (1992-1996). J Am Vet Med Assoc 2000;216(4):554–8.
3. Physick-Sheard PW, McGurrin MK. Ventricular arrhythmias during race recovery in Standardbred Racehorses and associations with autonomic activity. J Vet Intern Med 2010;24(5):1158–66.
4. Ryan N, Marr CM, McGladdery AJ. Survey of cardiac arrhythmias during submaximal and maximal exercise in Thoroughbred racehorses. Equine Vet J 2005;37(3):265–8.
5. Jose-Cunilleras E, Young LE, Newton JR, et al. Cardiac arrhythmias during and after treadmill exercise in poorly performing thoroughbred racehorses. Equine Vet J Suppl 2006;(36):163–70.
6. Buhl R, Peterson E, Lindholm M, et al. Cardiac arrhythmias in Standardbreds during and after racing - possible association between heart size, valvular regurgitations, and arrhythmias. J Equine Vet Sci 2013;33:590–6.
7. Buhl R, Meldgaard C, Barbesgaard L. Cardiac arrhythmias in clinically healthy showjumping horses. Equine Vet J Suppl 2010;(38):196–201.
8. Barbesgaard L, Buhl R, Meldgaard C. Prevalence of exercise-associated arrhythmias in normal performing dressage horses. Equine Vet J Suppl 2010;(38):202–7.
9. Slack J, Boston RC, Soma LR, et al. Occurrence of cardiac arrhythmias in Standardbred racehorses. Equine Vet J 2015;47(4):398–404.
10. Flethoj M, Kanters JK, Haugaard MM, et al. Changes in heart rate, arrhythmia frequency, and cardiac biomarker values in horses during recovery after a long-distance endurance ride. J Am Vet Med Assoc 2016;248(9):1034–42.

11. Flethoj M, Kanters JK, Pedersen PJ, et al. Appropriate threshold levels of cardiac beat-to-beat variation in semi-automatic analysis of equine ECG recordings. BMC Vet Res 2016;12(1):266.
12. Trachsel DS, Bitschnau C, Waldern N, et al. Observer agreement for detection of cardiac arrhythmias on telemetric ECG recordings obtained at rest, during and after exercise in 10 Warmblood horses. Equine Vet J Suppl 2010;(38):208–15.
13. Deem DA, Fregin GF. Atrial fibrillation in horses: a review of 106 clinical cases, with consideration of prevalence, clinical signs, and prognosis. J Am Vet Med Assoc 1982;180(3):261–5.
14. Reef VB, Levitan CW, Spencer PA. Factors affecting prognosis and conversion in equine atrial fibrillation. J Vet Intern Med 1988;2(1):1–6.
15. Holmes JR, Henigan M, Williams RB, et al. Paroxysmal atrial fibrillation in race-horses. Equine Vet J 1986;18(1):37–42.
16. Hiraga AK K. Two cases of paroxysmal atrial fibrillation during exercise in horses. Equine Vet Educ 1999;11:6–10.
17. Ohmura H, Hiraga A, Takahashi T, et al. Risk factors for atrial fibrillation during racing in slow-finishing horses. J Am Vet Med Assoc 2003;223(1):84–8.
18. Physick-Sheard PW. Seek and ye shall find: cardiac arrhythmias in the horse. Equine Vet J 2013;45(3):270–2.
19. Marr CM, Reef VB, Reimer JM, et al. An echocardiographic study of atrial fibrillation in horses: before and after conversion to sinus rhythm. J Vet Intern Med 1995;9(5):336–40.
20. Lyle CH, Turley G, Blissitt KJ, et al. Retrospective evaluation of episodic collapse in the horse in a referred population: 25 cases (1995-2009). J Vet Intern Med 2010;24(6):1498–502.
21. Verheyen T, Decloedt A, van der Vekens N, et al. Ventricular response during lungeing exercise in horses with lone atrial fibrillation. Equine Vet J 2013;45(3):309–14.
22. Buhl R, Carstensen H, Hesselkilde EZ, et al. Effect of induced chronic atrial fibrillation on exercise performance in Standardbred trotters. J Vet Intern Med 2018;32(4):1410–9.
23. Amada A, Kurita H. Five cases of paroxysmal atrial fibrillation in the racehorse. Exp Rep Equine Health Lab 1975;1975(12):89–100.
24. Holmes JR. Cardiac arrhythmias of the racehorse. In: Gillespe NE JR, editor. Equine exercise physiology 2. Davis (CA): ICEEP; 1986. p. 781–5.
25. Holmes JR, Darke PGG, Else RW. Atrial fibrillation in the horse. Equine Vet J 1969;1(5):212–22.
26. Miller MS, Gertsen KE, Dawson H. Paroxysmal atrial fibrillation: a case report. J Equine Vet Sci 1987;7(2):95–7.
27. Reef VB, Bonagura J, Buhl R, et al. Recommendations for management of equine athletes with cardiovascular abnormalities. J Vet Intern Med 2014;28(3):749–61.
28. Kriz NG, Hodgson DR, Rose RJ. Prevalence and clinical importance of heart murmurs in racehorses. J Am Vet Med Assoc 2000;216(9):1441–5.
29. Young LE, Wood JL. Effect of age and training on murmurs of atrioventricular valvular regurgitation in young thoroughbreds. Equine Vet J 2000;32(3):195–9.
30. Patteson MW, Cripps PJ. A survey of cardiac auscultatory findings in horses. Equine Vet J 1993;25(5):409–15.
31. Buhl R, Ersboll AK, Eriksen L, et al. Changes over time in echocardiographic measurements in young Standardbred racehorses undergoing training and racing and association with racing performance. J Am Vet Med Assoc 2005;226(11):1881–7.

32. Marr CM, Reef VB. Physiological valvular regurgitation in clinically normal young racehorses: prevalence and two-dimensional colour flow Doppler echocardiographic characteristics. Equine Vet J Suppl 1995;(19):56–62.
33. Young LE, Rogers K, Wood JL. Heart murmurs and valvular regurgitation in thoroughbred racehorses: epidemiology and associations with athletic performance. J Vet Intern Med 2008;22(2):418–26.
34. Young LE. Cardiac responses to training in 2-year-old thoroughbreds: an echocardiographic study. Equine Vet J Suppl 1999;(30):195–8.
35. Kriz NG, Hodgson DR, Rose RJ. Changes in cardiac dimensions and indices of cardiac function during deconditioning in horses. Am J Vet Res 2000;61(12): 1553–60.
36. Young LEW, Wood JLN. Effect of age and training on thoroughbred valvular competence. ACVIM Proc 2001;19:93–4.
37. Helwegen MM, Young LE, Rogers K, et al. Measurements of right ventricular internal dimensions and their relationships to severity of tricuspid valve regurgitation in national hunt thoroughbreds. Equine Vet J Suppl 2006;(36):171–7.
38. Trachsel DS, Schwarzwald CC, Bitschnau C, et al. Atrial natriuretic peptide and cardiac troponin I concentrations in healthy Warmblood horses and in Warmblood horses with mitral regurgitation at rest and after exercise. J Vet Cardiol 2013;15(2):105–21.
39. Lucke VM. Sudden death. Equine Vet J 1987;19(2):85–6.
40. Lyle CH, Uzal FA, McGorum BC, et al. Sudden death in racing Thoroughbred horses: an international multicentre study of post mortem findings. Equine Vet J 2011;43(3):324–31.
41. Lyle CH, Blissitt KJ, Kennedy RN, et al. Risk factors for race-associated sudden death in Thoroughbred racehorses in the UK (2000-2007). Equine Vet J 2012; 44(4):459–65.
42. Navas de Solis C. Exercising arrhythmias and sudden cardiac death in horses: review of the literature and comparative aspects. Equine Vet J 2016;48(4): 406–13.
43. Johnson BJ, Stover SM, Daft BM, et al. Causes of death in racehorses over a 2 year period. Equine Vet J 1994;26(4):327–30.
44. Boden LA, Charles JA, Slocombe RF, et al. Sudden death in racing Thoroughbreds in Victoria, Australia. Equine Vet J 2005;37(3):269–71.
45. Gelberg HB, Zachary JF, Everitt JI, et al. Sudden death in training and racing Thoroughbred horses. J Am Vet Med Assoc 1985;187(12):1354–6.
46. Kiryu K, Machida N, Kashida Y, et al. Pathologic and electrocardiographic findings in sudden cardiac death in racehorses. J Vet Med Sci 1999;61(8):921–8.
47. Platt H. Sudden and unexpected deaths in horses: a review of 69 cases. Br Vet J 1982;138(5):417–29.
48. Brown CM, Kaneene JB, Taylor RF. Sudden and unexpected death in horses and ponies: an analysis of 200 cases. Equine Vet J 1988;20(2):99–103.
49. Durando M. Exercise and stress testing. In: Marr CM, MBowen IM, editors. Cardiology of the horse. 2nd edition. Edinburgh (Scotland): Elsevier; 2010. p. 139–49.

Assessment of the Cardiovascular System in Horses During Prepurchase and Insurance Examinations

Virginia B. Reef, DVM

KEYWORDS

- Cardiac • Prepurchase examination • Insurance examination • Murmur • Arrhythmia

KEY POINTS

- Heart murmurs and arrhythmias are frequently detected in horses during a prepurchase examination.
- Differentiating normal arrhythmias and murmurs can be challenging but is an important part of the prepurchase examination.
- Most horses with murmurs and arrhythmias have a normal performance career and life expectancy.
- An echocardiogram should be performed in all horses with a grade 3/6 or louder midsystolic to late systolic, holosystolic, or pansystolic murmur or any holodiastolic murmur.
- Arrhythmias should be confirmed with a resting ECG; an exercising ECG is needed in performance horses.

INTRODUCTION

Cardiac evaluation is an important part of the prepurchase or insurance examination. A thorough auscultation of all 4 valve areas on both sides of the thorax should be performed in a quiet area. Any abnormalities in the cardiac rhythm should be described, along with any murmurs detected. The arterial pulses, peripheral pulses, and mucous membranes should be evaluated, along with auscultation of the lungs at rest and on deep inspiration. The heart should also be auscultated after exercise as part of a prepurchase examination of a performance horse. All abnormal findings should be recorded for the prepurchase or insurance examination. The functional significance of the abnormal cardiac findings should be described to the prospective buyer. Any recommended tests that were declined

Disclosure Statement: Nothing to disclose.
Section of Imaging, Department of Clinical Studies, New Bolton Center, University of Pennsylvania, 382 West Street Road, Kennett Square, PA 19348, USA
E-mail address: vreef@vet.upenn.edu

should be recorded. The impact of not performing the test should also be explained to the prospective purchaser. It is the responsibility of the buyer to determine the suitability of the horse for the intended purpose. The veterinarian's report is one of many factors the prospective purchaser considers when making a purchase decision.

Determining the significance of cardiac abnormalities detected can be challenging. Horses have normal arrhythmias and physiologic flow murmurs that, on occasion, are difficult to distinguish from murmurs associated with underlying pathology. Understanding the normal arrhythmias and murmurs is the first step in determining when further cardiac assessment is indicated. The impact of arrhythmias and heart murmurs associated with underlying cardiac pathology must be considered when assessing a horse for purchase or insurability. The challenge for the veterinarian in the prepurchase setting is considering not only the current impact of the abnormality detected but also predicting how this will change and affect the horse's function in the future. Recent recommendations for the suitability of horses with cardiovascular abnormalities for performance is a resource for advising clients about the possible impact of a cardiovascular abnormality detected.[1] In the insurance setting, the veterinarian is making assessments about the mortality risk or the impact of abnormalities detected on performance within the policy year (loss of use).

NORMAL FINDINGS
Cardiac Rhythm

A regular sinus rhythm with a resting heart rate ranging from 24 beats per minute (bpm) to 44 bpm is the most common rhythm detected in horses. The adult horse has high vagal tone present at rest, especially when fit, resulting in low normal resting heart rates and rhythm disturbances that disappear with excitement, exercise, or any intervention that increases sympathetic tone. The most common rhythm disturbance associated with high resting vagal tone is second-degree atrioventricular block (2°AVB), occurring in 15% to 18% of horses at rest and up to 44% of horses during a continuous 24-hour ECG.[2,3] Sinus arrhythmia usually coexists in horses with 2°AVB.[3] It is also often present alone or in conjunction with sinus bradycardia, sinoatrial block (SAB), or sinoatrial (SA) arrest.

A regularly irregular rhythm with the long pause equal to approximately 2 normal pauses (diastolic intervals) is auscultated in horses with 2°AVB or SAB. This pause is longer than 2 diastolic intervals in horses with SA arrest. An audible fourth heart sound may be heard in the long pause with 2°AVB. Periodic waxing and waning of the heart rate occurs with sinus arrhythmia. In horses with sinus bradycardia, a slow resting heart rate is detected, in conjunction with sinus arrhythmia.

Physiologic Flow Murmurs

Physiologic flow murmurs, occurring with normal blood flow, are common. Many lower-intensity murmurs, however, are associated with underlying cardiac pathology. Physiologic flow murmurs are low-intensity murmurs (≤grade 3/6); early systolic, mid-systolic, late systolic, or holosystolic; early diastolic or late diastolic; usually soft and blowing but may be squeaky and are localized with little or no radiation. Because both physiologic flow murmurs and murmurs associated with cardiac pathology can increase in intensity after exercise, a change in intensity with exercise cannot be used to differentiate them.[4]

ABNORMAL FINDINGS
Arrhythmias

Abnormal cardiac rhythms interrupt the underlying normal rhythm and may be associated with a change in resting heart rate. In some horses, arrhythmias detected at rest return rapidly after exercise and are present in the immediate postexercise auscultation. In others, arrhythmias are detected only in the postexercise examination. An exercising ECG is indicated to determine if these arrhythmias are present during exercise or are overdriven. With the widespread availability of an affordable smartphone-based handheld device, recording a horse's ECG has become something that is feasible in the field.[5] These devices do an excellent job of obtaining a tracing of the heart rhythm at rest (**Fig. 1**) or postexercise but not during exercise. Telemetry is needed to obtain an exercising ECG.

Bradyarrhythmias

Although occasional 2°AVB is normal when associated with high resting vagal tone, high-grade 2°AVB is not normal. 2°AVB is considered high-grade when the block is occurring more frequently (**Fig. 2**).

When a horse with high-grade 2°AVB, high-grade SA block, high-grade SA arrest, or profound sinus bradycardia is considered for purchase, a continuous 24-hour ECG is indicated to further characterize the severity of the arrhythmia. An exercising ECG is indicated to see if the high-grade bradyarrhythmia is overdriven with exercise and to determine if the heart rate increases appropriately for the work performed. An echocardiogram is also indicated to look for underlying structural heart disease.

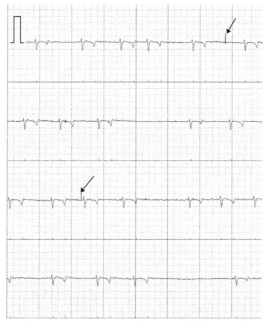

Fig. 1. Tracing of AF obtained with a smartphone-enabled recording device. Notice the irregularly irregular rhythm, the absence of P waves, and the baseline fibrillation waves. There are 2 artifacts (*arrows*) in the tracing.

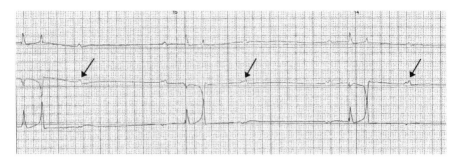

Fig. 2. Simultaneous rhythm tracings of advanced 2:1 2°AVB obtained during 24-hour continuous monitoring. There is 1 conducted P, QRS, and T complex followed by 1 P wave (*arrows*) that is blocked at the atrioventricular node.

Recommendations for a horse with high-grade second-degree atrioventricular block, sinoatrial block, sinoatrial arrest, or profound sinus bradycardia Even if these arrhythmias are overdriven during exercise, the horse is not suitable for a child rider, for hire, or to be used in a lesson program.[1] There is the risk that high-grade 2°AVB could progress to complete/third-degree AVB; however, the likelihood of that occurring is unknown.

Premature beats

Occasional premature complexes are detected in normal horses during routine continuous 24-hour ECG (Holter) monitoring.[2] Occasional atrial premature complexes (APCs) and ventricular premature complexes (VPCs) occur in normally performing horses in the immediate postexercise period, associated with the changing autonomic tone occurring as the heart rate slows.[6–13] Occasional APCs are present in horses during exercise, but exercising VPCs are much less common.[7–10]

Auscultation reveals a regularly irregular rhythm; the underlying rhythm is interrupted by a beat occurring earlier than normal. If the beat is originating from the ventricle, there is usually a longer than normal pause following the premature beat (compensatory pause) and the intensity of the premature beat is often increased. If the beat is originating from above the ventricle, there is usually no compensatory pause.

An ECG is necessary to definitively determine the origin of the premature beat (atrial or ventricular). The APC looks similar to the normal complex but usually has a different P-wave configuration (**Fig. 3**).[14] The VPC is widened and bizarre compared with the normal sinus beat with a QRS that is oriented in the opposite direction from the T wave (**Fig. 4**). VPCs are uniform, if they all have a similar configuration, and multiform, if their configurations vary. A continuous 24-hour ECG is indicated to determine the type and frequency of premature complexes. An exercising ECG is indicated to

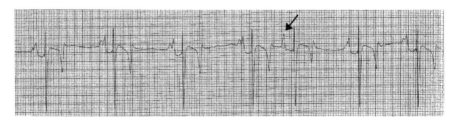

Fig. 3. Base-apex rhythm tracing of an APC (*arrow*). Notice the change in the P-wave morphology of the APC and the noncompensatory pause following the APC.

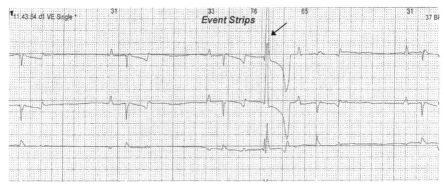

Fig. 4. Base-apex rhythm tracing of a VPC (*arrow*). This VPC is early enough to be interpolated between 2 normal sinus complexes.

determine their frequency during exercise or if they are overdriven during exercise. An echocardiogram is indicated in horses with frequent APCs or VPCs, looking for underlying structural heart disease.

Recommendations for a horse with atrial premature complex or ventricular premature complex Horses with occasional APCs that are overdriven during exercise or are occurring infrequently during exercise are as safe to use for performance as for their age-matched peers.[1] Horses with APCs have no increased risk for mortality during the year after the insurance examination. APCs do, however, increase the risk of atrial fibrillation (AF), but the magnitude of the risk is unknown.[1] This risk is a factor that should be considered in horses performing in high-intensity athletic events, particularly in horses with frequent APCs or APCs during exercise.

Horses with occasional uniform VPCs are more likely to have underlying structural heart disease, which could present a risk for the horse and rider. If the VPCs are overdriven during exercise, these horses can be ridden or driven by an informed adult rider but are not suitable for a child rider, for hire, or for use as a lesson horse.[1] VPCs that are multiform or associated with an R-on-T event (the QRS complex is originating out of the preceding T wave) are complex ventricular arrhythmias (VAs). Complex VAs are a reflection of underlying myocardial disease and are more likely to be associated with collapse or sudden cardiac death (SCD). The heart would be excluded for insurance coverage in these horses.

Atrial fibrillation

AF is the most common arrhythmia affecting performance in horses.[1,15,16] Horses with AF usually have a normal resting heart rate with an irregularly irregular rhythm and an absent fourth heart sound. Although the rhythm is irregular, there is often a periodicity of AF in the horse.[17] This patterned rhythm of some horses with AF may make it more difficult to distinguish from 2°AVB at rest. The exercising heart rate of horses with AF is usually 40 bpm to 60 bpm higher for each level of exercise than if that horse was in normal sinus rhythm.[15] The rhythm remains irregular during periods of excitement or after exercise, although the pauses between the irregular beats are much shorter and the rhythm may be erroneously perceived as regular.

AF is associated with underlying heart disease in horses, particularly those with mitral regurgitation (MR) and left atrial enlargement. Therefore, horses with AF should be carefully auscultated for any murmurs of valvular insufficiency. Although in many horses no underlying cause of AF can be determined (lone AF), it is likely that these horses have underlying atrial myocardial disease that is below the limit of clinical detection.

An ECG is indicated to confirm AF (**Fig. 5**, see also **Fig. 1**). An echocardiogram is indicated in all horses considered for purchase, looking for underlying structural heart disease. An exercising ECG should be performed in all horses with permanent AF considered for purchase, to determine the heart rate during exercise and to look for aberrant conduction or ventricular ectopy (**Fig. 6**) occurs in some exercising horses with AF.[18] The exercise stress test should be of an intensity that is equal to or slightly exceeds what the prospective purchaser expects from the horse.

Recommendations for horses with atrial fibrillation/historical atrial fibrillation If conversion of a horse with AF is desired in a horse considered for purchase, the prospective purchaser should be informed of the likely success of the cardioversion and the risk of recurrence. Horses with AF have a high likelihood of successful conversion, if there is no detectable underlying cardiac disease or the structural heart disease is mild, regardless of method of conversion.[1] Horses with a history of AF are at risk for experiencing a recurrence, particularly if the conversion occurred within the previous year.[16] Horses with historical AF are also at increased risk for experiencing a recurrence if they have left atrial enlargement, MR, or APCs.[1,16,19,20]

Although uncomplicated AF does not increase the risk of death during the year of a mortality insurance policy, it may prevent the horse from being able to do the job that the purchaser intends. An exercising heart rate of less than or equal to 220 bpm in AF when working slightly harder than expected is compatible with the horse being able to do the work expected (ridden, driven, or breeding exercise). Although uncommon, horses with AF can collapse and thus a horse with permanent AF should be used only by an informed adult rider or driver.[1] Horses with AF and aberrant conduction or ventricular ectopy during an exercise test or other sympathetic nervous system stimulation are a safety risk and should be converted to normal sinus rhythm or retired.[1] The heart of these horses is usually excluded when insurance is sought.

Accelerated idioventricular rhythm/ventricular tachycardia

Ventricular tachycardia (VT) is usually a rapid regular rhythm that is unlikely to be detected in a prepurchase or insurance setting. Horses with VT usually have loud booming heart sounds (bruit de canon) and frequent jugular pulsations. Heart sounds can vary in intensity and pulse deficits may be present. Accelerated idioventricular rhythm (AIVR) could be present, because this is a rhythm originating from the ventricle that is occurring at rate similar to the normal sinus rhythm.

If a horse with AIVR or a history of VT is considered for purchase, a baseline ECG, continuous 24-hour ECG, and exercising ECG should be performed looking for AIVR (**Fig. 7**) or any other ventricular ectopy. An echocardiogram is needed to look for evidence of structural heart disease. Areas of increased myocardial echogenicity consistent with a fibrous or fibrofatty scar (**Fig. 8**) are of concern because these are potential

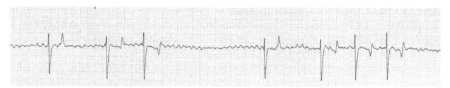

Fig. 5. Base-apex rhythm tracing of AF. Notice the irregularly irregular rhythm, the absence of P waves, and the baseline fibrillation waves.

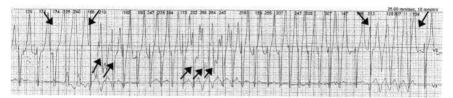

Fig. 6. Base-apex rhythm tracing of ventricular ectopy and rapid AF during excitement. Notice the different morphology of the QRS and T complexes. The lower angled arrows point to a ventricular complex with a different form. The arrows pointing to each other demonstrate short periods of torsades de pointes where the next abnormal QRS merges with the previous T wave (R-on-T).

substrates for re-entrant VAs. Measurement of cardiac troponin is also indicated to look for active myocardial injury.

Recommendations for horses with accelerated idioventricular rhythm or a history of ventricular tachycardia There is concern about underlying myocardial disease in a horse with AIVR, even when this rhythm is overdriven during exercise. The possibility remains of VAs occurring during exercise. Therefore, these horses should be ridden or driven only by an informed adult rider and are not suitable for use by a child, for hire, or in a lesson program.

VT is a rhythm that is more likely to be associated with underlying cardiac pathology and can be associated with SCD. Therefore, from an insurance perspective, a horse with a history of VT is at increased risk for mortality and the heart is not covered. If underlying myocardial disease is detected (see **Fig. 8**), rigorous athletic work is not recommended.[1] Abnormal myocardial thickness or function is also a concern, because this may affect the horse being able to perform its intended use. Although recurrence of uniform VT is uncommon, it is possible and something a purchaser must be made aware of. Horses with a history of multiform VT are more likely to have underlying myocardial disease. Although their actual likelihood of future VAs is unknown, the potential is higher due to the complexity of the VT they previously experienced.

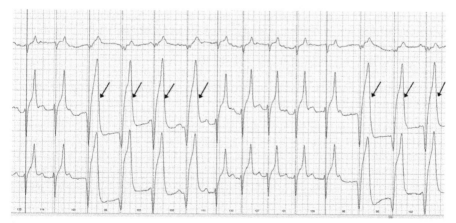

Fig. 7. Base-apex tracing of AIVR. Notice the large QRS and T complexes originating from the ventricle (*arrows*) that are occurring in a row at a slightly slower rate than the normal sinus complexes.

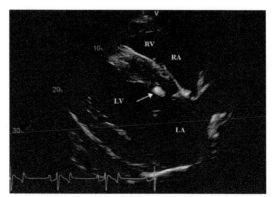

Fig. 8. Echocardiogram (right parasternal 4-chamber view) of an echoic area in the interventricular septum (*arrow*) consistent with a fibrous or fibrofatty infiltrate. LA, left atrium; LV, left ventricle; RA, right atrium; RV, right ventricle.

Murmurs

Murmurs are frequently detected at the time of a prepurchase or insurance examination. Murmurs associated with cardiac pathology are usually regurgitant murmurs, although ventricular septal defects (VSDs) are also detected in horses evaluated for sale or insurance purposes. Murmurs of MR and tricuspid regurgitation (TR) can be detected in horses of any age, whereas murmurs of aortic regurgitation (AR) are most commonly detected in older horses.[21–24] MR, TR, and AR all increase in prevalence with training and are often present in horses performing up to expectations.[25] TR is most likely to be detected in horses that train for long distances, such as National Hunt horses, steeplechasers, and Standardbred racehorses.[26] VSDs are usually evaluated in younger individuals; however, older horses with VSDs have been presented for a prepurchase examination.

Tricuspid regurgitation

TR murmurs are auscultated on the right side and are usually a grade 1 to 4/6. TR murmurs are usually soft and blowing, band-shaped or crescendo, and holosystolic. Murmurs of TR that are louder are associated with longer jets occupying a larger area.[27]

An echocardiogram is recommended as part of a prepurchase examination in all horses with a grade 3 to 6/6 right-sided systolic murmur to evaluate the tricuspid valve, right atrium and ventricle and to characterize the severity of the TR.[1] Structural changes to the tricuspid valve are uncommon. Horses with more severe TR jets detected with color flow Doppler echocardiography are likely to have larger right ventricular internal diameters detected.[26]

Recommendations for a horse with tricuspid regurgitation Horses with TR usually have a normal performance life, although horses with severe TR or major structural abnormalities may not be an elite competitor. They usually have a normal life expectancy, as long as there is normal right ventricular function. TR should not present a problem for insurability of the horse, unless there is severe tricuspid valve disease and/or right ventricular dysfunction.

Mitral regurgitation

Any loud systolic murmur auscultated on the left side is MR until proved otherwise. There are 3 types of MR murmurs, all loudest in the mitral to aortic valve area.[21]

The mitral valve prolapse (MVP) murmur is a midsystolic to late systolic or holosystolic crescendo murmur that is usually a grade 3 to 4/6. The murmur associated with degenerative valve disease can range from a grade 2 to 6/6, is more band shaped and holosystolic or pansystolic. Although louder murmurs are often associated with more advanced disease, there is no correlation between the murmur intensity and the severity of regurgitation. This murmur may radiate dorsally and cranially or caudally, depending on the direction of the regurgitant jet. Only rarely is this murmur heard on the right side. A ruptured chorda tendineae (RCT) normally produces a loud (grade 4–6/6), musical, honking, holosystolic, or pansystolic murmur that can become quieter over time. This murmur often radiates well to the right where it is similar in quality but quieter.

An echocardiogram is recommended as part of a prepurchase examination in all horses with a grade 3 to 6/6 left-sided systolic murmur to determine if mitral valve, left atrial, and left ventricular abnormalities are present and characterize the severity of the MR (**Fig. 9**).[1] Although in most horses, a structural abnormality of the mitral valve can be detected, this is not always the case.

Detecting the MVP is difficult because usually only part of the mitral valve bulges backwards into the atria (**Fig. 10**). Most horses with MVP have a normal-sized or mildly enlarged left atrium with a normal-sized left ventricle and normal left ventricular function. Color flow Doppler echocardiography usually detects one or more small jets of MR.

Although mitral valve thickening is subjective, generalized valvular thickening is often seen with degenerative valve disease and is usually associated with left atrial enlargement of varying degrees, often with concurrent left ventricular enlargement.

An RCT is also challenging to diagnose as the chorda tendineae everts into the left atrium during systole. These are more commonly imaged from the left parasternal window; however, detecting them requires a careful search of the mitral valve apparatus. When part or the entire leaflet is imaged everting into the left atrium during systole, or moving asynchronously during the cardiac cycle, a flail leaflet is present. Similar to the horse with degenerative valve disease, left atrial and left ventricular enlargement are usually present.

Recommendations for a horse with mitral regurgitation Nearly all horses with MR have 2 risk factors for AF: left atrial enlargement and MR. Even mild MR is a risk factor for the recurrence of AF.[20] This risk is probably higher in horses performing in high-

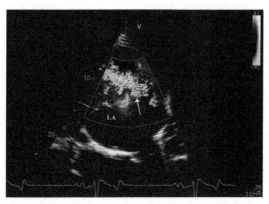

Fig. 9. Echocardiogram (left parasternal long-axis 2-chamber view) of a moderate-sized jet of MR (*arrow*) that extends toward the base of the left atrium (LA).

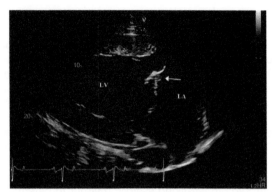

Fig. 10. Echocardiogram (left parasternal long-axis 2-chamber view) of MVP. Notice the small portion of the mitral valve, prolapsing (*arrow*) toward the left atrium (LA). LV, left ventricle.

intensity athletic events. Horses in disciplines, such as upper-level eventing and racing, are also likely to experience performance problems, should AF develop.

Most horses with MVP have an excellent prognosis for performance and for a normal life expectancy, competing successfully in all equine disciplines, even at the pinnacle of their sport. This is because, in most, there is only mild MR with a normal or mildly enlarged left atrium, normal-sized left ventricle, and normal left ventricular function. In these horses, the MR remains unchanged or only progresses slightly during the horse's life.[28] The main risk for MVP affecting performance is in disciplines where the horse is competing at high speed; and the risk is AF, making these horses not insurable for loss of use. Horses with MVP are not at increased risk for experiencing a cardiovascular death during the year of the policy and, therefore, mortality insurance is not a problem.

Horses with MR and mitral leaflet thickening are more likely to have progression of MR over time. A horse with mild left atrial enlargement, a normal-sized left ventricle, normal function, and mild MR is likely to do well for many years. This horse still could have a shortened performance life and life expectancy, particularly if it is relatively young when first diagnosed. Horses with moderate MR associated with mild valvular thickening or mild mitral valve dysplasia ultimately develop performance problems and have a shortened life expectancy as their MR worsens, but this progression is usually slow. Insurance is usually not a problem for a horse with MR until the regurgitation becomes moderate to severe; at that time, progression to congestive heart failure (CHF) is possible within the year of the mortality insurance policy.

Horses with RCT have a more guarded to poor prognosis. Small accessory leaflet RCT may result in only a small jet of MR. Although these horses are a risk for more rapid progression of their MR, many do fine for many years after a small accessory leaflet RCT. Rupture of a major chorda tendineae usually carries a poor prognosis with rapid progression to CHF. These horses are at risk for SCD if pulmonary artery enlargement, indicating pulmonary hypertension, is detected. Horses with severe mitral dysplasia, a flail leaflet, or healed endocarditis lesions must be given a guarded to poor prognosis because progression of the MR is likely.[1,21] These lesions are likely to shorten a horse's useful performance life and life expectancy.

A follow-up echocardiographic examination enables a more accurate progression of MR to be formulated; however, this is rarely available in the prepurchase setting. If a prior evaluation is available and there has been little or no change from the echocardiogram performed a year or more ago, the progression may be slow. If the left atrium and left ventricle are larger, however, the MR continues to progress. The magnitude of the change between the 2 examinations is a guide for how quickly the MR progresses. Annual echocardiographic re-examinations are recommended for horses purchased with MR.

Aortic regurgitation

Any holodiastolic murmur audible on the left side is AR until proved otherwise. Murmurs of AR are usually decrescendo, holodiastolic, or occasionally pandiastolic and vary from a grade 1 to 6/6. AR murmurs can be soft and blowing or loud and musical with a dive-bomber quality. AR murmurs are also usually heard on the right side, but are 1 to 2 grades softer. Although grades 1 to 2/6 holodiastolic blowing decrescendo murmurs usually indicate mild AR, the intensity does not correlate with severity. Bounding arterial pulses are an indication of a left ventricular volume overload and moderate or severe AR.[21,23]

An echocardiogram is recommended as part of a prepurchase examination in all horses with a grade 3 to 6/6 left-sided holodiastolic murmur or with bounding arterial pulses.[1] An echocardiogram determines the valvular abnormalities that are present and the effects the AR is having on the cardiac chambers and great vessels and characterizes the severity of the AR.

A parallel thickening of the left coronary cusp or nodular changes are common degenerative lesions of the aortic valve (**Fig. 11**). Often there is only mild left ventricular enlargement with a small jet of AR and a normal-sized aortic root when the murmur is first detected.

Horses with large nodular lesions, moderate aortic valve prolapse (AVP), fenestrated leaflet, or healed endocarditis lesion are likely to have more left ventricular and aortic root enlargement. An enlarged aortic root indicates some chronicity of the AR. A flail aortic leaflet is usually associated with severe AR.

Recommendations for horses with aortic regurgitation Most horses with AR have a normal performance life and life expectancy because the AR develops at an older age (usually in their teens) and progresses slowly when there is a degenerative lesion present on the aortic valve. Most horses with AR are retired, die, or are humanely euthanized for reasons other than their cardiac disease. Horses with mild AR

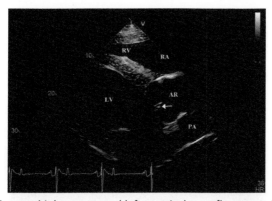

Fig. 11. Echocardiogram (right parasternal left ventricular outflow tract view) of degenerative change on the left coronary cusp of the aortic valve. Notice the echoic area parallel to the free edge of the cusp (*arrow*). AR, aortic root; LV, left ventricle; PA, pulmonary artery; RA, right atrium; RV, right ventricle.

associated with degenerative valve disease or mild AVP usually have a good prognosis for performance and for a normal life expectancy with the AR progressing slowly over many years. Horses with more significant valvular thickening, nodular changes, or fenestrations with moderate AR are likely to progress more rapidly. Moderate AR could affect performance and, ultimately, life expectancy, although this should occur over a period of years. If purchased, annual echocardiographic re-examinations should be performed to monitor the AR.

Horses with more severe valvular pathology, including markedly enlarged hyperdynamic or hypodynamic left ventricles and large AR jets, are a significant risk, because these horses are at increased risk for performance problems and experiencing a shortened life expectancy.[1] Prospective purchasers should be made aware of the risks associated with moderate to severe AR. All horses with moderate or severe AR should have an exercising ECG performed to be sure that exercising VAs are not present in these individuals, because these horses are at increased risk for SCD. If purchased, these horses should have biannual echocardiographic re-examinations and exercising ECGs. Horses with moderate to severe AR also develop left atrial enlargement and MR as the disease progresses. The development of AF in these horses is often an indication of a worsening of their regurgitation. Horses with severe AR are a cardiovascular risk for insurance purposes and the heart is normally excluded.

Ventricular septal defect

VSDs can be associated with a normal life expectancy if the defect is small.[29] Horses can even race successfully with small VSDs, although not at the pinnacle of their respective disciplines. Most horses with small to medium-sized VSDs develop MR as they age due to the left ventricular volume overload.

A loud grade 4 to 6/6 band-shaped pansystolic murmur is present in the tricuspid valve area with a softer crescendo-decrescendo murmur loudest in the pulmonic valve area. If the murmurs are loudest on the left, an outflow VSD or more complex congenital cardiac disease should be suspected.

An echocardiogram is indicated to determine the size and hemodynamic effect of the VSD (**Fig. 12**).[29] The size of the cardiac chambers, the myocardial function, and the peak velocity of the shunt need to be determined. Concurrent AVP, AR, and MR also influence the prognosis.

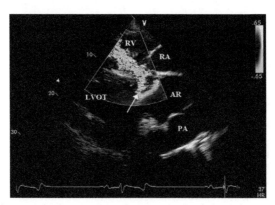

Fig. 12. Echocardiogram (right parasternal LVOT view) of the left-to-right shunt (*arrow*) associated with a perimembranous VSD. AR, aortic root; LVOT, left ventricular outflow tract; PA, pulmonary artery; RA, right atrium; RV, right ventricle.

Recommendations for horses with ventricular septal defect An adult horse with a single perimembranous VSD less than or equal to 2.5 cm in diameter, with a normal or only mildly enlarged left atrium and left ventricle, normal myocardial function, a peak shunt velocity of greater than or equal to 4.5 m/s, and no AVP, AR, or MR has a good prognosis for a normal life expectancy. This horse should be able to perform most ridden or driven exercise, although should not be expected to perform at the elite level in demanding disciplines.[21,29] When evaluating smaller equids, a VSD-to–aortic root ratio of less than or equal to 0.3 is associated with the VSD an incidental finding.[30] If purchased, these horses should have an annual echocardiographic re-examination. Horses with larger VSDs and cardiac chambers, poor myocardial function, lower shunt velocities, and significant AR or MR have a poorer prognosis for a normal life expectancy. The development of AF is often the beginning of their demise, leading to the development of CHF.

SUMMARY

The initial auscultatory findings are important in determining which horses need further cardiac evaluation as part of a prepurchase or insurance examination. Resting and exercising ECG and echocardiography are important tools in assessing the significance of arrhythmias and murmurs detected. These tests can help determine the functional significance of the abnormalities detected and their impact on performance, longevity, safety, and insurability.

REFERENCES

1. Reef VB, Bonagura J, Buhl R, et al. Recommendations for management of equine athletes with cardiovascular abnormalities. J Vet Intern Med 2014;28:749–61.
2. Reef VB. Frequency of cardiac arrhythmias and their significance in normal horses. Proc 7th Am College of Vet Intern Med Forum, San Diego (CA), May 26–28, 1989. p. 506–8.
3. Holmes JR, Alps BJ. Observations on partial atrio-ventricular heart block in the horse. Can Vet J 1966;7:280–90.
4. Kriz NG, Hodgson DR, Rose RJ. Prevalence and clinical importance of heart murmurs in racehorses. J Am Vet Med Assoc 2000;216:1441–5.
5. Vezzosi T, Sgorbini M, Bonelli F, et al. Evaluation of a smartphone electrocardiograph in healthy horses: comparison with standard base-apex electrocardiography. J Equine Vet Sci 2018;67:61–5.
6. Navas de Solis C, Sampson SN, McKay T, et al. Standardised exercise testing in 17 reining horses: musculoskeletal, respiratory, cardiac and clinicopathological findings. Equine Vet Educ 2018;30:262–7.
7. Navas de Solis C, Green C, Sides R, et al. Arrhythmias in thoroughbreds during and after treadmill and racetrack exercise. Equine Vet J 2014;46:24–5.
8. Barbesgaard L, Buhl R, Meldgaard C. Prevalence of exercise-associated arrhythmias in normal performing dressage horses. Equine Vet J 2010;42:202–7.
9. Buhl R, Meldgaard C, Barbesgaard L. Cardiac arrhythmias in clinically healthy showjumping horses. Equine Vet J 2010;42:196–201.
10. Buhl R, Petersen EE, Lindholm M, et al. Cardiac arrhythmias in standardbreds during and after racing—possible association between heart size, valvular regurgitations, and arrhythmias. J Equine Vet Sci 2013;33:590–6.
11. Jose-Cunilleras E, Young LE, Newton JR, et al. Cardiac arrhythmias during and after treadmill exercise in poorly performing thoroughbred racehorses. Equine Vet J 2006;(Suppls):163–70.

12. Martin BB Jr, Reef VB, Parente EJ, et al. Causes of poor performance of horses during training, racing, or showing: 348 cases (1992-1996). J Am Vet Med Assoc 2000;216:554–8.
13. Ryan N, Marr CM, McGladdery AJ. Survey of cardiac arrhythmias during submaximal and maximal exercise in Thoroughbred racehorses. Equine Vet J 2005;37:265–8.
14. Broux B, De Clercq D, Decloedt A, et al. Atrial premature depolarization-induced changes in QRS and T wave morphology on resting electrocardiograms in horses. J Vet Intern Med 2016;30:1253–9.
15. Buhl R, Carstensen H, Hesselkilde EZ, et al. Effect of induced chronic atrial fibrillation on exercise performance in Standardbred trotters. J Vet Intern Med 2018; 32(4):1410–9.
16. Reef VB, Levitan CW, Spencer PA. Factors affecting prognosis and conversion in equine atrial fibrillation. J Vet Intern Med 1988;2:1–6.
17. Meijler FL, Kroneman J, van der Tweel I, et al. Nonrandom ventricular rhythm in horses with atrial fibrillation and its significance for patients. J Am Coll Cardiol 1984;4:316–23.
18. Verheyen T, Decloedt A, van der Vekens N, et al. Ventricular response during lungeing exercise in horses with lone atrial fibrillation. Equine Vet J 2012;45:309–14.
19. Reef VB, Reimer JM, Spencer PA. Treatment of atrial fibrillation in horses: new perspectives. J Vet Intern Med 1995;9:57–67.
20. Decloedt A, Schwarzwald CC, De Clercq D, et al. Risk factors for recurrence of atrial fibrillation in horses after cardioversion to sinus rhythm. J Vet Intern Med 2015;29:946–53.
21. Reef VB. Heart murmurs in horses: determining their significance with echocardiography. Equine Vet J Suppl 1995;19:71–80.
22. Reef VB, Bain FT, Spencer PA. Severe mitral regurgitation in horses: clinical, echocardiographic and pathological findings. Equine Vet J 1998;30:18–27.
23. Reef VB, Spencer P. Echocardiographic evaluation of equine aortic insufficiency. Am J Vet Res 1987;48:904–9.
24. Ireland JL, Clegg PD, McGowan CM, et al. Disease prevalence in geriatric horses in the United Kingdom: veterinary clinical assessment of 200 cases. Equine Vet J 2012;44:101–6.
25. Young LE, Rogers K, Wood JL. Heart murmurs and valvular regurgitation in thoroughbred racehorses: epidemiology and associations with athletic performance. J Vet Intern Med 2008;22:418–26.
26. Helwegen MM, Young LE, Rogers K, et al. Measurements of right ventricular internal dimensions and their relationships to severity of tricuspid valve regurgitation in national hunt thoroughbreds. Equine Vet J 2006;Suppl:171–7.
27. Blissitt KJ, Bonagura JD. Colour flow Doppler echocardiography in horses with cardiac murmurs. Equine Vet J Suppl 1995;(19):82–5.
28. Imhasly A, Tschudi PR, Lombard CW, et al. Clinical and echocardiographic features of mild mitral valve regurgitation in 108 horses. Vet J 2010;183:166–71.
29. Reef VB. Evaluation of ventricular septal defects in horses using two-dimensional and Doppler echocardiography. Equine Vet J Suppl 1995;(19):86–95.
30. Marr CM. Cardiac murmurs: congenital heart disease. In: Marr CM, Bowen IM, editors. Cardiology of the horse. 2nd edition. London: Elsevier Ltd.; 2010. p. 193–205.

Cardiac Monitoring in Horses

Andre C. Shih, DVM

KEYWORDS

- Blood pressure • Cardiac output • Central venous pressure

KEY POINTS

- Monitoring variables of cardiac performance in horses is challenging owing to patient size, temperament, and anatomic peculiarities.
- Blood pressure is a major determinant of afterload, but it is not a reliable surrogate of cardiac performance and tissue perfusion.
- Cardiac output, together with arterial and venous oxygen content, provides insight as to the adequacy of delivery of blood and oxygen to the body as a whole and can be used to gauge fluid responsiveness and cardiovascular status of the patient.
- Measurement of intracardiac pressures serves to assess cardiac filling pressures, myocardial performance, and vascular resistance.

CLINICAL USE OF CARDIAC MONITORING

A thorough physical examination, complemented by basic monitoring (heart rate [HR], pulse quality, jugular filling, and mucous membranes), is sufficient to direct the care of most patients. There exists, however, a subset of patients for whom more direct cardiac monitoring (electrocardiogram, blood pressure [BP], cardiac output [CO], and systemic vascular resistance [SVR]) is essential to proper case management.[1] Advanced cardiac monitoring attempts to evaluate heart function through direct and indirect methods.[1,2] With advent of new technologies, this is also becoming reality in veterinary medicine. Horses have intrinsic characteristics (body size, temperament, and unique anatomic features) that make advanced cardiac monitoring a challenge.[2,3]

After HR, BP is one of the most common variables to monitor cardiovascular function.[3,4] Clinically, monitoring of BP helps the veterinarian to assess the cardiovascular status of a patient and have an acceptable understanding of the driving force of tissue perfusion at a specific moment. Hypotension, commonly observed in critically ill foals and a common complication of general anesthesia, is usually defined as mean arterial

This article is in memory of Dr Steeve Giguère, a true friend, great mentor, clinician, and researcher.
Capital Veterinary Specialist, 3001 Hartley Road, Jacksonville, FL, USA
E-mail address: Shih60@gmail.com

blood pressure (MAP) less than 70 mm Hg.[2] Both severe hypotension and hypertension should be prevented to avoid the negative affect of abnormal tissue perfusion. For example, renal, cerebral, and myocardial ischemia are often associated with severe hypotension[3,4] and retinal damage, kidney, heart, and brain injuries are associated with hypertension.[3,4] The clinical relevance of hypo- or hypertension depends on severity, duration and the underlying cause.[3,4]

It is important to remember that BP is the product of CO and SVR and therefore is *per se* not a surrogate of cardiac performance and tissue perfusion.[1,2] A low CO in a hypotensive patient will likely indicate hypovolemia or decreased cardiac function. Patients with low BP may experience high or optimal CO if SVR is low because of intense systemic vasodilation. Hence, a high CO in a hypotensive patient would suggest decreased vascular tone.[5] Patients with normal or high BP may experience low CO and poor tissue perfusion, if SVR is high because of severe systemic vasoconstriction.

Hence, in addition to BP, CO is one of the most important factors to assess cardiovascular function.[5] Unfortunately, measuring CO is challenging in equine medicine. Cardiac output, which is defined as the volume of blood pumped out by the heart in 1 minute,[1] indicates how well the heart is performing its pump function. It is typically measured in liters per minute (L/min). There is significant variation in CO dependent on patient size and age. A normal CO for neonatal foals ranges between 6.7 and 7.5 L/min, whereas a normal CO for a 400- to 500-kg adult horse is 32 to 40 L/min.[3] To make comparisons between individuals, CO is therefore typically indexed to body weight and termed cardiac index (CI = CO/BW [kg]).[3] The normal resting CI for an adult horse is 72 to 88 mL/kg/min.[6]

Horses are well-adapted athletic animals with significant cardiac reserve capacity. Blood pressure, HR, and CO vary dramatically from rest to exercise. Cardiac output during exercise can increase to more than 8 times its resting value.[3] Evaluation of CO at rest will therefore not determine if poor performance is caused by primary cardiac impairment, but knowledge of changes in CO and BP over time is essential for understanding of the physiology of exercise.[7]

With knowledge of CO and HR, one can calculate ventricular stroke volume. Systemic vascular resistance is calculated from the difference between MAP and central venous pressure (CVP), divided by CO. Measurement of BP and CO allow for calculation of many variables (**Box 1**). Most of the supportive care in critical care medicine aims to improve global *oxygen delivery to the tissues* (DO$_2$) (see **Box 1**).[1,2] Shock can be defined as an unbalance between oxygen delivery and consumption or a disturbance of oxygen utilization, leading to cellular and tissue hypoxia. Using CO monitoring and blood gas analyses, one should be able to optimize DO$_2$ and titrate therapy to match the need of the patient while reducing the risk of overzealous treatment.[8]

Standard therapy for most types of shock consists of aggressive fluid therapy and use of vasopressors to ensure adequate MAP.[1] However, not all hypovolemic patients respond to volume loading and overzealous fluid administration can be extremely harmful in a portion of the population.[9,10] Almost half of patients in human intensive care unit do not respond positively to fluid boli.[8] This emphasizes the need for identification of variables that reliably estimate volume status and fluid responsiveness (ie, that differentiate between patients who will benefit from fluid resuscitation and patients who will not).

Patients with *cardiogenic shock* have decrease in CO and are often hypotensive. They, however, tend to have an increase in preload and cardiac filling pressures. Administration of fluid boli, further accentuating excessive volume loading, and use of vasopressors, increasing afterload to the heart, would cause worsening of clinical

---

Box 1
Equations

$CO = HR \times SV$
$DO_2 = CaO_2 \times CO$
$C_aO_2 = 1.34 \times Hb \times S_aO_2 + 0.003 \times P_aO_2$
$C_vO_2 = 1.34 \times Hb \times S_vO_2 + 0.003 \times P_vO_2$
$VO_2 = (C_aO_2 - C_vO_2) \times CO$
$OER = VO_2/DO_2 = (C_aO_2 - C_vO_2)/C_aO_2 \approx (S_aO_2 - S_vO_2)/S_aO_2$
$SVR = (MAP - CVP) \times 80/CO$
$PVR = (PAP - PCWP) \times 80/CO$
Modified Stewart-Hamilton equation:
    $CO = \text{amount of indicator}/f \text{ (concentration indicator} \times \text{time)}$

Abbreviations: C_aO_2 (mL/dL), arterial oxygen content; CO (L/min), cardiac output; C_vO_2 (mL/dL), venous oxygen content; CVP (mm Hg), central venous pressure; DO_2 (mL/min), oxygen delivery; Hb (g/dL), hemoglobin concentration; HR (beats per minute), heart rate; MAP (mm Hg), mean arterial pressure; OER, oxygen extraction ratio; P_aO_2 (mm Hg), oxygen tension in the arterial blood; PAP (mm Hg), pulmonary artery pressure; PCWP, pulmonary capillary wedge pressure; P_vO_2 (mm Hg), oxygen tension in the venous blood; PVR (dynes/s/cm^{-5}), pulmonary vascular resistance; S_aO_2 (%), saturation of hemoglobin with oxygen in the arterial blood; SV (mL), stroke volume; S_vO_2 (%), saturation of hemoglobin with oxygen in the venous blood; SVR (dynes/s/cm^{-5}), systemic vascular resistance; VO_2 (mL/min), oxygen consumption.

---

signs. It is therefore important to differentiate between hypovolemic/distributive shock and cardiogenic shock. Cardiogenic shock patients usually present with tachycardia, weak arterial pulses, distended jugular veins, jugular pulses, peripheral edema, cardiac chamber enlargement, or dysfunction, and they can have clinical or echocardiographic evidence of right or left heart failure. An increase in CVP can be regarded as a surrogate for an increase in right atrial pressure, which is typically equivalent to ventricular filling pressure. Central venous pressure can be easily determined by jugular catheterization and attaching the catheter to a pressure transducer. Patients with cardiogenic shock would have low arterial BPs and a high CVP (ie, increased filling pressures). Central venous pressure higher than 15 mm Hg would indicate that a patient is fluid overloaded or in cardiogenic shock.

Unfortunately, variables traditionally used as indicators of preload to guide fluid resuscitation such as CVP, right atrial pressure, or pulmonary capillary wedge pressure (as a surrogate of left atrial pressure) have been repeatedly shown to be unreliable solo indicators of fluid status.[1,11,12] Neither the absolute values of CVP nor their relative changes can consistently predict the hemodynamic response to a fluid challenge.[11-15] Right atrial pressure and CVP can be falsely elevated with tricuspid regurgitation, positive pressure ventilation, or pleural effusion. One should only use CVP in conjunction with changes in CO or BP to achieve a reliable indicator of fluid responsiveness and cardiovascular status.[1] More reliable preload indicators would include size of the cardiac chambers determined by echocardiography, stroke volume variation (SVV), or pulse pressure variation (PPV).[14,15] In most cases of cardiogenic shock, preload indicators are essential to titrate inotropes, vasodilators, and diuretics.

Cardiac output monitoring also has prognostic value. In fact, studies in people revealed that the most commonly monitored indices (HR, body temperature, CVP, and urine output) were poor predictors of survival, whereas CO-derived hemodynamic parameters such as CI, SVR, and VO_2 showed good specificity and sensitivity with regards to predicting survival.[8] It was proposed that these values be incorporated in the goal-directed therapy for critically ill patients, helping to guide therapy, identify a patient's fluid responsiveness, and hopefully decrease morbidity and mortality.[13-15]

BP MEASUREMENT TECHNIQUES

The techniques available for the measurement of the BP can be divided in 2 major categories: invasive BP and non-invasive BP (NIPB) techniques.

Invasive Blood Pressure

The invasive method is the gold standard of BP measurement and provides accurate, beat-to-beat monitoring. In horses, the lateral dorsal metatarsal artery, the transverse facial artery and the facial artery are most commonly used for arterial catheterization.[10] This technique requires an intra-arterial catheter connected to a BP transducer via a non-compliant fluid-filled extension set.[10] The fluid extension set should be visually inspected for air bubbles, kinks, fluid leaks, obstructions, or clots, which can lead to damping the system response and erroneous BP measurements.

Non-invasive BP Techniques

The NIBP technique is considered suitable for the cardiovascular monitoring of stable patients,[10,16] although it is not well established for standing, awake horses. To correct for the effect of gravity, a correction of 0.74 mm Hg/cm of vertical distance between the site of cuff placement and the heart base needs to be added to (if the cuff is above heart base) or subtracted from (if the cuff is below heart base) the measured pressures. Normal values for NIBP in conscious, standing adult horses (corrected for vertical distance of cuff position above heart base) are around 135 ± 15, 110 ± 15, and 90 ± 15 mm Hg (mean $\pm$ SD) for systolic (SAP), mean (MAP), and diastolic arterial pressure (DAP), respectively, with a calculated pulse pressure of approximately 45 ± 6 mm Hg.[5,16–18]

In general, the techniques available for the NIBP monitoring can be subdivided into 2 major techniques: the ultrasonic Doppler flow detector and the oscillometric method.[18]

Ultrasonic Doppler flow detector

A cuff with a width of 30% to 40% of the circumference of the tail or limb is applied proximal to a Doppler flow detector that is placed over the respective artery. The cuff is attached to a sphygmomanometer, inflated until pulsation sounds disappear, and then gradually deflated until first pulsation sounds are detected. By definition, the sphygmomanometer pressure corresponding to reappearance of the sounds is the SAP.

Oscillometric blood pressure measurement

The oscillometric method is used in automated NIBP monitors. They use an inflatable cuff to first obstruct the blood flow from an area over a major peripheral artery. After cuff inflation and cuff pressure stabilization, the device deflates the cuff slowly, in a controlled manner. When cuff pressure is lower than SAP, the arterial pulse will resume and cuff pressure will start varying in a pulsatile manner. During cuff deflation, the amplitude of cuff pressure increases until blood flow returns to normal. The NIBP monitor will receive the cuff pressure mechanical signals, and the cuff pressure that is associated with the highest pulse amplitude is measured as MAP; SAP and DAP are then calculated by the aid of proprietary algorithms and results are displayed as BP.[5,17–21]

A cuff width-to-tail circumference ratio of 0.4 to 0.6 is commonly recommended and has been used in horses.[20,21] Wider cuffs tend to underestimate and smaller cuffs tend overestimate NIBP. Measurements may be less sensitive with severe hypotension and slow HR in horses, often accompanied by second-degree atrioventricular blocks or sinus arrhythmia, which often complicate or sometimes even prevent accurate and reliable NIBP measurements.[10,20–22]

CO MEASUREMENT TECHNIQUES

Despite the significant advantages of CO monitoring, its use is still limited in equine medicine (**Table 1**). This is likely because of the invasive nature of many available methods.[7,23] An excellent review of CO technologies as they pertain to horses was made by Corley and colleges in 2003[7]; however, newer methods for determination of CO have been established since. The choice of the monitoring system depends on the patient (species, size), and often on the devices and availability of expertise at a specific hospital or institution. The expertise and familiarity of the operator with the technique represents a critical factor to obtain reliable results with many of the

Table 1
Techniques for cardiac output measurement and their clinical application

Cardiac Output Measurement Technique	Company Manufacturing Equipment	Use in Foals	Use in Adults	Use during Exercise	Accuracy	Note
Pulmonary thermodilution	Edward Lifesciences LLC, Irvene, CA	Yes	Yes	Yes	Traditional reference standard	Requires pulmonary artery catheter
Transpulmonary thermodilution	Pulsion Medical systems/Phillips, Munich, Germany	Yes	No	No	Good correlation in foals	Requires central arterial catheter
Lithium dilution	LiDCO Ltd, Lake Villa, IL	Yes	Yes	Yes	Good correlation	Requires peripheral arterial catheter
Ultrasound velocity dilution	Transonic Inc, Ithaca, NY	Yes	No	No	Good correlation in foals	Requires peripheral arterial catheter
Fick's principle		Yes	No	Yes	Good correlation	Requires pulmonary artery catheter and measurement of oxygen consumption
Rebreathing CO_2	NICCO Respironic Inc/Phillips, Murrysville, PA	Yes	No	No	Good correlation in foals	Requires mechanical ventilation
Pulse contour analysis	Pulsion Medical Systems, Munich, Germany	Yes	Yes	?	Weak correlation	Requires calibration when changes in hemodynamic status occur
Echocardiogram		Yes	Yes	No	Moderate correlation	Requires large operator experience

CO-monitoring devices available. A typical example of high operator dependency is represented by echocardiography compared with other automatic devices that consistently produce results with low inter-operator variability.[7,24]

There are 4 basic methods of measuring CO: (1) indicator methods (such as pulmonary thermodilution and lithium dilution [LIDCO] techniques); (2) a derivation of Fick's principle; (3) arterial pulse wave analysis (pulse contour CO); and (4) imaging diagnostic techniques (transthoracic echocardiography, thoracic bio-impedance).[24,25]

Indicator Methods

Pulmonary artery dilution technique

The pulmonary artery (thermo)dilution (PAD) technique using a pulmonary arterial (PA) catheter (Swan-Ganz technique) remains an accepted clinical reference standard for CO measurement, although it is far from being a highly accurate and reliable gold standard. It is a commonly used method for CO monitoring in research settings. This technique is one of the few methods capable of determining CO in adult horses.

The Swan-Ganz PA catheter is a double lumen catheter with a thermistor in the tip. The placement of a PA catheter in an adult horse is straightforward and should be done in a standing position. Placement when the animal is in dorsal or lateral position is possible but far more challenging. An introducer kit is placed in the jugular vein and the Swan-Ganz catheter is fed through the introducer into the vein. The distal port is connected to a pressure transducer and the clinician can use the pressure waveform to monitor the catheter advancement from the jugular vein to the right atrium, the right ventricle, and finally confirm placement in proximal PA. Most PA catheters have an inflatable balloon located near the tip of the catheter to facilitate passage from the ventricle to the PA and for measurement of pulmonary capillary wedge pressure. Once positioned, the proximal port should sit in the right atrium and the distal port should sit in the PA. Regular 110-cm Swan-Ganz catheters designed to fit a human heart can be used for foals and up to average size adult horses, but may be too short for adults of very large breeds.[26] Also, in adult horses the proximal port of standard human catheters is usually located in the right ventricle rather than the right atrium, and a separate catheter needs to be placed in the right atrium for indicator injection.

The PAD method involves using thermal energy as an indicator. A small bolus of cold, isotonic solution (5% dextrose or 0.9% saline) is injected into the patient's right atrium and the dilution of the indicator is followed continuously in the pulmonary artery. Plotting a graph of the concentration of the indicator (ie, the blood temperature) against time will produce a concentration-time curve, and the area under the curve is calculated. CO is inversely proportional to the area under the curve, as determined by the Stewart-Hamilton principle (see **Box 1**).

The use of a PA catheter carries some risks, including arrhythmias, damage to the cardiac endothelium, infection, and pulmonary thromboembolism.[26,27] For those reasons, PAD is not routinely used in clinical veterinary medicine. There has, therefore, been growing interest in less-invasive techniques for CO measurement, such as transpulmonary thermodilution, LiDCO, and ultrasound velocity dilution (UDCO) techniques. These other indicator methods are, in principle, a modification of PAD and also follow the Stewart-Hamilton principle.

Lithium dilution and ultrasound velocity dilution

The LiDCO method has demonstrated excellent agreement when compared with PAD in animal models.[27,28] It is capable of measuring CO in adult horses (including measurements during exercise),[26,28] and is currently one of the most commonly used methods of determining CO in anesthetized foals.[25]

The LiDCO technique (LiDCO Ltd, Lake Villa, IL) requires injection of lithium chloride (0.003 mmol/kg) via a central vein. Subsequently, arterial blood is withdrawn by means of a peristaltic pump and guided through a lithium sensor placed near arterial catheter. Cardiac output is then derived from the lithium concentration-over-time curve by the Stewart-Hamilton principle.[25]

For an adult horse, blood removed for one LiDCO determination is minimal (20–40 mL per measurement). Nonetheless, blood loss associated with repeated LiDCO measurements is a drawback of this technique.[29] Also, accumulation of the indicator (lithium) in the body, leading to erroneous measurements and potential risks of other undesirable effects, needs to be considered.[25] Lithium sensors can also react with some drugs commonly used during anesthesia, such as alpha-2 agonists and neuro-muscular blockers (ie, atracurium), resulting in unreliable readings.[30,31]

Ultrasound velocity dilution (COstatus, Transonic Inc, Ithaca, NY) is a novel technique for determining CO.[32] Ultrasound velocity dilution is minimally invasive, does not involve blood loss, and uses a physiologic non-cumulative signal (saline solution).[32] This technique has been used in anesthetized foals and juvenile horses with good success.[32] To determine CO using the UDCO technique, an arterio-venous loop is made by attaching tubing between metatarsal (peripheral) arterial and central venous catheters, creating an extracorporeal circuit.[32] An ultrasound velocity sensors is placed upstream from the venous catheter and an arterial flow sensor is placed downstream from the arterial catheter. A bolus of isotonic saline (0.5–1 mL/kg) is injected into the venous circulation, creating a transient hemodilution and resulting in a change in the velocity of ultrasound in this blood. The CO is calculated as a function of the volume of isotonic saline and the consequent decrease in ultrasound velocity. In adult horses, UDCO would require a large amount of fluid (0.5 mL/kg) to be rapidly administered through the small, high-resistance arterio-venous loop. Therefore, it is not currently viable for use in animals larger than 250 kg.[32]

The Fick Method

This technique is one of the oldest methods of measuring CO and it was validated in horses in 1890.[3] According to Fick's principle, $CO = V_{O_2}/(C_aO_2 - C_vO_2)$, whereby V_{O_2} is oxygen uptake in the tissues. Arterial oxygen content (C_aO_2) and venous oxygen content (C_vO_2) are calculated by measuring, with a blood gas analyzer, the partial pressure of oxygen in the arterial (P_aO_2) and venous blood (P_vO_2), saturation of hemoglobin with oxygen in the arterial (S_aO_2) and venous blood (S_vO_2), and hemoglobin concentration (Hb), using the formulas: $C_aO_2 = (1.34 \times Hb \times S_aO_2) + (0.003 \times P_aO_2)$ and $C_vO_2 = (1.34 \times Hb \times S_vO_2) + (0.003 \times P_vO_2)$, respectively.[8] Fick's method has some drawbacks for clinical use. Mixed venous blood sampling (to measure C_vO_2) requires placement of a PA catheter, with all the complications stated above. Blood samples from the right atrium and jugular vein are easier to collect but will introduce some degree of error. Furthermore, oxygen uptake is calculated as $V_{O_2} = VE \times (FIO_2 - FEO_2)$, whereby VE is the expired minute ventilation volume and FIo_2 and FEO_2 represent the fractional concentrations of oxygen in inspired and expired gas, respectively. Accurate determination of expired minute ventilation volume requires a specially designed tight-fit mask and a cooperative horse.[1,7]

Pulse Contour Analysis

Calculation of CO based on the contour of the arterial pulse wave, *if accurate*, would offer the advantage of providing minimally invasive, continuous, beat-to-beat CO measurements. Arterial pulse wave analysis monitors also display volumetric preload variables, such as SVV and PPV. Both SVV and PPV have predictive value for the patient's fluid responsiveness.[7,33] The stroke volume correlates well with the area of the arterial wave before the dicrotic notch; however, the arterial pressure waveform is also dependent on multiple factors, including changes in aortic impedance, SVR and waveform damping, all of which prevent this from being a straightforward relationship.[7,33] Changes in SVR and volemic state of the patient render pulse contour technology less accurate.[33]

Imaging Techniques

Echocardiography

Echocardiography is one of the truly non-invasive techniques available for measurement of CO in juvenile and adult horses.[34] A great advantage of echocardiography over other monitoring techniques is the large amount of structural, functional, and hemodynamic information that can be obtained beyond just CO. Systolic and diastolic ventricular function and chamber filling can be rapidly assessed, and valves, myocardium, and pericardium can be directly visualized.[29,34–38]

Cardiac output can be determined with echocardiography using non-Doppler or Doppler-based methods.[29,35–37] Non-Doppler techniques are based on various geometric models to calculate volumetric estimates of the left ventricular size. The most common method is based on bi-plane or modified (single-plane) Simpson's model, wherein the left ventricle is divided into a series of disks stacked from base to apex, and left ventricular volume is calculated by summing up the approximated volumes of the individual disks.[25,39] Stroke volume is calculated by determining the difference in left ventricle volume between diastole and systole.[25,39] The non-Doppler technique can provide rapid CO estimation in emergency situations. However, difficulty with endocardial border definition and erroneous foreshortening of the ventricle can produce inaccurate results.

Measurement of blood flow velocity using spectral Doppler ultrasound and aortic or pulmonary artery diameter, respectively, also allow estimation of stroke volume and CO. However, accurate measurement of vessel diameter and proper alignment of the Doppler beam with blood flow to measure velocity in the great vessels is very challenging in horses. Measurements are time-consuming and prone to large errors.[25,39] Doppler-based methods are therefore not routinely used in clinical patients. Although CO by echocardiography represents significantly less risk to the patient and is less time-consuming than other methods of CO determination, this method requires expensive equipment and highly trained personnel to minimize operator error.[38,39]

SUMMARY

In conclusion, frequent and accurate cardiac monitoring can be extremely useful to guide therapy and improve clinical outcome. In critically ill patients, it can be used to gauge fluid responsiveness and more accurately determine cardiovascular status and therefore appropriate therapy. In anesthetized patients, it can be used to detect deteriorating cardiovascular status earlier than is possible with other, more commonly monitored variables. Although monitoring the cardiovascular status is important, no hemodynamic monitoring technique can improve outcome by itself. It is important to understand that, while BP, CO, and DO_2 provide insight as to the adequacy of delivery of blood and oxygen to the body as a whole,[40] it does not does not allow direct assessment of adequacy of microcirculation. A good BP and normal CO therefore do not necessarily indicate adequate tissue perfusion. Cardiac monitoring should always be interpreted together with a thorough physical examination and other auxiliary microcirculatory monitoring.

REFERENCES

1. Mellema M. Cardiac output monitoring. In: Silverstein D, Hopper K, editors. Small animal critical care medicine. St Louis (MO): Saunders Elsevier; 2009. p. 894–8.
2. Valverde A, Giguere S, Sanchez LC, et al. Effects of dobutamine, norepinephrine, and vasopressin on cardiovascular function in anesthetized neonatal foals with induced hypotension. Am J Vet Res 2006;67:1730–7.
3. Evans DL. Cardiovascular adaptations to exercise and training. Vet Clin North Am Equine Pract 1985;1:513–31.
4. Grimm A, Lamont LA, Robertson SA, et al. Vet anest analg. Ames (IA): Wiley Blackwell; 2015.
5. Parry B, McCarthy MA, Anderson GA. Survey of resting blood pressure values in clinically normal horses. Equine Vet J 1984;16:53–8.
6. Bonagura J, Reef V. Cardiovascualar diseases. In: Reed S, WM B, editors. Equine internal medicine. 1st edition. Philadelphia: WB Saunders; 1998. p. 290–370.
7. Corley KT, Donaldson LL, Durando MM, et al. Cardiac output technologies with special reference to the horse. J Vet Intern Med 2003;17:262–72.
8. Pinsky MR, Payen D. Functional hemodynamic monitoring. Crit Care 2005;9: 566–72.
9. Corley KT. Inotropes and vasopressors in adult and foals. Vet Clin North Am Equine Pract 2004;20:77–106.
10. Magdesian KG. Monitoring the critically ill equine patient. Vet Clin North Am Equine Pract 2004;20:11–39.
11. Durairaj L, Schmidt GA. Fluid therapy in resuscitated sepsis: less is more. Chest 2008;133:252–63.
12. Kumar A, Anel R, Bunnell E, et al. Pulmonary artery occlusion pressure and central venous pressure fail to predict ventricular filling volume, cardiac performance, or the response to volume infusion in normal subjects. Crit Care Med 2004;32:691–9.
13. Shippy CR, Appel PL, Shoemaker WC. Reliability of clinical monitoring to assess blood volume in critically ill patients. Crit Care Med 1984;12:107–12.
14. Godje O, Peyerl M, Seebauer T, et al. Central venous pressure, pulmonary capillary wedge pressure and intrathoracic blood volumes as preload indicators in cardiac surgery patients. Eur J Cardiothorac Surg 1998;13:533–9 [discussion: 539–40].
15. Marik PE, Baram M, Vahid B. Does central venous pressure predict fluid responsiveness? A systematic review of the literature and the tale of seven mares. Chest 2008;134:172–8.
16. Johnson JH, Garner HE, Hutcheson DP. Ultrasonic measurement of arterial blood pressure in conditioned Thoroughbreds. Equine Vet J 1976;8:55.
17. Heliczer N, Lorello O, Casoni D, et al. Accuracy and precision of noninvasive blood pressure in normo-, hyper-, and hypotensive standing and anesthetized adult horses. J Vet Intern Med 2016;30:866.
18. Olsen E, Pedersen TLS, Robinson R, et al. Accuracy and precision of oscillometric blood pressure in standing conscious horses. J Vet Emerg Crit Care (San Antonio) 2016;26:85.
19. ScheerB, Perel A, Pfeiffer U. Clinical review: complications and risk factors of peripheral arterial catheters used for haemodynamic monitoring in anaesthesia and intensive care medicine. Crit Care 2002;6:199–204.
20. Branson KR. A clinical evaluation of an oscillometric blood pressure monitor on anesthetized horses. J Equine Vet Sci 1997;17:537.

21. Hatz LA, Hartnack S, Kummerle J, et al. A study of measurement of noninvasive blood pressure with the oscillometric device, Sentinel, in isoflurane-anaesthetized horses. Vet Anaesth Analg 2015;42:369.

22. Tünsmeyer J, Hopster K, Feige K, et al. Agreement of high definition oscillometry with direct arterial blood pressure measurement at different blood pressure ranges in horses under general anaesthesia. Vet Anaesth Analg 2015;42:286.

23. Vincent JL, Rhodes A, Perel A, et al. Clinical review: update on hemodynamic monitoring - a consensus. Crit Care 2011;15:229.

24. Hoffman GM, Ghanayem NS, Tweddell JS. Noninvasive assessment of cardiac output. Semin Thorac Cardiovasc Surg Pediatr Card Surg Annu 2005;12–21. https://doi.org/10.1053/j.pcsu.2005.01.005.

25. Giguere S, Bucki E, Adin DB, et al. Cardiac output measurement by partial carbon dioxide rebreathing, 2-dimensional echocardiography, and lithium-dilution method in anesthetized neonatal foals. J Vet Intern Med 2005;19:737–43.

26. Linton RA, Jonas MM, Tibby SM, et al. Cardiac output measured by lithium dilution and transpulmonary thermodilution in patients in a paediatric intensive care unit. Intensive Care Med 2000;26:1507–11.

27. Connors AF Jr, Speroff T, Dawson NV, et al. The effectiveness of right heart catheterization in the initial care of critically ill patients. SUPPORT Investigators. JAMA 1996;276:889–97.

28. Durando MM, Corley KT, Boston RC, et al. Cardiac output determination by use of lithium dilution during exercise in horse. Am J Vet Res 2008;8:1054–62.

29. Uehara Y, Koga M, Takahashi M. Determination of cardiac output by echocardiography. J Vet Med Sci 1995;57:401–7.

30. Beaulieu JM, Sotnikova TD, Yao WD, et al. Lithium antagonizes dopamine-dependent behaviors mediated by an AKT/glycogen synthase kinase 3 signaling cascade. Proc Natl Acad Sci U S A 2004;101:5099–104.

31. Corley KT, Donaldson LL, Furr MO. Comparison of lithium dilution and thermodilution cardiac output measurements in anaesthetised neonatal foals. Equine Vet J 2002;34:598–601.

32. Shih A, Giguere S, Vigani A, et al. Determination of cardiac output by ultrasound velocity dilution in normovolemia and hypovolemia in dogs. Vet Anaesth Analg 2011;38:279–85.

33. Shih AC, Giguere S, Sanchez LC, et al. Determination of cardiac output in anesthetized neonatal foals by use of two pulse wave analysis methods. Am J Vet Res 2009;70:334–9.

34. Cheung AT, Savino JS, Weiss SJ, et al. Echocardiographic and hemodynamic indexes of left ventricular preload in patients with normal and abnormal ventricular function. Anesthesiology 1994;81:376–87.

35. Thys DM, Hillei Z. Left ventricular performance indices by transesophageal Doppler. Anesthesiology 1988;69:728–33.

36. Madan AK, UyBarreta VV, Aliabadi-Wahle S, et al. Esophageal Doppler ultrasound monitor versus pulmonary artery catheter in the hemodynamic management of critically ill surgical patients. J Trauma 1999;46:607–12.

37. Marr CM, Patteson MW. Echocardiogram. In: Marr CM, Bowen M, editors. Cardiology of the horse. 2 edition. Philadelphia: Saunders Elsevier; 1999. p. 105–24.

38. Young LE, Blissit KJ, Clutton RE. Feasibility of transoesophageal echocardiography for evaluation of left ventricular performance in anesthetized horses. Equine Vet J 1995;19(S1):63–70.

39. McConachie E, Barton MH, Rapoport G, et al. Doppler and volumetric echocardiographic methods for cardiac output measurement in standing adult horses. J Vet Intern Med 2013;27:324–30.
40. Vigani A, Shih A, Queiroz P, et al. Quantitative response of volumetric variables measured by a new ultrasound dilution method in a juvenile model of hemorrhagic shock and resuscitation. Resuscitation 2012;88:1031–7.

Cardiac Therapeutics in Horses

Adam Redpath, BVMS(Hons), PGCert(VetMed), MRCVS*,
Mark Bowen, BVetMed, MMedSci(MedEd), PhD, CertVA, CertEM(IntMed), PFHEA, FRCVS

KEYWORDS

- Equine arrhythmia • Cardiac therapeutics • Congestive heart failure
- Antiarrhythmic agents

KEY POINTS

- Quinidine remains the drug of choice for the pharmacologic cardioversion of atrial fibrillation. Medications such as amiodarone have established evidence available for their use in specific situations. The role of other agents, such as flecainide, sotalol, and the angiotensin-converting enzyme (ACE) inhibitors, are under increasing scrutiny for their usefulness in the management of atrial fibrillation.
- Management of acute tachyarrhythmias is achieved through a variety of pharmacologic agents. Lidocaine, magnesium, and procainamide remain the most commonly used first-line medications for ventricular tachyarrhythmias. However, the administration of other agents can be useful in refractory cases.
- Management of acute onset congestive heart failure relies on the use of diuretics and vasodilators. The use of ACE inhibitors is growing in the management of such cases, although evidence of their efficacy or robust criteria for the selection are lacking.
- Medication to delay the progression of asymptomatic heart disease in the horse are the subject of an emerging field of research, but clinical evidence of benefit based on longitudinal data is lacking.

INTRODUCTION

Many cardiac therapeutics lack significant evidence of benefit in the horse, and in many cases their use is based on extrapolation of evidence from other species or based on isolated clinical case reports or limited case series in the horse. Most agents are not approved for use in horses and several medicines described historically, such as quinidine gluconate, have limited availability, even in human medicine, whereas others, such as bretylium, have been discontinued. The aim of this article is to provide evidence-based guidance on the use of cardiac therapeutics for the treatment of

Disclosure Statement: None.
Oakham Veterinary Hospital, University of Nottingham, School of Veterinary Medicine and Science, Sutton Bonington, LE12 5RD, UK
* Corresponding author.
E-mail address: adam.redpath@nottingham.ac.uk

cardiac disease and, where known, describe their pharmacology relevant to equine clinical practice. Evidence for current dosing recommendations are based on pharmacologic studies or, where lacking, based on the literature or authors experience (**Table 1**).

ANTIARRHYTHMIC AGENTS

Classically the antiarrhythmic agents have been divided into 4 main classes based on their predominant actions on cardiac tissues using the Vaughan-Williams classification system.[1] Although this classification system is useful for considering how these drugs impact on formation and propagation of the cardiac action potential (**Fig. 1**), the categorization of agents is not absolute, with many antiarrhythmic drugs having actions across more than one group. More relevant to the equine practitioner is how each drug is chosen for the treatment of different supraventricular and ventricular arrhythmias. Many indications for antiarrhythmics are based on limited evidence; therefore, if rhythm control is not achieved with initial choice of antiarrhythmic agents, clinicians are encouraged to consider alternative agents (**Table 2**). As well as possessing antiarrhythmic effects, many, especially the class I and III agents, have the potential to be proarrhythmic and therefore should be used with care and for the management of arrhythmias that are clinically significant (**Box 1**). Criteria for the selection of cases for management of AF are covered elsewhere (See Gunther van Loon's article "Cardiac Arrhythmias in Horses," in this issue.)

Class I Antiarrhythmic Agents (Na Channel Blockers)

Class I antiarrhythmic agents block voltage-gated sodium channels of the myocardium, with their actions being mediated predominantly through non-nodal tissue, thus slowing the propagation of action potentials. They are use dependent, so binding is preferential to activated or inactivated sodium channels, and drugs dissociate from channels in the closed state. These agents can be further subdivided based on their kinetics for dissociation from the sodium channels.

Class Ia antiarrhythmic agents

Class Ia agents block fast sodium channels and prolong the action potential (class III activity), lengthening the effective refractory period. These drugs are also potentially proarrhythmic because they cause QT interval prolongation, promoting re-entry. They are useful for the treatment of supraventricular and ventricular tachyarrhythmias.

Quinidine Enteral quinidine sulfate is the most established therapy for the treatment of AF.[2] Quinidine gluconate has been used intravenously for the treatment of ventricular tachycardia (VT) and recent onset AF of less than 7 days duration, but is largely of historical interest since its production was discontinued in 2017.

Quinidine has a variety of cardiovascular and non-cardiac effects. Its class Ia and III activities slow impulse conduction and prolong the effective refractory period. The vagolytic activity results in accelerated atrioventricular (AV) nodal conduction. It also possesses α-adrenoreceptor antagonistic effects, resulting in hypotension and a reflex increase in sympathetic outflow, potentiating its proarrhythmic effects.

Plasma concentrations of quinidine following oral administration are unpredictable owing to highly variable pharmacokinetics between individuals. The time to peak concentrations ranging from 1 to 4 hours and the standard deviation for both bioavailability and plasma half-life, representing approximately 50% of the mean of each factor, with bioavailability being further impacted by feeding.[3,4] The reason for the variability in

Table 1
Commonly used cardiac therapeutics including indications and typical doses used for these indications

Drug	Indication	Dose
Acepromazine	Vasodilation to decrease afterload in congestive heart failure	0.1–1.0 mg/kg p.o. bid or tid[a] 0.01–0.06 mg/kg i.m. tid or qid[a] Dose to effect—monitor NIBP
Amiodarone	Atrial fibrillation Refractory ventricular tachycardia[a] Oral maintenance dosing has been described following i.v. infusions	5 mg/kg/h i.v. for 1 h, then 0.83 mg/kg/h for 23 h then 1.9 mg/kg/h for 30 h or to effect 10 mg/kg p.o. sid[a]
Atropine	Bradycardia of vagal origin Lower doses can be associated with paradoxical parasympathomimetic effect worsening bradycardia	10–20 µg/kg i.v., i.m. or s.c.
Benazepril	Congestive heart failure, to induce vasodilation and decrease of sodium and fluid retention Putative agent to delay progression of asymptomatic heart disease[a]	0.5–1.0 mg/kg p.o. sid-bid
Digoxin	Congestive heart failure, for positive inotropic effects and baroreceptor sensitization Control of ventricular response rate in atrial fibrillation or supraventricular tachycardia (usually alongside other medications)	2.2 µg/kg i.v., bid or as required 11 µg/kg p.o. bid Therapeutic drugs monitoring essential
Esmolol	Rate control in ventricular and supraventricular tachycardia	200–500 µg/kg over 2–5 min, followed by a CRI of 25–100 µg/kg/min, titrate to effect[a]
Diltiazem	Management of rapid ventricular response rate during quinidine management of atrial fibrillation	0.125 mg/kg slow i.v. every 10 min, titrate to effect up to a maximum of 1.25 mg/kg
Dobutamine	Acute heart failure or severe hypotension, for positive inotropic effects and vasoconstriction	1–5 µg/kg/min i.v.
Flecainide	Supraventricular and ventricular arrhythmias refractory to other therapy[a] Safe dosing strategies have not been fully documented—use with extreme caution and consider combining with a β-blocker[a]	1–2 mg/kg i.v. at a rate of 0.2 mg/kg/min

(continued on next page)

Table 1
(continued)

Drug	Indication	Dose
Furosemide	Congestive heart failure, diuresis, and reduction of sodium and fluid retention	Acute diuresis: 1–3 mg/kg i.v. or i.m. tid or qid or 1–2 mg/kg i.v. loading dose followed by 0.12 mg/kg/h CRI Chronic diuresis: 1–2 mg/kg i.m. bid
Glycopyrrolate	Bradycardia of vagal origin	5–10 µg/kg i.v.
Hydralazine	Vasodilation to decrease afterload in congestive heart failure	0.5 mg/kg i.v. q4 h
Lidocaine	Ventricular tachycardia	0.25–0.5 mg/kg i.v. q5 min; total not to exceed 2 mg/kg in the conscious horse or 1.3 mg/kg loading dose, then 50 µg/kg/min CRI
Magnesium sulfate	Ventricular arrhythmias, especially torsades de pointes and refractory ventricular tachycardia	2–5 mg/kg i.v. q2 min to a maximum of 50 mg/kg total
Milrinone	Inodilation for acute management of congestive heart failure[a]	5–10 µg/kg/min i.v.
Norepinephrine	Severe refractory cardiogenic shock Hypotension and shock associated with excessive peripheral vasodilation (after adequate fluid loading)	0.1–0.3 µg/kg/min i.v.
Phenylephrine	Severe refractory cardiogenic shock Hypotension and shock associated with excessive peripheral vasodilation (after adequate fluid loading)	0.1–0.2 µg/kg/min i.v.; not to exceed 0.01 mg/kg
Phenytoin	Digoxin-induced ventricular tachycardia Other ventricular arrhythmias Isolated premature ventricular depolarizations[a]	7.5 mg/kg i.v. 20 mg/kg p.o. bid for 3–4 doses then 10–15 mg/kg p.o. bid
Pimobendan	Putative inodilator in congestive heart failure[a]	0.25 mg/kg i.v. bid Oral doses not established
Procainamide	Supraventricular and ventricular arrhythmias[a]	1 mg/kg/min i.v. Total dose not to exceed 20 mg/kg
Propafenone	Refractory supraventricular and ventricular arrhythmias[a]	0.5–2.0 mg/kg i.v. over 5 min

(continued on next page)

Table 1
(continued)

Drug	Indication	Dose
Propranolol	Refractory ventricular and supraventricular tachycardia	0.03–0.16 mg/kg i.v.[b]
	Management of rapid ventricular response rate during quinidine management of atrial fibrillation	0.38–0.78 mg/kg p.o. tid
Quinidine gluconate[b]	Acute onset atrial fibrillation Ventricular tachycardia	2.2 mg/kg i.v. every 10 min, 12 mg/kg maximum dose
Quinidine sulfate	Atrial fibrillation Potentially for other supraventricular and ventricular arrhythmias	22 mg/kg by nasogastric tube every 2 h for 4–6 doses
Ramipril	Congestive heart failure, to induce vasodilation and decrease of sodium and fluid retention Putative agent to delay progression of asymptomatic heart disease[a]	0.05–0.2 mg/kg[a]
Scopalamine	Bradycardia of vagal origin	0.1–0.2 mg/kg i.v. Short duration of action
Sotalol	Reduction in conversion threshold for atrial fibrillation, prevention of early recurrence of atrial fibrillation after treatment[a] Putative therapy for supraventricular and ventricular arrhythmias[a]	2–3 mg/kg p.o. bid
Spironolactone	Diuretic and mineralocorticoid receptor antagonist, usually combined with furosemide for more pronounced, potassium-sparing diuresis in congestive heart failure[a]	2–4 mg/kg p.o. sid[a]

Abbreviations: CRI, constant rate infusion; i.m., intramuscular; i.v., intravenous; NIBP, non-invasive blood pressure; p.o., oral; s.c., subcutaneous.

[a] Indicates weak evidence for this dosing strategy in the horse and not used as first-line management.

[b] Indicates regional drug availability limits use via this route.

pharmacokinetic parameters has not been described but is reported in other species and may reflect variable gastric emptying due to the presence of food and the limited water solubility of quinidine sulfate. Plasma protein binding, and therefore free concentrations of quinidine, is affected by plasma pH. Plasma alkalinization promotes binding, which may be useful in the management of adverse effects, but further contributes to the variable kinetics that contribute to both treatment failure and adverse events when following standard dosing recommendations. Therapeutic drug monitoring, taken 1 hour after administration, is ideal for estimating appropriate dosing, although QRS

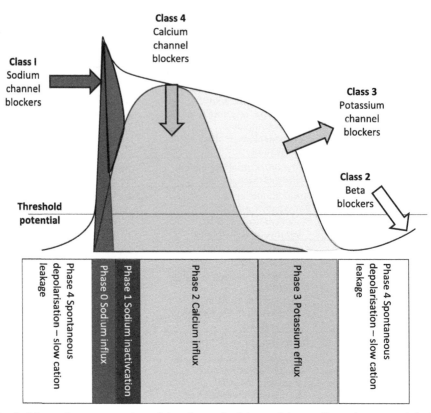

Fig. 1. Schematic representation of the electrophysiology of the cardiac action potential of myocardial tissue illustrating the 5 phases of the cardiac action potential and the Vaughan-Williams classification of antiarrhythmic therapies. Phase 4 represents spontaneous depolarization of pacemaker cells through slow leakage of sodium and potassium until the threshold potential is reached (represented by the horizontal line) and is slowed by use of class 2 antiarrhythmic agents (the β-blockers). Phase 0 represents opening of fast sodium channels resulting in cellular depolarization and is slowed by the use of class 1 antiarrhythmic agents. Phase 2 causes the plateau phase of the action potential caused by calcium influx resulting in cellular contraction and is reduced by the use of class 4 antiarrhythmic agents. Phase 3, repolarization is caused by potassium efflux and slowed by the use of class 3 antiarrhythmic agents.

prolongation by 25% over baseline is often used as a proxy to predicting animals in which the therapeutic range of 2–5 μg/mL is being exceeded.[5] Quinidine is metabolized in the liver and should be used with care in animals with liver dysfunction. There are significant drug interactions with quinidine and other protein-bound drugs, such as digoxin. Quinidine toxicity can manifest in cardiac and non-cardiac adverse effects, demonstrating the wide-ranging effects on ion channels, physiologic receptors, and direct effects of this agent. The management of these are discussed in detail in Gunther van Loon's article, "Cardiac Arrhythmias in Horses," in this issue.

Procainamide Intravenous procainamide has been used for the acute management of VT and the management of acute onset AF in horses.[6] Although a class Ia agent, it has an improved safety profile compared with quinidine; it does not induce QRS prolongation and is a less potent vagolytic agent than quinidine. Prolongation of the QT interval

Table 2
Clinical application of the antiarrhythmic agents for different classes of arrhythmia in the horse

Arrhythmia	First-Line Treatments	Alternative/Refractory Cases	Comments
Persistent arrhythmias			
Supraventricular tachycardia	Rate control Digoxin Esmolol Rhythm control Quinidine gluconate[a] Procainamide	Rate control Diltiazem Propranolol Rhythm control Sotalol Quinidine sulfate	Treat cases where rate >100 bpm or evidence of poor perfusion using rate control
Ventricular tachycardia	Magnesium sulfate Lidocaine Where available: Quinidine gluconate[a] Procainamide	Sotalol Propafenone Amiodarone Phenytoin (digoxin-induced arrhythmias) Propranolol (where other treatments fail, eg, resistant VT following quinidine administrations)	Treat if evidence of poor perfusion or malignant arrhythmia (HR >100 bpm, multiform/polymorphic complexes, R-on-T phenomenon)
Atrial fibrillation	Acute onset (<7 d): Quinidine gluconate [a] Acute onset or longstanding/chronic disease: Quinidine sulfate Transvenous electrical cardioversion	Amiodarone Procainamide Amiodarone	Treat if causing (or predicted to cause) clinical signs of poor performance/epistaxis or associated with tachyarrhythmia or ventricular complexes/ventricular aberrancy at exercise
Ventricular fibrillation	Not amenable to pharmacologic manipulation. Bretylium previously described for use in foals now discontinued from supply. Consider DC cardioversion		
Intermittent arrhythmias			
Isolated ventricular premature complexes	Sotalol	Phenytoin	Consider and address primary cause (electrolytes, myocardial disease, toxins, SIRS) before initiating antiarrhythmic therapy
Isolated supraventricular premature complexes	Treatment rarely indicated	Sotalol	Consider primary cause (electrolytes, myocardial disease, toxins, SIRS)

Indication for treatment should be based on electrocardiographic evidence predicting worsening of rhythm (malignant rhythm) including rates over 100 bpm, multiform arrhythmia, or for ventricular tachycardia the presence of an R-on-T phenomenon.

[a] Indicates regional drug availability limits used via this route. Evidence for use of these medicines is frequently based on anecdotal reports, single cases reports, or occasional case series.

Box 1
Criteria for the pharmacologic management of acute tachyarrhythmias.

Pharmacologic management of acute tachyarrhythmias are indicated when:
1. There is evidence of poor cardiac function manifesting with either clinical signs (eg, depression, weakness, collapse, syncope, severe systemic hypotension) OR
2. There are laboratory parameters indicating poor peripheral perfusion (azotemia or hyperlactatemia) OR
3. A malignant arrhythmia is present that may worsen if left untreated, including:
   a. Rates over 100 bpm (in the adult horse) OR
   b. Multiform or polymorphic complexes OR
   c. The presence of the R-on-T phenomenon

---

occurs following intravenous (i.v.) administration and may account for its proarrhythmic effect at higher doses.[7] Mild peripheral vasodilation can occur leading to hypotension.[8] Procainamide undergoes acetylation in plasma to N-acetylprocainamide (NAPA) and renal elimination. NAPA is an active metabolite with class III antiarrhythmic activity that has a half-life twice the duration of the parent drug.[7]

Class Ib antiarrhythmic agents

Class Ib antiarrhythmic agents are useful for the management of ventricular arrhythmias. They are ineffective at managing atrial arrhythmias, owing to the rapid association-dissociation characteristics with activated sodium channels, meaning they are ineffective during the shorter atrial action potential, but can be used for ventricular arrhythmias whereby the action potential is longer. These agents shorten the action potential without causing QT prolongation. They preferentially bind to refractory sodium channels and thus act primarily on damaged myocardial cells to prevent re-entry pathways.

Lidocaine Intravenous lidocaine is a first-line drug in the treatment of VT. It should be administered as i.v. bolus doses of 0.5 mg/kg every 5 minutes, up to a total dose of 4 mg/kg, although it should be used with caution above cumulative doses of 2 mg/kg in conscious horses because the plasma concentrations associated with toxicity can be highly variable.[8,9] Continuous rate infusions of 50 μg/kg/min can be used after loading doses to provide prolonged therapeutic concentrations. CNS adverse effects include nystagmus, muscle twitching, disorientation, excitement, and convulsions. Usually such signs begin with mild excitement reactions and are short-lived because of the rapid hepatic metabolism of the drug, and usually only associated with single bolus doses of lidocaine exceeding 2 mg/kg. Diazepam can be administered at 0.05 mg/kg to control seizures if necessary. Lipid infusions have been used as part of the management of cardiovascular collapse in a foal after administration an unknown quantity of lidocaine, resulting in asystole.[10] However, given the short half-life of lidocaine, the value of this intervention is as yet unproven. Greater care should be exercised when administering to animals with liver dysfunction or reduced hepatic blood flow; fasting will prolong hepatic clearance of lidocaine because of the resultant reduction in hepatic blood flow and via other intrinsic mechanisms.[11] Lidocaine is less effective in hypokalemia, and therefore electrolyte imbalance should be corrected before treatment with lidocaine. Hemodynamic effects are rare, and lidocaine rarely alters nodal conduction except at extreme doses.[9,10] Lidocaine undergoes a high level of first-pass metabolism when given orally; absorption is variable following intramuscular administration and, therefore, only i.v. administration is recommended.

Phenytoin (diphenylhydantoin) Phenytoin is primarily used for the acute treatment of cardiac glycoside-induced arrhythmias.[12] It may have a role in the management of intermittent ventricular ectopy but requires ongoing maintenance administration to maintain sinus rhythm and the evidence for efficacy is limited.[13] There is a narrow therapeutic index, and sedation, recumbency, and even excitement reactions at extreme doses may be observed.[13] The dosage for phenytoin in the horse is 10 to 20 mg/kg po bid for 3 to 4 doses followed by a maintenance dose of 10 to 15 mg/kg po bid, but accurate dosing should be informed based on therapeutic drug monitoring to avoid adverse events. Phenytoin has poor oral bioavailability (35% ± 9%) because of extensive first-pass metabolism. Hepatic enzymes may be induced by the use of phenytoin, thereby impacting on the metabolism of other drugs, including lidocaine.

Other class 1b agents Other class Ib agents including tocainide and mexiletine are administered orally for treatment of ventricular arrhythmias in humans and dogs, but have not yet been evaluated for use in the horse and cannot currently be recommended.

Class Ic antiarrhythmic agents

Class Ic agents are potent inhibitors of the fast sodium channel with differential blockade within the Purkinje fibers with little impact on the surrounding myocardium, making them potentially valuable for the management of ventricular arrhythmias. They also exert some class III effects, resulting in QT prolongation.[14] Initial studies in human patients after acute myocardial infarction demonstrated increased mortality in patients in whom both flecainide and encainide were used to suppress ventricular ectopy.[15] Class 1c drugs should not be used in patients with documented structural heart disease or myocardial damage.

Flecainide Flecainide has undergone several studies to investigate its potential use in the management of AF and VT.[16–21] However, at this stage, it cannot be recommended in the horse given its narrow safety profile, with reports documenting the development of supraventricular tachycardia, VT, and, in one horse, fatal ventricular fibrillation. It is ineffective in chronic AF,[17] but, with further dose optimization, it may have a future role in the management of acute onset AF.[21]

Propafenone Despite being classified as a class Ic agent, propafenone also has class II and IV effects. It has been associated with increased mortality in humans.[22] Its effects on action potential vary with the species and it is used for the treatment of sustained supraventricular, VT, and ventricular premature complexes in humans. Oral administration of propafenone in horses has not been effective at doses extrapolated from human medicine.[23] Intravenous use has been described for the successful management of sustained VT in a single horse at a dose rate of 0.5–1.0 mg/kg for more than 5–10 min.[6] However, it seems to have no value in the management of AF using a loading dose followed by a constant rate infusion.[24] Following i.v. administration, propafenone has a rapid distribution and plasma concentrations decrease below the therapeutic concentrations required in other species (500 ng/mL) within 30 minutes of administration of a bolus of 2 mg/kg, suggesting that a continuous rate infusion may be more appropriate than intermittent dosing.[25] Elimination is by hepatic and renal routes, and this may be affected by co-administration of quinidine. Propafenone reduces clearance of warfarin and digoxin.

Class II Antiarrhythmic Agents (β-Adrenoceptor Antagonists)

β-Adrenoreceptor antagonists (β-blockers) prolong phase 4 of the cardiac action potential, suppressing sinoatrial pacemaker activity and AV nodal conduction, thereby slowing the heart rate. They also exert negative inotropic and antiarrhythmic effects. There are 3 subtypes of β-adrenoreceptors: stimulation of β_1-adrenoreceptors in the heart affects the force and rate of cardiac contraction, the automaticity of the pacemaker sites, and conduction through the AV node. The β_2-adrenoreceptors are located within the blood vessels and bronchioles and their activation leads to bronchodilation and vasodilation. β_2-Adrenoreceptors are also located in the sinoatrial and AV nodes, activation of which causes increased automaticity and AV nodal conduction, resulting in an increase in rate (eg, after i.v. administration of clenbuterol). β_3-Adrenoreceptors have been identified in the human and canine myocardium, in which they cause a reduction in myocardial contractility but have not been identified in the equine myocardium. In human patients, β-blockers have been shown to increase survival in human patients with ischemic and non-ischemic heart failure.[26] Furthermore they have been shown to improve survival in asymptomatic or mildly symptomatic human patients with ventricular arrhythmias following myocardial ischemia; a population in which other antiarrhythmic medication was considered harmful.[27]

Propranolol

Propranolol is a non-specific β-adrenoceptor antagonist acting on both β_1- and β_2-adrenoreceptors, and which causes dose-dependent suppression of myocardial contractility, although this is not usually seen at therapeutic doses. Propranolol should be reserved for the treatment of supraventricular tachycardias and VTs that are refractory to other therapeutic agents because of its deleterious effects on cardiac performance. Because it has no effect on phase 1 of the cardiac action potential, it can be used for the treatment of quinidine-induced ventricular tachyarrhythmias. The negative inotropic and chronotropic properties of the drug can lead to sinus bradycardia and hypotension. If this occurs, it should be treated with an acute inotrope such as dobutamine.

Propranolol is only effective when administered intravenously in horses, and the i.v. formulation has limited availability in certain regions. Rapid first-pass metabolism results in low bioavailability and therapeutic plasma concentrations are rarely achieved after oral administration.[8] It undergoes rapid hepatic metabolism giving it a short plasma half-life in the horse (2 hours). Plasma concentrations may be increased if hepatic blood flow is reduced; for example, by significant cardiac disease or in the significant hepatic dysfunction.

Sotalol

Sotalol has both class II and class III antiarrhythmic effects. It is widely used in human and small-animal medicine for chronic oral antiarrhythmic therapy, in which it is effective for both ventricular and supraventricular arrhythmias. The pharmacokinetics of sotalol have recently been evaluated in horses, and it is a potentially useful drug when long-term oral antiarrhythmic therapy is required. Sotalol may also be a useful adjunctive therapy for horses undergoing transvenous electrocardioversion (TVEC) from AF, requiring lower energies for conversion and reducing recurrence of early recurrence of AF.[28,29] Experience suggests that sotalol is ineffective as a monotherapy for conversion of AF to normal sinus rhythm in horses, despite its use in this setting in human patients. It has not been evaluated in combination with other pharmacologic agents in the horse to determine whether a dose-reducing effect would be seen with pharmacologic conversion, as with TVEC.

Sotalol is potentially useful for rate control in horses that develop exercise-induced tachyarrhythmias, in particular those with AF that are not suitable candidates for rhythm control. However, further work is required to document the safety of sotalol in this setting because it is not recommended for long-term rate control in human medicine because of the risk of torsades de pointes and sudden cardiac death.

Sotalol has moderate oral bioavailability (48%) with maximal absorption achieved approximately 1 hour after administration and a mean elimination half-life of 15 hours.[30] Intravenous administration results in a significant prolongation of QT interval but no significant changes in other electrocardiographic and echocardiographic parameters. QT interval prolongation may occur to a lesser extent when the drug is given orally.[28,30] Transient sweating and mild colic have been observed following i.v. administration, but no significant adverse effects were noted following oral administration at a dose of 2 mg/kg po bid, although the authors have observed sweating when administered at higher dose rates (5 mg/kg po).

Other β-blockers

The use of more receptor-specific β-blockers, such as atenolol, have not been evaluated in horses, despite their widespread use in small-animal cardiology. Their receptor specificity would suggest an improved safety profile compared with propranolol and sotalol. Esmolol, a short-acting i.v. β-blocker, is potentially valuable in the control of ventricular response rates for management of supraventricular tachycardia and VT.[31] Doses of 200–500 μg/kg followed by a continuous rate infusion of 25 μg/kg/min have been recommended before oral therapy, although no pharmacologic data exist to support this dosing regimen.

Class III Antiarrhythmic Agents (K-Channel Blockers)

Class III agents suppress the inward potassium current, prolonging phase 3 of the action potential and the refractory period. They are used for the treatment of VT in humans. However, prolongation of the action potential and hence of the QT interval may result in a proarrhythmic effect.

Amiodarone

Amiodarone has been evaluated for the treatment of AF in the horse using a continuous rate infusion; however, it has been associated with a variety of adverse effects, including gastrointestinal, neurologic, cardiac, and dermatologic signs.[32–34] Amiodarone is a highly lipophilic drug with a slow onset of action and long tissue half-life. It has poor bioavailability and is excreted in urine.[32,35]

Amiodarone is a potential treatment of horses with VT that are resistant to other medications. However, so far there is only one report in which it has been used to successfully treat a horse with sustained VT that had failed to convert following administration of magnesium sulfate, lidocaine, and propafenone; this included several weeks of oral dosing despite its reported poor oral bioavailability.[34] Reliable cost-effective protocols for using amiodarone in VT would be beneficial given the adverse CNS effects of lidocaine and the poor availability of other suitable products.

Class IV Antiarrhythmic Agents (Calcium Channel Blockers)

Class IV agents are calcium channel blockers and, therefore, act on phase 2 of the cardiac action potential. They primarily act on nodal tissues and are used for the treatment of supraventricular arrhythmias in humans and dogs but have not been critically evaluated in horses. There is limited data regarding the use of diltiazem in horses, but other drugs in this class including verapamil have not been assessed and no recommendations can be made about their use.

Diltiazem

Diltiazem is highly protein bound and has been proposed as a suitable treatment of digitalis-induced arrhythmias. Because of its inhibitory effects on AV nodal conduction it has been proposed to reduce the ventricular response rate in the management of AF in dogs. Despite a lack of published evidence in naturally occurring AF, experimental studies suggest that diltiazem is a potentially useful alternative medication for acute ventricular rate control in horses undergoing pharmacologic conversion of AF with quinidine.[36,37]

Diltiazem can be used for the management of hypertension in other species, although is not indicated in the treatment of primary hypertension, in which drugs acting on vascular calcium channels are preferred to induce vasodilation. The role of hypertension in equine disease is poorly understood and is occasionally observed in horses with equine metabolic syndrome;[38] however, there is no evidence that these agents would provide clinical benefit in such cases. Furthermore, there are no data about its oral bioavailability of diltiazem to make any dosing recommendations.

Other Antiarrhythmic Drugs

Magnesium sulfate

Magnesium sulfate can be effective at terminating refractory ventricular arrhythmias, even in patients with normomagnesemia and can reduce the occurrence of ventricular ectopy and VT in human patients with congestive heart failure (CHF).[39] Its mechanism of action is not fully understood but, as magnesium ions act as cofactors in the Na^+/K^+ ATPase system, hypomagnesemia may result in hypokalemia, predisposing to arrhythmias. In apparently normomagnesemic patients, magnesium ions may exert their effect through a calcium channel-blocking effect;[40] however, this role is difficult to document because magnesium ions are largely intracellular, compromising assessment of magnesium status based on plasma concentrations, even when measuring its ionized form. In human patients, magnesium is the treatment of choice for quinidine-induced torsades de pointes, and can be effectively used for the same condition in the horse. Given its lack of adverse effects, it is the authors' first-line treatment for the management of VT. It can be safely combined with antiarrhythmic agents and may potentiate the effects of lidocaine given its effects on Na^+/K^+ ATPase transporters in patients with hypokalemia.

Anticholinergic agents

Anticholinergic agents are only effective in controlling vagal-mediated bradyarrhythmias and are predominantly used to treat or prevent life-threatening drug-induced bradycardia. All anticholinergic agents competitively inhibit the binding of acetylcholine to the postganglionic synapses in the heart, thus blocking vagally induced slowing of the heart rate. Low doses of atropine (less than 5 μg/kg) can be associated with a paradoxical parasympathomimetic effect, which may exacerbate bradycardia, especially when administered intravenously. This is mediated through effects within the CNS. However, the phenomenon can also be observed with low doses of glycopyrrolate, suggesting a peripheral effect by blockade of inhibitory presynaptic muscarinic receptors. Anticholinergic agents also cause ileus and decreased salivary secretions.

Atropine Atropine is a tertiary amine and crosses the blood-brain barrier and may occasionally give rise to adverse CNS effects in addition to the paradoxical parasympathomimetic effects discussed above, such as excitement and sedation, especially when administered intravenously. The gastrointestinal effects of atropine last up to 12 hours.

Glycopyrrolate Glycopyrrolate does not cross the blood-brain barrier and, therefore, results in fewer CNS adverse effects. It causes a dose-dependent reduction in gastrointestinal motility that can persist for up to 24 hours.[41,42] Glycopyrrolate can effectively increase systemic blood pressure in anesthetized horses with bradycardia-related hypotension,[43] but, given the gastrointestinal effects, it should be used only when life-threatening bradyarrhythmias occur.

Butyl scopolamine (hyoscine) Scopolamine is an anticholinergic agent used widely in equine practice for the treatment of spasmodic colic and has been shown to inhibit romifidine-induced bradyarrhythmias.[44] Unlike atropine, scopolamine does not induce an initial bradycardia following administration, and the reduction in gastrointestinal motility lasts only 20–30 minutes in horses.[45] However, scopolamine administration provides a short-lived increase in heart rate and blood pressure, and further work is required to establish appropriate infusion rates for maintaining this effect.[46] Its use in the face of life-threatening bradycardias in horses has not been established.

MANAGEMENT OF HORSES WITH CONGESTIVE HEART FAILURE

Recognition and clinical signs of CHF are detailed in John D. Bonagura's article, "Overview of the Equine Heart in Health and Disease," in this issue. There are no data to recommend any specific therapy for the management of horses with asymptomatic heart disease, or whether any such interventions would reduce the progression of disease or have added benefit. However, studies have demonstrated significant prolongation of life expectancy and quality of life in medicated dogs with myxomatous mitral valve disease (MVD), and the value of pre-emptive therapy in the horse may develop a robust evidence base in the future.[47–49]

In many cases, the long-term prognosis for symptomatic CHF is poor; thus, before embarking on therapy, clear expectations should be established especially if the horse owner expects to be able to continue ridden exercise. There is a clear rationale for treating horses with symptomatic CHF in which the primary cause can be addressed (eg, monensin or oleander toxicities, CHF secondary to arrhythmias, ruptured chordae tendinea, pericardial or acquired myocardial disease) to optimize cardiac output and tissue oxygen delivery over a limited time frame. In the acute cardiac crisis, the function of cardiac therapeutics can be optimized by increasing oxygen content through inhaled oxygen therapy.

Stroke volume, the amount of blood ejected by the left ventricle in each cardiac cycle, is the product of cardiac contractility, preload (end-diastolic left ventricular volume), and afterload (ventricular wall tension, largely influenced by systemic blood pressure). These factors form the primary targets for both acute and chronic management of CHF. A clinically applicable algorithm for the management of symptomatic CHF in the horse is shown in **Fig. 2**.

Preload Reduction

Reducing preload reduces cardiac work and remains one of the most important aspects of management of CHF. It involves the use of diuretics. Diuretics reduce clinical signs of CHF and may slow progression of cardiac chamber dilation by causing a reduction in left ventricular filling pressure.

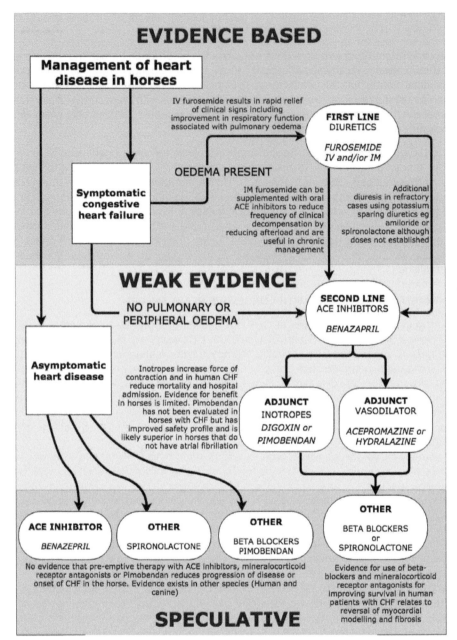

Fig. 2. Treatment algorithm for the management of symptomatic and asymptomatic congestive heart failure (CHF) in the horse demonstrating evidence-based decision making for use in such cases. Treatment modalities are presented in order of selection for horses with evidence or absence of edema and stratified based on available evidence in green (reliable evidence base), amber (weak or limited evidence), or red (speculative therapy) based on therapeutics used in other species but have not been evaluated in a systematic way in the horse. ACE, angiotensin-converting enzyme.

Furosemide

Furosemide is a loop diuretic that inhibits the reabsorption of electrolytes in the thick ascending loop of Henle, resulting in the increased excretion of sodium, chloride, potassium ions, and water. The resultant decrease in plasma volume, ventricular end-diastolic pressure, and atrial pressure reduces pulmonary and systemic venous hydrostatic pressure. This in turn diminishes systemic congestion, peripheral and pulmonary edema, and reducing the work of ventilation.[50] It is the most commonly used diuretic in the horse and is usually given parentally, because oral bioavailability is poor and does not induce significant diuresis.[51]

Furosemide can be administered intravenously to achieve rapid diuresis; however, it is short acting, with urine flow returning to normal within 2 hours.[52] Constant rate infusions (0.12 mg/kg/h, preceded by a loading dose of 1–2 mg/kg i.v.) result in more rapid fluid loss than intermittent dosing (1 mg/kg i.v. q8 h), although resulting in the same fluid loss over a 24-hour period.[53] Chronic diuresis can be achieved after the initial stabilization with the use of intramuscular injections (1–2 mg/kg q6–12 h).[53] Long-term or high-dose furosemide administration may lead to hypokalemia, hyponatremia, hypomagnesemia, and metabolic acidosis. Therefore, serum electrolyte concentrations should be monitored during long-term furosemide treatment.

Alternative/additional diuretics

Potassium-sparing diuretics can be divided into 2 categories. Diuretics, such as amiloride, inhibit sodium-selective channels in the late distal convoluted tubule and the cortical collecting duct. The other category of potassium-sparing diuretics are inhibitors of type 1 mineralocorticoid receptors and act as aldosterone antagonists, such as spironolactone. The mineralocorticoid receptor antagonists have benefits in addition to their weak diuretic effects because they act on the terminal mediator of the renin-angiotensin-aldosterone system and are discussed in more detail in the subsequent section.

Thiazide diuretics inhibit the sodium/chloride symporter in the renal epithelial cell of the distal convoluted tubule, increasing the loss of sodium, chloride, and water. Excessive sodium and fluid in the distal nephron enhance the secretion of potassium and hydrogen ions. Alone, these diuretics are only useful in mild heart failure. However, when combined with loop diuretics, they exhibit synergism, which may be useful in patients resistant to loop diuretics. Pharmacokinetics and dosage for the thiazide diuretics have not been established in the horse.

Afterload Reduction

CHF results in activation of the renin-angiotensin-aldosterone system and increased sympathetic activity in response to a decrease in cardiac output, and results in venous and arterial vasoconstriction. Afterload reduction, through the use of vasodilators, increases stroke volume and can have a marked reduction in valvular regurgitation by promoting forward blood flow, but data on their impact on CHF in horses are limited. Venodilators provide an increase in venous capacitance and decrease ventricular filling pressures, wall stress, and preload.

Inhibitors of the renin-angiotensin-aldosterone system

The renin-angiotensin-aldosterone system (RAAS) is an important homeostatic mechanism for maintaining hemodynamics. Drugs that target RAAS bring about therapeutic benefits through vasodilation and through reducing the tissue effects of these mediators. The complex cascade of mediators and enzymes responds to low blood pressure, low sodium concentrations, and low peripheral oxygen content, resulting in vasoconstriction and sodium and water retention, and thus an increase in

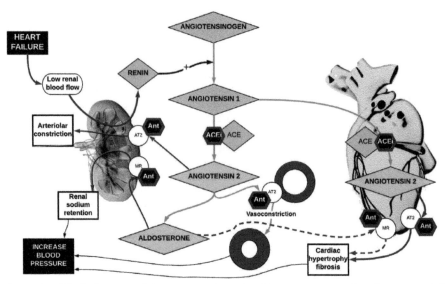

Fig. 3. Simplified schematic of the renin-angiotensin-aldosterone system identifying potential therapeutic targets. Release of renin from the kidneys initiates the production of angiotensin 1, which is converted through circulating and tissue angiotensin-converting enzymes (ACEs) to produce biologically active angiotensin 2 and subsequently the release of biologically active aldosterone from the adrenal glands. Angiotensin 2 is a potent vasoconstrictor, although aldosterone causes renal reabsorption of sodium and hence increases circulating volume, both increasing systemic blood pressure. Both agents result in cardiac modeling, hypertrophy, and, ultimately, cardiac fibrosis. Putative pharmacologic targets (*bordered black hexagons*) include the ACE inhibitors (ACEi) that are widely used in veterinary practice. Specific receptor antagonists (Ant) for aldosterone, the mineralocorticoid receptor (MR) antagonists, such as spironolactone, and the angiotensin 2 receptor antagonists have not been evaluated in the horse. Circulating or tissue factors are represented by diamond boxes. Receptor targets *AT2* (angiotensin 2 receptors) and *MR* (mineralocorticoid) are represented by unfilled circles.

circulating volume that mediates hypertension associated with early heart failure (**Fig. 3**). RAAS activation also mediates cardiac modeling and myocardial fibrosis.[54] The most widely exploited therapeutic targets in the management of cardiac disease are the angiotensin-converting enzyme inhibitors (ACEi) that block the conversion of angiotensin 1 to angiotensin 2, thereby theoretically blocking the entire cascade, as well as acting locally to inhibit tissue, specifically myocardial, production of angiotensin 2, a key mediator in myocardial remodeling. Angiotensin 2 receptor antagonists have received little attention in veterinary cardiology, although they have potent disease-modifying effects in human patients. Aldosterone, the final step in the RAAS can also be inhibited using mineralocorticoid receptor antagonists, such as spironolactone.

ACE inhibitors ACEi have been shown to be effective in managing CHF and delaying progression of both symptomatic and asymptomatic heart disease in other species.[55–59] There is growing evidence that the RAAS may play a role in atrial structural and electrical remodeling leading to AF,[60,61] which may lead to future therapeutic protocols that prevent the development of AF in horses with MVD. Of the ACEi evaluated in the horse, benazepril is the authors' current ACEi of choice in the horse and may be valuable for the treatment of symptomatic CHF. This recommendation is based in superior oral bioavailability[62] and evidence of reduction in cardiac chamber dimensions (using 2D echocardiography) in horses with clinically relevant mitral and aortic valve regurgitation[63] Further evidence is required before recommendations about their use in delaying the progression of cardiac dysfunction caused by valvular heart disease in asymptomatic patients can be made. The evidence for the use of other ACEi is questionable[64–68]

Spironolactone Spironolactone is a competitive mineralocorticoid receptor antagonist that has been shown to have beneficial effects when added to conventional therapy for CHF in humans and MVD in dogs.[69,70] Aldosterone induces myocardial and perivascular fibrosis and alters the endothelial function of vessels, which may be counteracted by the use of aldosterone antagonists.[71] Its use has not yet been evaluated in horses, but it is a potentially useful component in multi-modal therapy for CHF.

Direct-acting vasodilators

Hydralazine Hydralazine is a direct-acting arteriodilator. Its mechanism of action is still debated, but it is dependent on intact endothelium and is thought to involve calcium channels.[72] It has been shown to increase stroke volume and decrease ventricular wall stress in human patients with aortic regurgitation.[73,74] In normal horses, hydralazine produces a sympathetically mediated reflex increase in heart rate.[75] Hydralazine increases renal perfusion by reducing renal vasculature resistance and, therefore, may be useful in patients with marginal renal function who cannot tolerate ACEi. There are no data to support the oral administration of hydralazine to horses because it undergoes hepatic metabolism in most species resulting in poor oral bioavailability. i.v. administration (0.5 mg/kg i.v. q4 h) may be useful in the initial management of severe CHF but has not been critically evaluated in horses with CHF.

Nitrates: nitroglycerin (glyceryl trinitrate) Nitrate vasodilators result in the generation of nitric oxide within tissues, resulting in vasodilation through cyclic guanosine monophosphate pathways. There are no data to support their use in the management of CHF in horses. Glyceryl trinitrate (GTN) is a percutaneous gel that is approved for the prevention of angina in humans; however, its absorption has not been robustly established following transdermal administration to horses, although there is some evidence of a biological effect in the digital vasculature in the horse.[76] The absorption of GTN is affected by the characteristics of the skin, and, when applied to the clipped lateral thorax of normal dogs, there was no change in arterial blood pressure, pulmonary artery pressure, or cardiac output.[77] The oral nitrates have not been evaluated in veterinary species; although agents such as isosorbide dinitrate have benefits in human CHF when used in combination with other vasodilators.[78]

Miscellaneous vasodilators

Acepromazine is an α-adrenoceptor and 5-hydroxytryptamine (serotonin) receptor antagonist that induces vasodilation in the horse.[6] Given its low cost and availability in equine practice it is the authors' first-line vasodilator in horses with CHF, but should be used with care to prevent severe hypotension. Moderate doses should be used initially (0.01–0.02 mg/kg) and titrated to effect based on response to therapy using blood pressure monitoring. Other vasodilators, including the calcium channel blocker, amlodipine, and the indirectly acting vasodilators, prazosin and isoxsuprine, have not been evaluated for the management of equine cardiovascular disease and cannot be recommended. Sildenafil, a phosphodiesterase (PDE) subtype-5 inhibitor, has been proposed as a treatment of persistent pulmonary hypertension (PH) in the neonatal human patients,[79,80] and may have a role in the management of PH in foals and cor pulmonale in adult horses with lung pathology, although it cannot be recommended at this time.[81]

Positive Inotropes

Positive inotropes function through increasing the force of myocardial contraction by increasing intracellular calcium concentrations or by sensitizing the myocardium to the effects of calcium. However, they can be detrimental both through direct effects and through increasing the myocardial oxygen demand. Therefore, afterload reduction may be more beneficial in animals with myocardial failure, because the failing heart is largely influenced by afterload. The use of positive inotropes may be controversial in atrioventricular valve insufficiency as they may increase regurgitant flow in addition to increasing forward flow. Both acute and chronic inotropes may be useful in specific cases of CHF in the horse.

The cardiac glycosides

The cardiac glycosides, once considered potent inotropes, have been shown to have important indirect effects on cardiac output and are therefore considered separately to the classic inotropes. Digoxin is the most commonly used cardiac glycoside. Its positive inotropic effects result from the inhibition of Na^+/K^+ ATPase, which increases intracellular sodium concentrations, slowing down calcium extrusion from the cell via the Na^+/Ca^{2+} exchanger, increasing intracytoplasmic calcium concentrations. It can also be used to slow the ventricular response rate in supraventricular tachyarrhythmias such as AF.[82]

Digoxin has a narrow therapeutic index, with toxic effects seen when plasma concentrations exceed 2 ng/mL.[83] Pharmacokinetics are highly variable and therefore plasma concentrations are difficult to predict, further complicated by protein binding, such that co-administration of drugs such as quinidine will increase free concentrations of both agents. Excretion can also be affected by the administration of other drugs through renal (eg, quinidine) and non-renal (eg, propafenone and amiodarone) routes.[82] Peak concentrations occur 1–2 hours following administration,[83,84] yet a second peak has been reported resulting from enterohepatic recycling resulting high plasma concentrations 9–15 hours after administration.[83] The plasma half-life of digoxin is also variable (16.8–28.8 hours).[83,85] These variable kinetics and complex drug interactions highlight the importance of therapeutic drug monitoring to prevent toxicity and to validate the efficiency of the dose of digoxin. Therapeutic drug monitoring should be performed after five half-lives (3–6 days) once steady-state digoxin concentrations have been achieved. Serum should be obtained 1–2 hours (peak) and 12 hours (trough) after dosing, and concentrations should be in the range of 0.5–2.0 ng/mL (1.0–2.6 nmol/L).[83] Toxicity can cause depression, anorexia, and cardiac arrhythmias. Cardiac effects of digoxin toxicity are either related to the negative chronotropic actions of the drug or the production of tachyarrhythmias.[86] Tachyarrhythmias often occur in hypokalemia because inhibition of the Na^+/K^+-ATPase exacerbates the hypopolarization of the myocardium.

Acute inotropes and vasopressors

Acute inotropes are predominantly used for resuscitation of the critically ill or in anesthetized horses with hypotension. However, they may be useful in promoting cardiac output in animals with acute CHF, especially when it is the result of primary myocardial diseases in which contractility is reduced. Since these agents increase myocardial oxygen demand they should be used with care, and avoided in animals with chronic CHF or with concurrent tachyarrhythmias. The actions of inotropes are mediated largely through α- and β-adrenoceptors, and the lack of receptor specificity of these agents results in a differential effect on receptors at increasing doses, resulting in both inotropic and chronotropic effects.

Dobutamine Dobutamine is the most widely used positive inotrope (β-adrenergic) in the horse with weak positive chronotropic (β-adrenergic) and vasoconstrictive effects (α-adrenergic). The effects on heart rate are seen with increasing concentrations, although tachycardia is common when used at lower infusion rates in horses that have already received anticholinergic agents such as atropine.[87] It can also be used to increase heart rate, because of its β_1-adrenergic effects, in horses with pathologic bradyarrhythmias.[88] It has a very short half-life (2 minutes) and undergoes metabolism via conjugation. Steady-state concentrations are usually achieved within 10 minutes of initiating a constant i.v. infusion. Dobutamine is useful for short-term circulatory support of patients with acute heart failure. Because of the development of tolerance and lack of an enteral formulation, dobutamine is not appropriate for long-term therapy.

Incremental doses of dobutamine (1–5 μg/kg/min i.v.) have been described following atropine administration (35 μg/kg i.v.) in the horse as part of a pharmacologic stress test. In normal horses, heart rate increased during the infusion to a maximum of 157 ± 13 bpm and systolic ventricular function (determined by calculation of fractional shortening) increased from 35% ± 4% to 51% ± 3%.[89] There are no published data on the use of dobutamine stress testing in horses with cardiac disease to determine its value in documenting myocardial dysfunction at this time, and it is therefore currently not recommended for clinical use. Pronounced distress was observed in one Thoroughbred racehorse during the infusion that prevented infusion rates higher than 3 μg/kg/min; however, colic has not been observed in any case despite the high systemic doses of atropine being used.

Other positive inotropes and vasopressors Other positive inotropes are reserved for the management of non-responsive hypotension in the horse, especially for the management of drug-resistant hypotension in adults and foals with sepsis, and a normal or high cardiac output. In such cases, the combination of peripheral vasoconstriction and increased contractility caused by norepinephrine can be effective in maintaining peripheral circulation, although perfusion is not improved in the normal horse with normal vasomotor tone.[90] No evidence for its use in horses with cardiogenic shock are available, and the increase in afterload could have deleterious effects if not offset by peripheral vasodilators. There is no value in the use of dopamine, or its synthetic analogue dopexamine, in equine cardiac or renal disease; indeed adverse effects of dopamine on peripheral perfusion are well documented.[90] Phenylephrine is a vasopressor increasing peripheral blood pressure without increasing cardiac output,[90,91] and has no place in the management of acute cardiac disease and is inferior to norepinephrine in the management of hypotension in sepsis.

Inodilators
The so-called inodilators combine the positive effects of increased myocardial contractility and peripheral vasodilation, causing afterload reduction. PDE inhibitors are the prototypical agents contained in this group.

Milrinone Milrinone has not been evaluated fully in the equine clinical setting but produces a dose-dependent increase in heart rate, cardiac output, arterial blood pressure, and ejection fraction, and a reduction in right atrial, pulmonary arterial pressures, and systemic vascular resistance in normal anesthetized horses.[92] As such, it has the potential to provide short-term support of circulation in advanced CHF.

Pimobendan Pimobendan has been used in dogs for the management of heart failure due to myxomatous valvular disease and dilated cardiomyopathy, in which it has been shown to improve survival in affected animals, delay the onset of clinical signs in asymptomatic animals, and reduce cardiac enlargement.[47–49,93] Data are lacking regarding its use in horses with CHF, but it has been shown to have positive chronotropic and inotropic effects in healthy mature horses when given intravenously.[94] This is a promising drug for the management of chronic cardiac disease in horses in the future, although oral bioavailability has not been fully established.

REFERENCES

1. Vaughan Williams EM. Classification of antidysrhythmic drugs. Pharmacol Ther B 1975;1:115–38.
2. Glendinning SA. The use of quinidine sulphate for the treatment of atrial fibrillation in twelve horses. Vet Rec 1965;77:951–60.
3. Bouckaert S, Voorspoels J, Vandenbossche G, et al. Effect of drug formulation and feeding on the pharmacokinetics of orally administered quinidine in the horse. J Vet Pharmacol Ther 1994;17:275–8.
4. McGuirk SM, Muir WW, Sams RA. Pharmacokinetic analysis of intravenously and orally administered quinidine in horses. Am J Vet Res 1981;42:938–42.
5. Reef VB. Arrhythmias. In: Marr CM, editor. Cardiology of the horse. 1st edition. London: Saunders; 1999. p. 179–202.
6. Marr CM, Reef VB. Caerdiac arrhythmias. In: Kobluk CN, Arnes TR, Geor RJ, editors. The horses: disease and clinical management. Philadelphia: Saunders; 1995. p. 137–56.
7. Ellis EJ, Ravis WR, Malloy M, et al. The pharmacokinetics and pharmacodynamics of procainamide in horses after intravenous administration. J Vet Pharmacol Ther 1994;17:265–70.
8. Muir WW 3rd, McGuirk S. Cardiovascular drugs. Their pharmacology and use in horses. Vet Clin North Am Equine Pract 1987;3:37–57.
9. Meyer GA, Lin HC, Hanson RR, et al. Effects of intravenous lidocaine overdose on cardiac electrical activity and blood pressure in the horse. Equine Vet J 2001;33:434–7.
10. Vieitez V, Gomez de Segura IA, Martin-Cuervo M, et al. Successful use of lipid emulsion to resuscitate a foal after intravenous lidocaine induced cardiovascular collapse. Equine Vet J 2017;49:767–9.
11. Engelking LR, Blyden GT, Lofstedt J, et al. Pharmacokinetics of antipyrine, acetaminophen and lidocaine in fed and fasted horses. J Vet Pharmacol Ther 1987;10:73–82.
12. Wijnberg ID, van der Kolk JH, Hiddink EG. Use of phenytoin to treat digitalis-induced cardiac arrhythmias in a miniature Shetland pony. Vet Rec 1999;144:259–61.
13. Wijnberg ID, Ververs FF. Phenytoin sodium as a treatment for ventricular dysrhythmia in horses. J Vet Intern Med 2004;18:350–3.

14. Haugaard MM, Pehrson S, Carstensen H, et al. Antiarrhythmic and electrophysiologic effects of flecainide on acutely induced atrial fibrillation in healthy horses. J Vet Intern Med 2015;29:339–47.

15. Echt DS, Liebson PR, Mitchell LB, et al. Mortality and morbidity in patients receiving encainide, flecainide, or placebo. The Cardiac Arrhythmia Suppression Trial. N Engl J Med 1991;324:781–8.

16. Ohmura H, Nukada T, Mizuno Y, et al. Safe and efficacious dosage of flecainide acetate for treating equine atrial fibrillation. J Vet Med Sci 2000;62:711–5.

17. van Loon G, Blissitt KJ, Keen JA, et al. Use of intravenous flecainide in horses with naturally-occurring atrial fibrillation. Equine Vet J 2004;36:609–14.

18. Birettoni F, Porciello F, Rishniw M, et al. Treatment of chronic atrial fibrillation in the horse with flecainide: personal observation. Vet Res Commun 2007;31(Suppl 1): 273–5.

19. Risberg AI, McGuirk SM. Successful conversion of equine atrial fibrillation using oral flecainide. J Vet Intern Med 2006;20:207–9.

20. Dembek KA, Hurcombe SD, Schober KE, et al. Sudden death of a horse with supraventricular tachycardia following oral administration of flecainide acetate. J Vet Emerg Crit Care (San Antonio) 2014;24:759–63.

21. Takahashi Y, Ishikawa Y, Ohmura H. Treatment of recent-onset atrial fibrillation with quinidine and flecainide in Thoroughbred racehorses: 107 cases (1987–2014). J Am Vet Med Assoc 2018;252:1409–14.

22. Siebels J, Cappato R, Ruppel R, et al. Preliminary results of the Cardiac Arrest Study Hamburg (CASH). CASH investigators. Am J Cardiol 1993;72:109F–13F.

23. Bowen IM, Marr CM, Elliott J. Drugs acting on the cardiovascular system. In: Betone JJ, Horspool LJI, editors. Equine clinical pharmacology. Philadelphia: Saunders; 2004. p. 193–215.

24. De Clercq D, van Loon G, Tavernier R, et al. Use of propafenone for conversion of chronic atrial fibrillation in horses. Am J Vet Res 2009;70:223–7.

25. Puigdemont A, Riu JL, Guitart R, et al. Propafenone kinetics in the horse. Comparative analysis of compartmental and noncompartmental models. J Pharmacol Methods 1990;23:79–85.

26. Packer M, Coats AJ, Fowler MB, et al, Carvedilol Prospective Randomized Cumulative Survival Study Group. Effect of carvedilol on survival in severe chronic heart failure. N Engl J Med 2001;344:1651–8.

27. Kennedy HL, Brooks MM, Barker AH, et al. beta-Blocker therapy in the cardiac arrhythmia suppression trial. CAST investigators. Am J Cardiol 1994;74:674–80.

28. Decloedt A, Broux B, De Clercq D, et al. Effect of sotalol on heart rate, QT interval, and atrial fibrillation cycle length in horses with atrial fibrillation. J Vet Intern Med 2018;32:815–21.

29. Prutton J, Hallowell GD, Bowen IM, et al. The use of transvenous electrical cardioversion for the treatment of atrial fibrillation in a British equine hospital population. J Vet Intern Med 2012;26:430.

30. Broux B, De Clercq D, Decloedt A, et al. Pharmacokinetics of intravenously and orally administered sotalol hydrochloride in horses and effects on surface electrocardiogram and left ventricular systolic function. Vet J 2016;208:60–4.

31. House AM, Giguere S. How to diagnose and treat ventricular tachycardia. Lexington (KY): American Association of Equine Practitioners; 2009. p. 308–12.

32. De Clercq D, van Loon G, Baert K, et al. Intravenous amiodarone treatment in horses with chronic atrial fibrillation. Vet J 2006;172:129–34.

33. De Clercq D, van Loon G, Baert K, et al. Effects of an adapted intravenous amio-darone treatment protocol in horses with atrial fibrillation. Equine Vet J 2007;39: 344–9.

34. De Clercq D, van Loon G, Baert K, et al. Treatment with amiodarone of refractory ventricular tachycardia in a horse. J Vet Intern Med 2007;21:878–80.

35. Trachsel D, Tschudi P, Portier CJ, et al. Pharmacokinetics and pharmacodynamic effects of amiodarone in plasma of ponies after single intravenous administration. Toxicol Appl Pharmacol 2004;195:113–25.

36. Schwarzwald CC, Bonagura JD, Luis-Fuentes V. Effects of diltiazem on hemody-namic variables and ventricular function in healthy horses. J Vet Intern Med 2005; 19:703–11.

37. Schwarzwald CC, Hamlin RL, Bonagura JD, et al. Atrial, SA nodal, and AV nodal electrophysiology in standing horses: normal findings and electrophysiologic ef-fects of quinidine and diltiazem. J Vet Intern Med 2007;21:166–75.

38. Heliczer N, Gerber V, Bruckmaier R, et al. Cardiovascular findings in ponies with equine metabolic syndrome. J Am Vet Med Assoc 2017;250:1027–35.

39. Ceremuzynski L, Gebalska J, Wolk R, et al. Hypomagnesemia in heart failure with ventricular arrhythmias. Beneficial effects of magnesium supplementation. J Intern Med 2000;247:78–86.

40. Agus ZS, Kelepouris E, Dukes I, et al. Cytosolic magnesium modulates calcium channel activity in mammalian ventricular cells. Am J Physiol 1989;256:C452–5.

41. Singh S, Young SS, McDonell WN, et al. Modification of cardiopulmonary and in-testinal motility effects of xylazine with glycopyrrolate in horses. Can J Vet Res 1997;61:99–107.

42. Teixeira Neto FJ, McDonell WN, Black WD, et al. Effects of glycopyrrolate on cardiorespiratory function in horses anesthetized with halothane and xylazine. Am J Vet Res 2004;65:456–63.

43. Dyson DH, Pascoe PJ, McDonell WN. Effects of intravenously administered gly-copyrrolate in anesthetized horses. Can Vet J 1999;40:29–32.

44. Marques JA, Teixeira Neto FJ, Campebell RC, et al. Effects of hyoscine-N-butylbromide given before romifidine in horses. Vet Rec 1998;142:166–8.

45. Roelvink ME, Goossens L, Kalsbeek HC, et al. Analgesic and spasmolytic effects of dipyrone, hyoscine-N-butylbromide and a combination of the two in ponies. Vet Rec 1991;129:378–80.

46. Borer KE, Clarke KW. The effect of hyoscine on dobutamine requirement in spon-taneously breathing horses anaesthetized with halothane. Vet Anaesth Analg 2006;33:149–57.

47. Haggstrom J, Boswood A, O'Grady M, et al. Effect of pimobendan or benazepril hydrochloride on survival times in dogs with congestive heart failure caused by naturally occurring myxomatous mitral valve disease: the QUEST study. J Vet Intern Med 2008;22:1124–35.

48. Boswood A, Haggstrom J, Gordon SG, et al. Effect of pimobendan in dogs with preclinical myxomatous mitral valve disease and cardiomegaly: the EPIC Study - a randomized clinical trial. J Vet Intern Med 2016;30:1765–79.

49. Boswood A, Gordon SG, Haggstrom J, et al. Longitudinal analysis of quality of life, clinical, radiographic, echocardiographic, and laboratory variables in dogs with preclinical myxomatous mitral valve disease receiving pimobendan or pla-cebo: the EPIC study. J Vet Intern Med 2018;32:72–85.

50. Muir WW, Milne DW, Skarda RT. Acute hemodynamic effects of furosemide administered intravenously in the horse. Am J Vet Res 1976;37:1177–80.

51. Johansson AM, Gardner SY, Levine JF, et al. Pharmacokinetics and pharmacody-namics of furosemide after oral administration to horses. J Vet Intern Med 2004; 18:739–43.

52. Tobin T, Roberts BL, Swerczek TW, et al. The pharmacology of furosemide in the horse. III. Dose and time response relationships, effects of repeated dosing. and performance effects. J Equine Med Surg 1978;2:216–26.

53. Johansson AM, Gardner SY, Levine JF, et al. Furosemide continuous rate infusion in the horse: evaluation of enhanced efficacy and reduced side effects. J Vet Intern Med 2003;17:887–95.

54. Kurdi M, Booz GW. New take on the role of angiotensin II in cardiac hypertrophy and fibrosis. Hypertension 2011;57:1034–8.

55. Group CTS. Effects of enalapril on mortality in severe congestive heart failure. Re-sults of the Cooperative North Scandinavian Enalapril Survival Study (CONSENSUS). N Engl J Med 1987;316:1429–35.

56. Ettinger SJ, Benitz AM, Ericsson GF, et al. Effects of enalapril maleate on survival of dogs with naturally acquired heart failure. The Long-Term Investigation of Vet-erinary Enalapril (LIVE) Study Group. J Am Vet Med Assoc 1998;213:1573–7.

57. Swedberg K, Kjekshus J. Effects of enalapril on mortality in severe congestive heart failure: results of the Cooperative North Scandinavian Enalapril Survival Study (CONSENSUS). Am J Cardiol 1988;62:60A–6A.

58. Francis GS, Benedict C, Johnstone DE, et al. Comparison of neuroendocrine acti-vation in patients with left ventricular dysfunction with and without congestive heart failure. A substudy of the Studies of Left Ventricular Dysfunction (SOLVD). Circulation 1990;82:1724–9.

59. Atkins CE, Keene BW, Brown WA, et al. Results of the veterinary enalapril trial to prove reduction in onset of heart failure in dogs chronically treated with enalapril alone for compensated, naturally occurring mitral valve insufficiency. J Am Vet Med Assoc 2007;231:1061–9.

60. Nakashima H, Kumagai K, Urata H, et al. Angiotensin II antagonist prevents elec-trical remodeling in atrial fibrillation. Circulation 2000;101:2612–7.

61. Li D, Shinagawa K, Pang L, et al. Effects of angiotensin-converting enzyme inhi-bition on the development of the atrial fibrillation substrate in dogs with ventricular tachypacing-induced congestive heart failure. Circulation 2001;104:2608–14.

62. Afonso T, Giguere S, Rapoport G, et al. Pharmacodynamic evaluation of 4 angiotensin-converting enzyme inhibitors in healthy adult horses. J Vet Intern Med 2013;27:1185–92.

63. Afonso T, Giguere S, Brown SA, et al. Preliminary investigation of orally adminis-tered benazepril in horses with left-sided valvular regurgitation. Equine Vet J 2018;50:446–51.

64. Tillman LG, Moore JN. Serum angiotensin converting enzyme activity and response to angiotensin I in horses. Equine Vet J Suppl 1989;(7):80–3.

65. Sleeper MM, McDonnell SM, Ely JJ, et al. Chronic oral therapy with enalapril in normal ponies. J Vet Cardiol 2008;10:111–5.

66. Gardner SY, Atkins CE, Sams RA, et al. Characterization of the pharmacokinetic and pharmacodynamic properties of the angiotensin-converting enzyme inhibi-tor, enalapril, in horses. J Vet Intern Med 2004;18:231–7.

67. Davis JL, Kruger K, LaFevers DH, et al. Effects of quinapril on angiotensin con-verting enzyme and plasma renin activity as well as pharmacokinetic parameters of quinapril and its active metabolite, quinaprilat, after intravenous and oral administration to mature horses. Equine Vet J 2013;46:729–33.

68. Gehlen H, Vieht JC, Stadler P. Effects of the ACE inhibitor quinapril on echocardiographic variables in horses with mitral valve insufficiency. J Vet Med A Physiol Pathol Clin Med 2003;50:460–5.

69. Pitt B, Zannad F, Remme WJ, et al. The effect of spironolactone on morbidity and mortality in patients with severe heart failure. Randomized Aldactone Evaluation Study Investigators. N Engl J Med 1999;341:709–17.

70. Bernay F, Bland JM, Haggstrom J, et al. Efficacy of spironolactone on survival in dogs with naturally occurring mitral regurgitation caused by myxomatous mitral valve disease. J Vet Intern Med 2010;24:331–41.

71. Lijnen P, Petrov V. Induction of cardiac fibrosis by aldosterone. J Mol Cell Cardiol 2000;32:865–79.

72. Bang L, Nielsen-Kudsk JE, Gruhn N, et al. Hydralazine-induced vasodilation involves opening of high conductance Ca^{2+}-activated K^+ channels. Eur J Pharmacol 1998;361:43–9.

73. Wilson JR, St John Sutton M, Schwartz JS, et al. Determinants of circulatory response to intravenous hydralazine in congestive heart failure. Am J Cardiol 1983;52:299–303.

74. Lin M, Chiang HT, Lin SL, et al. Vasodilator therapy in chronic asymptomatic aortic regurgitation: enalapril versus hydralazine therapy. J Am Coll Cardiol 1994;24:1046–53.

75. Bertone JJ. Cardiovascular effects of hydralazine HCl administration in horses. Am J Vet Res 1988;49:618–21.

76. Hinckley KA, Fearn S, Howard BR, et al. Nitric oxide donors as treatment for grass induced acute laminitis in ponies. Equine Vet J 1996;28:17–28.

77. Kittleson M, Kienle R. Management of heart failure. In: Kittleson MD, Kienle RD, editors. Small animal cardiovascular medicine. New York: Mosby; 1998. p. 192–248.

78. Thadani U, Jacob RG. Isosorbide dinitrate/hydralazine: its role in the treatment of heart failure. Drugs Today (Barc) 2008;44:925–37.

79. Binns-Loveman KM, Kaplowitz MR, Fike CD. Sildenafil and an early stage of chronic hypoxia-induced pulmonary hypertension in newborn piglets. Pediatr Pulmonol 2005;40:72–80.

80. Baquero H, Soliz A, Neira F, et al. Oral sildenafil in infants with persistent pulmonary hypertension of the newborn: a pilot randomized blinded study. Pediatrics 2006;117:1077–83.

81. Palmer JE. Ventilatory support of the critically ill foal. Vet Clin North Am Equine Pract 2005;21:457–86, vii-viii.

82. Muir WW, McGuirk SM. Pharmacology and pharmacokinetics of drugs used to treat cardiac disease in horses. Vet Clin North Am Equine Pract 1985;1:335–52.

83. Button C, Gross DR, Johnston JT, et al. Digoxin pharmacokinetics, bioavailability, efficacy, and dosage regimens in the horse. Am J Vet Res 1980;41:1388–95.

84. Sweeney RW, Reef VB, Reimer JM. Pharmacokinetics of digoxin administered to horses with congestive heart failure. Am J Vet Res 1993;54:1108–11.

85. Pedersoli WM, Ravis WR, Belmonte AA, et al. Pharmacokinetics of a single, orally administered dose of digoxin in horses. Am J Vet Res 1981;42:1412–4.

86. Francfort P, Schatzmann HJ. Pharmacological experiments as a basis for the administration of digoxin in the horse. Res Vet Sci 1976;20:84–9.

87. Hinchcliff KW, McKeever KH, Muir WW 3rd. Hemodynamic effects of atropine, dobutamine, nitroprusside, phenylephrine, and propranolol in conscious horses. J Vet Intern Med 1991;5:80–6.

88. Richardson DW, Kohn CW. Uroperitoneum in the foal. J Am Vet Med Assoc 1983; 182:267–71.
89. Vasu MA, O'Keefe DD, Kapellakis GZ, et al. Myocardial oxygen consumption: effects of epinephrine, isoproterenol, dopamine, norepinephrine, and dobutamine. Am J Physiol 1978;235:H237–41.
90. Dancker C, Hopster K, Rohn K, et al. Effects of dobutamine, dopamine, phenylephrine and noradrenaline on systemic haemodynamics and intestinal perfusion in isoflurane anaesthetised horses. Equine Vet J 2018;50:104–10.
91. Lee YH, Clarke KW, Alibhai HI, et al. Effects of dopamine, dobutamine, dopexamine, phenylephrine, and saline solution on intramuscular blood flow and other cardiopulmonary variables in halothane-anesthetized ponies. Am J Vet Res 1998; 59:1463–72.
92. Muir WW. The haemodynamic effects of milrinone HCl in halothane anaesthetised horses. Equine Vet J Suppl 1995;(19):108–13.
93. Vollmar AC, Fox PR. Long-term outcome of Irish wolfhound dogs with preclinical cardiomyopathy, atrial fibrillation, or both treated with pimobendan, benazepril hydrochloride, or methyldigoxin monotherapy. J Vet Intern Med 2016;30:553–9.
94. Afonso T, Giguere S, Rapoport G, et al. Cardiovascular effects of pimobendan in healthy mature horses. Equine Vet J 2016;48:352–6.

Moving?

Make sure your subscription moves with you!

To notify us of your new address, find your **Clinics Account Number** (located on your mailing label above your name), and contact customer service at:

Email: journalscustomerservice-usa@elsevier.com

800-654-2452 (subscribers in the U.S. & Canada)
314-447-8871 (subscribers outside of the U.S. & Canada)

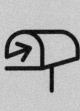

Fax number: 314-447-8029

Elsevier Health Sciences Division
Subscription Customer Service
3251 Riverport Lane
Maryland Heights, MO 63043

*To ensure uninterrupted delivery of your subscription, please notify us at least 4 weeks in advance of move.

ELSEVIER

Printed and bound by CPI Group (UK) Ltd, Croydon, CR0 4YY

03/10/2024

01040480-0005